Materials for the Direct Restoration of Teeth

Related titles

Non-Metallic Biomaterials for Tooth Repair and Replacement
(ISBN 978-0-85709-244-1)

Dental Biomaterials: Imaging, Testing and Modelling
(ISBN 978-1-84569-296-4)

Biocompatibility of Dental Materials
(ISBN 978-0-08-100884-3)

Woodhead Publishing Series in Biomaterials: Number 116

Materials for the Direct Restoration of Teeth

John Nicholson
Dental Institute, Queen Mary University of London and Bluefield Centre for Biomaterials, London, UK

Beata Czarnecka
Department of Biomaterials and Experimental Dentistry, University of Medical Sciences, Poznań, Poland

ELSEVIER

AMSTERDAM • BOSTON • CAMBRIDGE • HEIDELBERG
LONDON • NEW YORK • OXFORD • PARIS • SAN DIEGO
SAN FRANCISCO • SINGAPORE • SYDNEY • TOKYO
Woodhead Publishing is an imprint of Elsevier

WP
WOODHEAD PUBLISHING

Woodhead Publishing is an imprint of Elsevier
The Officers' Mess Business Centre, Royston Road, Duxford, CB22 4QH, UK
50 Hampshire Street, 5th Floor, Cambridge, MA 02139, USA
The Boulevard, Langford Lane, Kidlington, OX5 1GB, UK

Library of Congress Cataloging-in-Publication Data
A catalog record for this book is available from the Library of Congress

British Library Cataloguing-in-Publication Data
A catalogue record for this book is available from the British Library

ISBN: 978-0-08-100491-3 (print)
ISBN: 978-0-08-100494-4 (online)

For information on all Woodhead publications
visit our website at www.elsevier.com

Publisher: Matthew Deans
Acquisition Editor: Laura Overend
Editorial Project Manager: Lucy Beg
Production Project Manager: Poulouse Joseph
Designer: Victoria Pearson

Contents

Woodhead Publishing Series in Biomaterials

1 **Sterilisation of tissues using ionising radiations**
Edited by J. F. Kennedy, G. O. Phillips and P. A. Williams
2 **Surfaces and interfaces for biomaterials**
Edited by P. Vadgama
3 **Molecular interfacial phenomena of polymers and biopolymers**
Edited by C. Chen
4 **Biomaterials, artificial organs and tissue engineering**
Edited by L. Hench and J. Jones
5 **Medical modelling**
R. Bibb
6 **Artificial cells, cell engineering and therapy**
Edited by S. Prakash
7 **Biomedical polymers**
Edited by M. Jenkins
8 **Tissue engineering using ceramics and polymers**
Edited by A. R. Boccaccini and J. Gough
9 **Bioceramics and their clinical applications**
Edited by T. Kokubo
10 **Dental biomaterials**
Edited by R. V. Curtis and T. F. Watson
11 **Joint replacement technology**
Edited by P. A. Revell
12 **Natural-based polymers for biomedical applications**
Edited by R. L. Reiss et al
13 **Degradation rate of bioresorbable materials**
Edited by F. J. Buchanan
14 **Orthopaedic bone cements**
Edited by S. Deb
15 **Shape memory alloys for biomedical applications**
Edited by T. Yoneyama and S.Miyazaki
16 **Cellular response to biomaterials**
Edited by L. Di Silvio
17 **Biomaterials for treating skin loss**
Edited by D. P. Orgill and C. Blanco
18 **Biomaterials and tissue engineering in urology**
Edited by J.Denstedt and A. Atala
19 **Materials science for dentistry**
B. W. Darvell
20 **Bone repair biomaterials**
Edited by J. A. Planell, S. M. Best, D. Lacroix and A. Merolli

21 **Biomedical composites**
Edited by L. Ambrosio
22 **Drug–device combination products**
Edited by A. Lewis
23 **Biomaterials and regenerative medicine in ophthalmology**
Edited by T. V. Chirila
24 **Regenerative medicine and biomaterials for the repair of connective tissues**
Edited by C. Archer and J. Ralphs
25 **Metals for biomedical devices**
Edited by M. Niinomi
26 **Biointegration of medical implant materials: Science and design**
Edited by C. P. Sharma
27 **Biomaterials and devices for the circulatory system**
Edited by T. Gourlay and R. Black
28 **Surface modification of biomaterials: Methods analysis and applications**
Edited by R. Williams
29 **Biomaterials for artificial organs**
Edited by M. Lysaght and T. Webster
30 **Injectable biomaterials: Science and applications**
Edited by B. Vernon
31 **Biomedical hydrogels: Biochemistry, manufacture and medical applications**
Edited by S. Rimmer
32 **Preprosthetic and maxillofacial surgery: Biomaterials, bone grafting and tissue engineering**
Edited by J. Ferri and E. Hunziker
33 **Bioactive materials in medicine: Design and applications**
Edited by X. Zhao, J. M. Courtney and H. Qian
34 **Advanced wound repair therapies**
Edited by D. Farrar
35 **Electrospinning for tissue regeneration**
Edited by L. Bosworth and S. Downes
36 **Bioactive glasses: Materials, properties and applications**
Edited by H. O. Ylänen
37 **Coatings for biomedical applications**
Edited by M. Driver
38 **Progenitor and stem cell technologies and therapies**
Edited by A. Atala
39 **Biomaterials for spinal surgery**
Edited by L. Ambrosio and E. Tanner
40 **Minimized cardiopulmonary bypass techniques and technologies**
Edited by T. Gourlay and S. Gunaydin
41 **Wear of orthopaedic implants and artificial joints**
Edited by S. Affatato
42 **Biomaterials in plastic surgery: Breast implants**
Edited by W. Peters, H. Brandon, K. L. Jerina, C. Wolf and V. L. Young
43 **MEMS for biomedical applications**
Edited by S. Bhansali and A. Vasudev
44 **Durability and reliability of medical polymers**
Edited by M. Jenkins and A. Stamboulis

45 **Biosensors for medical applications**
Edited by S. Higson
46 **Sterilisation of biomaterials and medical devices**
Edited by S. Lerouge and A. Simmons
47 **The hip resurfacing handbook: A practical guide to the use and management of modern hip resurfacings**
Edited by K. De Smet, P. Campbell and C. Van Der Straeten
48 **Developments in tissue engineered and regenerative medicine products**
J. Basu and J. W. Ludlow
49 **Nanomedicine: Technologies and applications**
Edited by T. J. Webster
50 **Biocompatibility and performance of medical devices**
Edited by J-P. Boutrand
51 **Medical robotics: Minimally invasive surgery**
Edited by P. Gomes
52 **Implantable sensor systems for medical applications**
Edited by A. Inmann and D. Hodgins
53 **Non-metallic biomaterials for tooth repair and replacement**
Edited by P. Vallittu
54 **Joining and assembly of medical materials and devices**
Edited by Y. (Norman) Zhou and M. D. Breyen
55 **Diamond-based materials for biomedical applications**
Edited by R.Narayan
56 **Nanomaterials in tissue engineering: Fabrication and applications**
Edited by A. K. Gaharwar, S. Sant, M. J. Hancock and S. A. Hacking
57 **Biomimetic biomaterials: Structure and applications**
Edited by A. J. Ruys
58 **Standardisation in cell and tissue engineering: Methods and protocols**
Edited by V. Salih
59 **Inhaler devices: Fundamentals, design and drug delivery**
Edited by P. Prokopovich
60 **Bio-tribocorrosion in biomaterials and medical implants**
Edited by Y. Yan
61 **Microfluidic devices for biomedical applications**
Edited by X-J. James Li and Y. Zhou
62 **Decontamination in hospitals and healthcare**
Edited by J. T. Walker
63 **Biomedical imaging: Applications and advances**
Edited by P. Morris
64 **Characterization of biomaterials**
Edited by M. Jaffe, W. Hammond, P. Tolias and T. Arinzeh
65 **Biomaterials and medical tribology**
Edited by J. Paolo Davim
66 **Biomaterials for cancer therapeutics: Diagnosis, prevention and therapy**
Edited by K. Park
67 **New functional biomaterials for medicine and healthcare**
E.P. Ivanova, K.Bazaka and R. J. Crawford
68 **Porous silicon for biomedical applications**
Edited by H. A. Santos

69 **A practical approach to spinal trauma**
Edited by H. N. Bajaj and S. Katoch
70 **Rapid prototyping of biomaterials: Principles and applications**
Edited by R.Narayan
71 **Cardiac regeneration and repair Volume 1: Pathology and therapies**
Edited by R-K. Li and R. D. Weisel
72 **Cardiac regeneration and repair Volume 2: Biomaterials and tissue engineering**
Edited by R-K. Li and R. D. Weisel
73 **Semiconducting silicon nanowires for biomedical applications**
Edited by J.L. Coffer
74 **Silk biomaterials for tissue engineering and regenerative medicine**
Edited by S. Kundu
75 **Biomaterials for bone regeneration: Novel techniques and applications**
Edited by P.Dubruel and S. Van Vlierberghe
76 **Biomedical foams for tissue engineering applications**
Edited by P. Netti
77 **Precious metals for biomedical applications**
Edited by N. Baltzer and T. Copponnex
78 **Bone substitute biomaterials**
Edited by K. Mallick
79 **Regulatory affairs for biomaterials and medical devices**
Edited by S. F. Amato and R. Ezzell
80 **Joint replacement technology Second edition**
Edited by P. A. Revell
81 **Computational modelling of biomechanics and biotribology in the musculoskeletal system: Biomaterials and tissues**
Edited by Z. Jin
82 **Biophotonics for medical applications**
Edited by I. Meglinski
83 **Modelling degradation of bioresorbable polymeric medical devices**
Edited by J. Pan
84 **Perspectives in total hip arthroplasty: Advances in biomaterials and their tribological interactions**
S. Affatato
85 **Tissue engineering using ceramics and polymers Second edition**
Edited by A. R. Boccaccini and P. X. Ma
86 **Biomaterials and medical-device associated infections**
Edited by L. Barnes and I. R. Cooper
87 **Surgical techniques in total knee arthroplasty (TKA) and alternative procedures**
Edited by S. Affatato
88 **Lanthanide oxide nanoparticles for molecular imaging and therapeutics**
G. H. Lee
89 **Surface modification of magnesium and its alloys for biomedical applications Volume 1: Biological interactions, mechanical properties and testing**
Edited by T. S. N. Sankara Narayanan, I. S. Park and M. H. Lee
90 **Surface modification of magnesium and its alloys for biomedical applications Volume 2: Modification and coating techniques**
Edited by T. S. N. Sankara Narayanan, I. S. Park and M. H. Lee

91 **Medical modelling: the application of advanced design and rapid prototyping techniques in medicine Second Edition**
Edited by R. Bibb, D. Eggbeer and A. Paterson
92 **Switchable and responsive surfaces and materials for biomedical applications**
Edited by Z. Zhang
93 **Biomedical textiles for orthopaedic and surgical applications: fundamentals, applications and tissue engineering**
Edited by T. Blair
94 **Surface coating and modification of metallic biomaterials**
Edited by C. Wen
95 **Hydroxyapatite (HAP) for biomedical applications**
Edited by M. Mucalo
96 **Implantable neuroprostheses for restoring function**
Edited by K. Kilgore
97 **Shape memory polymers for biomedical applications**
Edited by L. Yahia
98 **Regenerative engineering of musculoskeletal tissues and interfaces**
Edited by S.P. Nukavarapu, J.W. Freeman and C.T. Laurencin
99 **Advanced cardiac imaging**
Edited by K. Nieman, O. Gaemperli, P. Lancellotti and S. Plein
100 **Functional Marine Biomaterials: Properties and Applications**
Edited by SK. Kim
101 **Shoulder and elbow trauma and its complications: Volume 1: The Shoulder**
Edited by R. M. Greiwe
102 **Nanotechnology-Enhanced Orthopedic Materials: Fabrications, Applications and Future Trends**
Edited by L. Yang
103 **Medical devices: Regulations, standards and practices**
Edited by S. Ramakrishna, L. Tian, C. Wang, S. L. and T. Wee Eong
104 **Biomineralisation and biomaterials: fundamentals and applications**
Edited by C. Aparicio and M. Ginebra
105 **Shoulder and elbow trauma and its complications: Volume 2: The Elbow**
Edited by R. M. Greiwe
106 **Characterisation and Design of Tissue Scaffolds**
Edited by P. Tomlins
107 **Biosynthetic Polymers for Medical Applications**
Edited by L. Poole-Warren, P. Martens and R.Green
108 **Advances in Polyurethane Biomaterials**
Edited by S.L. Cooper
109 **Nanocomposites for Musculoskeletal Tissue Regeneration**
Edited by H.Liu
110 **Thin Film Coatings for Biomaterials and Biomedical Applications**
Edited by H.J. Griesser
111 **Laser surface modification of biomaterials**
Edited by R. Vilar
112 **Biomaterials and regenerative medicine in ophthalmology Second edition**
Edited by T.V. Chirila and D. Harkin
113 **Extracellular Matrix-derived Medical Implants in Clinical Medicine**
Edited by D. Mooradian

114 **Wound Healing Biomaterials: Volume 1: Therapies and Regeneration**
Edited by M. S. Ågren
115 **Wound Healing Biomaterials: Volume 2: Functional biomaterials**
Edited by M. S. Ågren
116 **Materials for the Direct Restoration of Teeth**
J. Nicholson and B. Czarnecka
117 **Science and principles of biodegradable and bioresorbable medical polymers**
Edited by X. Zhang

Clinical aspects of tooth repair

1

1.1 Introduction

The teeth play an important part in human health, both physical and psychological [1,2]. At the physical level, they are essential in the mastication of food, with different teeth having different structures, which reflect their specialized purpose within the cycle of mastication of food. On the psychological level, the appearance of the teeth influences how individuals perceive themselves. People with missing or damaged teeth are typically self-conscious and may show lack of confidence or other signs of distress about their appearance [3].

Human teeth are small, calcified structures that are found in the mouth in distinctive positions relative to each other. Their location reflects their function, so that incisors are found at the front of the mouth and have sharp edges that fit them for the function of cutting food as it is taken into to the mouth. Molars are found towards the back of the mouth, and they have a flattened morphology that makes them suitable for crushing food immediately before swallowing and subsequent digestion [1,2].

In addition, there are canine teeth alongside the incisors, which share some of the functions of cutting and tearing food. Next to them come the pre-molars, which share some of the functions of crushing of the molars.

Teeth are typically long-lasting structures, capable of remaining functional in service for many years. In adults, there are 32 teeth and in children 20 teeth. These children's teeth are lost around the age 7 onwards, and described as 'deciduous'. The adult teeth, by contrast, are described as 'permanent'.

The healthy tooth is covered with a thin layer of enamel (Fig. 1.1), the hardest substance in the human body [1,2]. It is highly mineralized, containing distinct crystalline phases of the calcium phosphate mineral hydroxyapatite $Ca_{10}(PO_4)_6(OH)_2$. It also contains traces of the protein collagen, which has important effects on the mechanical properties of the enamel. Specifically, the protein causes the enamel to be tougher than it would otherwise be, and hence more resistant to crack propagation through it [4]. It also reduces the permeability of the enamel, thus increasing its resistance to acid attack [4].

Beneath the layer of enamel is a structure called dentine. It is a permeable pale yellow material that consists of approximately 70% hydroxyapatite, 20% organic matter (mainly collagen) and 10% water by mass.

Anatomically, the dentine has a tubular structure, with microscopic tubules radiating outwards from the central pulp cavity. These tubules range in diameter between 0.9 and 2.5 μm, with the diameter being widest near the pulp and becoming reduced as the tubule extends towards the dentino-enamel junction [2]. These tubules are filled with odontoblast processes.

The inner part of the tooth comprises a cavity, which contains soft connective tissue known as the dental pulp. It consists of blood vessels and nerve fibres and these enter the tooth via a small opening at the end of the tooth root called the apex.

Materials for the Direct Restoration of Teeth. http://dx.doi.org/10.1016/B978-0-08-100491-3.00001-5

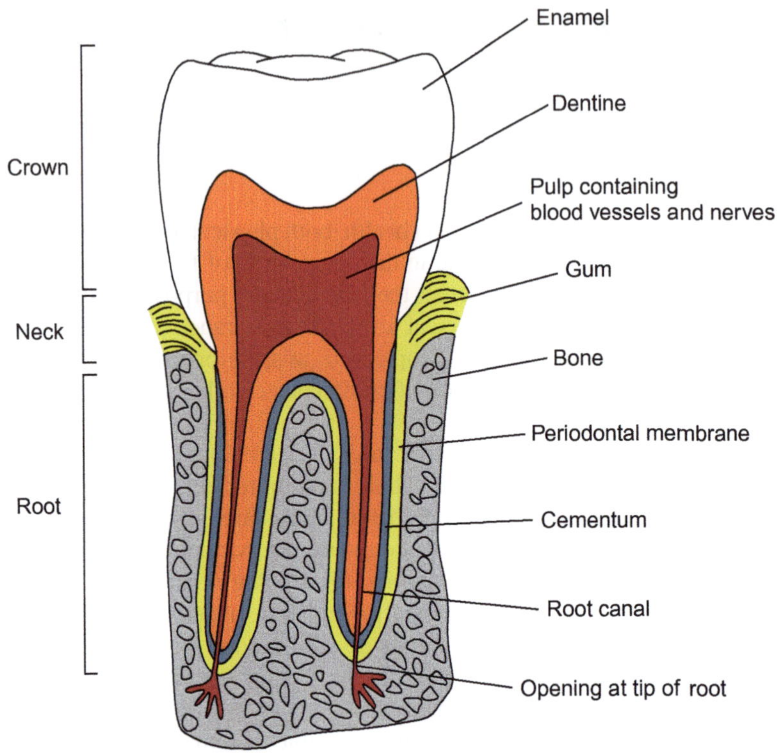

Fig. 1.1 Structure of a typical tooth.

The outer layer of the pulp, adjacent to the dentine, contains dentine-producing cells known as odontoblasts. These cells produce dentine throughout the whole of life and are capable of providing a degree of repair to dentine that has been damaged by either trauma or bacterial activity. Also, in case of damage to the odontoblasts, in young patients, connective tissue cells from the pulp, the fibroblasts, can become transformed into odontoblasts, and these can then start the process of repairing the dentine. Because of these morphological and physiological connections between the dentine and the pulp, this tissue can be regarded as a single entity, the pulpo-dentinal complex.

The pulp contains sensitive cells which can be damaged by extensive mechanical trauma to the tooth, or by chemical assault from substances released from materials used to repair the tooth. The pulp can also become infected and transmit that infection to the rest of the body through the circulatory system. For this reason, the bacterially mediated disease of dental caries is potentially serious and should not be left untreated [5].

The tooth root is covered with a substance called cementum. This is a specialized tissue that shows some resemblance to bone [2] and has the approximate composition 455 hydroxyapatite, 33% protein (collagen) and 22% water by mass. Cementum occurs in two forms, acellular, which covers about two-thirds to the root, and cellular, which covers the remaining one-third closer to the tip of the tooth root. This form is more permeable than the acellular cementum.

The tooth is anchored within the bone of either the mandible or the maxilla by means of the periodontal ligament or membrane. The mechanical properties of this membrane are such that the tooth is supported during its use in mastication with a cushion of viscoelastic material and periodontal liquid within the more rigid supporting frame of alveolar bone [6]. This biomechanical structure thus contributes to the overall function of the tooth, while allowing a very small degree of movement within the tooth socket. This behaviour of the periodontal ligament can be attributed to its structure, which consists mainly on type 1 collagen fibres arranged in tight aligned bundles [7]. The periodontal ligament and the tooth are attached through the layer of cementum.

In service, teeth have to resistant a variety of assaults while maintaining their function. These include possible trauma, attack by acidic foodstuffs and beverages, biomechanical stresses of chewing and grinding and the effects of acidic metabolic products from the commonly occurring oral biofilm. Consequently, throughout life, teeth become damaged. The various types of damage are considered in the rest of this chapter. The remainder of the book is concerned with the materials available to the clinician to repair teeth that have been affected by these various damaging factors.

1.2 Dental caries

Tooth decay (dental caries) is one of the most common diseases in humans [8]. It has been defined as 'a chronic, dietomicrobial, site-specific disease caused by a shift from protective factors favouring tooth remineralization to destructive factors leading to demineralization' [9]. The specific factors leading to destruction of the mineral phase of the tooth are the presence of oral bacteria, mainly *Streptococcus mutans* [10], and the availability of fermentable carbohydrates from the diet. This combination leads to the production of organic acids as a result of the metabolic process of the bacteria, of which the main one is lactic acid, though other weak acids, such as ethanoic and propanoic can also occur [11]. These acids dissolve the mineral component of the tooth, leading to loss of structure.

The process of the disease of dental caries has been studied in depth for many years, and the details of its progress are now reasonably well understood [12]. The role of acidogenic bacteria in the mouth has long been known to be critical, and their ability to generate organic acids is well established as the mechanism by which they cause damage to the tooth.

Organic acids attack the mineral phase of the tooth, causing dissolution and loss of structure. Weak organic acids have a particularly severe effect on the tooth, as they have a strong affinity for calcium, and thereby attack the mineral phase readily [12]. In extreme cases, this attack leads to the formation of a distinct cavity within the tooth. Such a cavity mechanically weakens the tooth, and must be repaired in order to restore the tooth to its fully functioning state. A repair of this type must also remove the bacterial infection and ensure that the affected tooth does not become the locus of further systemic infection for the patient.

The development of caries has been studied in detail and the essential steps identified [13]. They are:

1. key bacteria on the oral plaque ferment dietary carbohydrates, as a result of which organic acids are produced. As already mentioned, the main acid produced is lactic acid, but others such as formic, ethanoic and propionic acids have also been found to occur to variable extents at different times within the caries process [11];
2. these organic acids diffuse into the enamel or cementum, and later can spread to the dentine [12,14]. As they do, they attack the mineral phase in the subsurface layers, dissolving it and carrying its components away [15];
3. the mineral from the tooth, ie, the lightly carbonated hydroxyapatite phase, diffuses out of the tooth in soluble form. In time this leads to the development of cavities within the tooth, a situation known as dental caries. These cavities appear as discoloured zones, which are mechanically softer than the intact tooth, as leathery collagen fibrils are more abundant in affected dentine than in caries-free dentine. Also, cavities spread more rapidly within the dentine, causing them to balloon out when they reach this tissue, having passed through the enamel.

Several different types of dental caries have been described by clinicians. Specifically these are: smooth-surface caries, pit and fissure caries, enamel caries, dentinal caries, secondary caries, early childhood caries and root caries [12]. All occur by the same essential mechanism, as described above, and all arise as a consequence of a disturbance to the demineralization–remineralization balance. Attack by organic acids produced by bacteria in the plaque favours demineralization, but the natural remineralization processes of the mouth can reverse this. Certain dietary and hygiene behaviours as well as clinical treatments can enhance this natural remineralization provided they occur early enough in the demineralization part of the process. For example, complexes of casein phosphopeptide with amorphous calcium phosphate have been shown in various studies to be capable of enhancing the remineralization step under certain conditions and in specific groups of individuals [16,17]. These are now available commercially as an anticaries treatment for patients.

Remineralization can occur at the tooth surface by the diffusion of calcium and phosphate ions from the saliva into the tooth surface, followed by precipitation. This precipitation occurs at nucleation sites on the surfaces of the remaining crystals within the tooth and occurs because the saliva is saturated with respect to calcium and phosphate ions [12]. Remineralization is enhanced by the presence of fluoride and results in a new mineral phase, which contains a small amount of fluoride ion. The resulting lightly fluoridated mineral phase is more resistant to acid attack than the native carbonated hydroxyapatite [12].

Fluoride is known to be important as a species to combat dental caries in the mouth [18,19]. Three mechanisms have been proposed to account for this anticaries effect, namely:

- **(i)** combination with the tooth mineral to form the less soluble mineral fluorapatite from the naturally occurring hydroxyapatite phase [20–23];
- **(ii)** promotion of remineralization processes at the surface of the hydroxyapatite phase [24–26]; and
- **(iii)** reduction of the solvating ability of the saliva through forming strong hydrogen bonds with the water [27,28].

Of these, the most important appears to be the promotion of remineralization [24–26]. This process is the opposite of demineralization and occurs when crystals of hydroxyapatite are induced to grow by precipitation of Ca^{2+} and PO_4^{3-} ions from saliva [27]. It has a complex mechanism and involves not only the tooth and the saliva, but also the pellicle and the plaque [12]. Fluoride ions have an influence on this activity since they enhance the rate of deposition of hydroxyapatite. In doing so, they are incorporated into the new mineral, phase though this does not appear to be their primary role [28].

Although fluoride enhances the remineralization process, it is not essential for the process to occur. There is a considerable body of evidence to show that, in a healthy mouth, both demineralization and remineralization take place in a balanced way, with each occurring several times a day. The overall effect is that the tooth is maintained in a sound, undamaged state.

For a full cavity to develop, the process of demineralization has to occur at a faster rate than remineralization, and to be able to continue unchecked [29–32]. The pathological factors that promote this include the continued presence of acidogenic bacteria, repeated consumption of fermentable carbohydrates and also, in some patients, reduced salivary function [32].

The nature of the oral micro-organisms is critical to the way in which caries progresses. The acid-producing bacteria represent a very small proportion of the total within the plaque, typically less than 1%. The major species involved are *S. mutans* and also *S. sobrinus*, as well as various lactobacilli species [29]. Several other bacterial types are known, including *Veillonella parvula*, *Prevotella melaninogenica* and *Fusobacterium periodonticum* [30], and in total, over 700 individual species of bacteria have been reported as being able to exist within the human oral cavity [30]. The majority of these are not acidogenic, and do not pose any threat of caries.

However, the acidogenic bacteria are more serious because, not only do they generate acid as a result of their metabolic processes, they also live preferentially under conditions of low pH. In other words, they are not only acidogenic, they are also aciduric [29]. Consequently, as caries develops, the population of bacteria at the tooth surface changes and the proportion of acid-producing bacteria within the biofilm increases. This means that the conditions within the plaque become more acidic with time; hence the caries becomes more aggressive. This change in microbial ecology is important in controlling the rate at which caries develops [29,31].

The teeth have an essentially mechanical role in the cutting, tearing and crushing of food as it enters the gastro-intestinal tract. To discharge this role effectively requires the combined effect of the mineralized tissue (both enamel and dentine) and also of the collagen [33].

Fibrils of this latter substance within the dentine act as a scaffold for the mineral crystallites. These crystallites reinforce the dentine matrix and the whole structure acts as a support for the enamel. The mineralized dentine has the important biomechanical function of preventing cracks propagating from the enamel, which is very brittle, through the dentino-enamel junction into the dentine [34]. This prevents the enamel crown from fracturing when loaded.

As dental caries progresses, it reaches the dentine and it moves much more rapidly through this tissue than through the enamel [35,36]. This substantially alters the mechanical properties of the enamel and with it the properties of the overall tooth [37,38]. The tooth becomes weakened and no longer capable of carrying out its role in the mastication of food without potential fracture. These weakening effects are exacerbated by changes in the organic phase of the tooth following partial demineralization. The remaining collagen fibrils have a leathery, compliance texture, and in the absence of mineral crystallites, they collapse and become more compacted [33,39]. Water is more capable of infiltrating them in this state than when part of an undamaged mineralized structure. Consequently, demineralized dentine has an increased capacity for holding water, making it able to hold more than the nominal 20% of sound dentine [4]. The net effect is to create a damaged dentine layer that is highly deformable when loaded, unlike fully mineralized dentine [40].

Remineralization of such affected dentine may not necessarily restore the mechanical function of the original dentine [33]. If the architecture of the remineralized dentine is poor, the resulting tissue will not act as a reinforced structure capable of fulfilling the required biomechanical function [41,42]. There is evidence that remineralized dentine contains larger hydroxyapatite crystallites than unaffected dentine [42] and that the mineral phase crystallites are of a different quality from those in native dentine [41]. Achieving sound and useful remineralization in clinical dentistry is thus a difficult task.

Early non-cavitated carious lesions only may be repaired by remineralization processes. However partly because of the uncertainty in outcome, and partly because results are more reliable, the method of choice for the repair of a tooth damaged by caries is surgical removal of the carious region, followed by repair with some sort of synthetic material. The act of cutting out damaged tooth material (enamel and dentine) is known to compromise the mechanical properties of the tooth [43], as shown by the results in Table 1.1. In this study, a set of 10 non-carious teeth was used per experimental set. They were mounted in dental stone and tested in compression, with the load at failure in kilograms recorded.

First, cavities were cut in a set of teeth, and these were mounted in dental stone and tested to failure in compression. Lastly, two types of repair were prepared in teeth, namely horizontally or obliquely cut, and these were repaired with light-cured composite resin. These teeth were then mounted in dental stone and tested in compression. Results are shown in Table 1.1. They show that repairing the tooth brings the strength

Table 1.1 Compressive loads at failure for drilled and repaired teeth

Sample	Load at failure (kg)	% of original
Original	104.69 (13.59)	100
With drilled cavity	48.88 (6.25)	46.7
Restored horizontally	63.46 (7.98)	60.6
Restored obliquely	84.05 (14.03)	80.3

Standard deviations in parentheses.
Source: T.P.N. Bhardwaj, P. Solmon, A. Parameswaran, Tooth restored with composite resin – a comparative analysis, Trends Biomater. Artif. Organs 15 (2002) 57–60.

back to a reasonable level so that, although the overall strength in compression is less than that of an undamaged tooth, the tooth is capable of functioning in this state. Clinically, repaired teeth rarely fail mechanically, showing that in general such repair is effective in maintaining a functioning dentition.

1.3 Dental trauma

Dental trauma is also a public dental health problem that typically occurs at a young age [44]. There is some evidence that its incidence is increasing, as young people take part in more dangerous sports and other pass-times, and so are more prone to inflict injuries on their teeth [45]. Treatment to repair the damage caused by trauma is expensive, and some sort of maintenance and possibly upgrade of the treatment may be necessary for the rest of the patient's life [44].

Determining the number of patients who experience the effects of dental trauma is complicated, and two statistics are used, namely prevalence and incidence. Prevalence is the measure of the total number of experiences of dental trauma within a given population and once such an event has occurred, it remains within the population as long as the individual in question remains within that population. By contrast, the incidence refers to the number of new patients experiencing dental trauma within a given period of time, typically 1 year [44].

Estimates of the prevalence of traumatic dental injury vary. Some typical examples from different countries are shown in Table 1.2.

Statistics from most countries and regions of the world show that about one-third of all pre-school children have suffered some sort of traumatic injury to their primary dentition. Statistics vary for injuries to the permanent dentition, but numbers are still striking. About a quarter of all school children and one-third of all adults have suffered damage to their permanent teeth [44]. Variations are considerable between countries, and these may arise in part for cultural reasons. For example, the relatively high prevalence of traumatic dental injury in Nigerian pre-school children has been attributed to the fact that such children are typically looked after by children who are themselves only a few years older [52].

Table 1.2 Prevalence of traumatic dental injuries to permanent teeth in different countries [44]

Country/region	Year	Age	Prevalence (%)	References
North America	1996	6–20	18.4	[46]
North America	2004	6–20	16.0	[47]
Canada	2005	14	18.5	[48]
United Kingdom	2001	14	23.7	[49]
United Kingdom	2002	14	43.8	[50]
Israel	2005	9–13	29.6	[51]

There are several factors, which influence the prevalence of dental trauma. A highly significant one is gender, with boys being almost twice as likely to suffer dental injury as girls [44]. However, this is changing, especially in Western societies, where girls are taking an increasing interest in sport [53]. With this change in activity, girls are being exposed to the same risk factors as boys, and the incidence and prevalence of dental trauma are changing accordingly [54,55].

Age is another important risk factor in traumatic dental injury [44]. School children and teenagers are at greatest risk and studies have shown that over 70% of all reported dental injuries occur before that age of 19 years [56–59]. There is now also evidence of growing numbers of dental injuries in older patients [44]. This arises because such patients are increasingly likely to retain their teeth into old age, and these teeth can be damaged, for example in falls. In a study in New Zealand, it was shown that dental trauma in the elderly had the highest rate in males aged 65–74 [60], and that this was part of a pattern of increased numbers of injuries in the elderly as a result of falls.

Among the general population, including the young, with their greater susceptibility to traumatic dental injury, the majority of incidents involve the anterior teeth [44]. The most commonly affected teeth are the maxillary central and lateral incisors. Injury typically affects a single tooth, though certain traumatic events, such as sports injuries, violent incidents and road traffic accidents, may result in injuries to several teeth at once. In such cases, it is not uncommon for both of the maxillary incisors to be damaged, and so to need repair.

Dental traumatic injury often results in fracture of the affected tooth, an injury that necessitates substantial repair. This fracture can vary in severity, from involving the enamel only, through involving both enamel and dentine, to involving both tissues and also exposure of the pulp. Trauma can also affect the root of the tooth, which can themselves be fractured as a result of the incident [44]. Complications involving the root can often follow traumatic events, and may require endodontic treatment prior to repair of the fractured tooth crown. Certain patients may damage an already traumatized tooth, and this can inhibit the healing process in the tooth and lead to a variety of complications [61].

Repair of a tooth damaged in dental traumatic injury is most often achieved using dental composite resins of various types [62]. Modern repairs are carried out using flowable or universal composites [63,64], and both chemically cured [62] and light-cured materials [65] have been used. Modern materials are generally light-cured, so that the use of these is preferred in contemporary clinical practice. As the geometry of the fracture usually does not favour retention of the restorative material, it is critical that a reliable bonding system is used, which gives high bond strengths to both dentine and enamel.

A repair may involve either complete fabrication with a synthetic material or re-attachment of a broken fragment [66]. Like full repair with a composite resin, reattachment of a broken fragment requires the use of bonding techniques, specifically acid-etching, and typically includes some use of a dental composite resin. If this can be done, it has the advantages of being less time-consuming, and gives a repair with good strength and aesthetics [66]. By contrast, undertaking the repair entirely in composite resin provides a restoration of reduced mechanical properties, and one that may discolour or otherwise change its appearance over time.

1.4 Abfraction, abrasion and erosion

As well as lesions caused by the effects of dental caries and mechanical damage caused by trauma, teeth can suffer damage due to non-carious lesions. These typically occur in the cervical region of the tooth and for many years were attributed to the effects of abrasion from toothbrushing [67]. However, the current view is that these lesions are caused by biomechanical effects, and they are now generally known as *abfraction lesions* [67,68].

Abfraction is defined as the pathological loss of materials from the tooth caused by biomechanical loading forces [69]. These loading forces cause flexure of the tooth that result in failure of the enamel and the dentine in a direction away from that of the loading. The concept of abfraction is primarily based on engineering considerations that assume stress concentration at the cervical region of the tooth.

Non-carious cervical lesions were previously designated erosion or abrasion lesions [70]. It was not until the later 1970s that the possibility that these lesions might originate from occlusal loading first emerged [71–73]. The term 'abfraction' has been applied to this phenomenon since the early 1990s [74], some time after the role of toothbrush abrasion in the development of the cervical lesion was first questioned [71,75]. Rather than toothbrushing causing erosion, it was suggested that bruxism might be the cause of the characteristic angled notches of the cervical lesion [71,76].

It was Grippo in 1991 who first proposed the mechanism of abfraction [67]. His idea was that there was flexure at the cemento-enamel junction of the tooth, and that this resulted in damage to the enamel rods. He went on to suggest that this initial damage was followed by loosening and a flaking away of part of the tooth structure in the cervical region. Grippo suggested that this mechanism of abfraction is the cause of all non-carious cervical lesions in teeth.

However, this view has been challenged. For example, Lee and Eakle [77] suggested that they arise from a combination of factors, of which occlusal stress is one, but with abrasion and erosion also playing a part. Similarly, Spranger [78] has proposed a combination of factors in the development of cervical lesions, and that the phenomenon is related to the tooth anatomy, occlusion and parafunction, all of which contribute to elastic deformation forces at the neck of the tooth and which are augmented by wear phenomena [78].

It is worth considering the results of subsequent studies of the mechanical forces on the tooth, not only during bruxism but also during normal mastication. Studies of normal mastication have shown that, when the tooth is hyper-occluded, forces are transmitted to the tooth and this results in energy being transferred to the cervical region [79–82]. However, the force exerted during mastication and swallowing is only about 40% of the maximum bite force [83]. Tooth contact during consumption of food is extremely brief, typically only 194 ms during mastication itself and 683 ms during swallowing [84].

Although these contacts are transient, they do result in distinct forces on the tooth. The tooth is known to undergo tiny lateral displacements when loaded and this results in compressive stress on the side towards which the tooth bends and tensile stress on the other side [82,85]. These stresses lead to micro-fractures in the enamel or dentine in the cervical region, which propagate in a perpendicular direction to the long axis of the tooth [82,85]. The result is a localized defect around the cemento-enamel junction.

Non-carious cervical lesions of the tooth are typically wedge-shaped and show loss of tooth tissue mainly on the buccal surfaces of the tooth close to the cemento-enamel junction. This is the case, regardless of the tooth affected [72]. When the tooth is loaded asymmetrically, there are typically flexing stresses, and these produce tension on one side of the tooth and compression on the other. Both types of force are located close to the cemento-enamel junction [86]. The result is that tooth mineral fractures in this region, and falls away, causing a non-carious lesion to develop. These lesions typically involve exposure of the dentine [72].

Direct clinical evidence for the mechanism of formation of non-carious cervical lesions is lacking. Instead a variety of indirect and modelling studies have been carried out, and they provide evidence for its plausibility. For example, the stress distribution in teeth that have been loaded appropriately has been studied, and results show that when the cusps are loaded obliquely, stress concentrates at the cervical regions of the tooth [87,88].

The teeth most likely to develop non-carious cervical lesions are the maxillary pre-molars, and in a study of the loading of these teeth, applying force was shown to lead to tooth flexing [89]. Force applied to the cusps led to concentration of stress in the cervical regions of the buccal sides of the tooth, which is consistent with the observation that non-carious cervical lesions occur most frequently on this side of the affected teeth [89].

Studies have shown that tensile stress at the cervical region is capable of disrupting the bonds between the enamel and the dentine, causing the eventual separation of these two tissues [90–93]. There is also evidence that central loading of the tooth can cause damage in the cervical region, and lead to loss of crystalline material and formation of lesions [94]. Specifically such loading causes compressive stress to develop and these result in the tooth undergoing a barrelling deformation by way of reaction. Once again, the effect of this deformation is most pronounced at the cervical region of the tooth [94].

Several finite-element studies have been carried out to model the effects of loading of the tooth [95–98]. Results have been striking and, for example, normal chewing loads of 100 N have been found to generate maximum principal stresses in the cervical enamel in excess of 80 MPa, the fracture stress value for enamel. In other words, sound teeth subjected to normal masticatory loads distribute stress in such a way that the cervical enamel is likely to be damaged. Patients who exhibit bruxism can exceed normal chewing loads by some way; hence their enamel is subject to exceptionally high stresses, well above the level required to fracture the crystallites and permanently damage the tooth.

Repairs of a tooth may make problems of cervical lesions more serious. For example, it has been shown that mesial occlusal distal (MOD) cavity preparations result in tooth cusps becoming effectively cantilever beams that deflect when the tooth is subject to occlusal loading [60,95–99]. Deeper cavity preparation causes longer cantilever beams to be created. Because the deflection varies as the length of the beam cubed, it follows that doubling the depth of the cavity causes cuspal deflection to increase by a factor of eight [100]. The peak tensile and shear stresses were found to be a maximum at the cervical region furthest away from the point of loading, due to the effect of the lever arm [90].

Repair of such non-carious lesions is not straightforward. The repair of such a class V cavity leads to increased stresses around the prepared cavity, and these may lead to retention problems for repair materials placed in the cavity. For example, bonded composite resin repairs have been shown to be susceptible to failure as a result of bruxism and other forms of occlusal loading [101]. There is also evidence that cervical debonding and leakage can occur in class V restorations when the teeth are subject to loading [102].

1.4.1 Erosion and abfraction

In addition to the effects of biomechanical loading causing the formation of non-carious cervical lesions, there may also be a role for erosion in their formation. Dental erosion is the loss of material from the tooth surface by the effect of strong acid but without the involvement of bacteria [103,104]. In other words, the acid involved does not arise from the metabolic activity of key bacteria in the oral biofilm but from the stomach (hydrochloric acid) or from components of the diet. These may be beverages of various kinds (cola, fruit juices) [105], or fruit or vinegar-based preserves eaten at or between meal-times.

It has been suggested that erosion of this type may contribute to the development of non-carious cervical lesions because erosive agents enter the surface of the enamel through internal channels. Having done so, they would weaken the enamel by chemical attack from within. The resulting affected enamel would then be more susceptible to wear (tooth brush erosion) and fracture when loaded than unaffected enamel. This erosion might influence the formation of cervical lesions without having a primary role in their occurrence.

This combined effect might also help to explain why non-carious cervical lesions most often appear on the labial and buccal surfaces of the tooth and are very rare on the lingual side [106]. There is much greater salivary flow along the lingual side of the tooth, and this would result in more rapid clearance of acidic foods and beverages than along the buccal sides. Hence the enamel would be attacked to a much smaller extent, if at all. It therefore retains its strength and this thereby more able to resist fracture as a result of occlusal loading.

1.4.2 Erosion without abfraction

It is also possible to have tooth erosion (sometimes called tooth wear) without the formation of non-carious cervical lesions, and these appear to be a growing clinical problem. There have been several studies to show this, with consumption of acidic beverages by younger people being considered the major causative agent [107–109]. Typical findings have been that 5.7% of tooth surfaces in a particular patient cohort were found to eroded to an unacceptable degree in patients aged 15–26 years in a study of over 1000 individuals in the United Kingdom [110]. A much smaller cohort (100 patients) in Helsinki showed a similar proportion affected to an unacceptable extent [111].

Eating disorders are also associated with tooth erosion [112]. Specifically, bulimic patients are likely to suffer from erosion, with the palatal surfaces of the maxillary incisors, canines and pre-molars being most serious affected [113]. This is because of their behavioural pattern of regurgitating food, which is acidified by strong acid from the stomach (HCl). Bulimics, who are typically young females, generally have low salivary flow rates, and are frequently found to have increased tooth sensitivity both to low temperatures and to touch [113].

Similar effects can occur in patients who suffer from oesophageal reflux as part of a wider range of medical problems, including hiatus hernia [114]. Once again, the low pH of the reflux causes erosion of the mineral phase of the tooth enamel, with specific inner surfaces of the maxillary teeth being the most affected.

In all cases, the affected teeth need to be cared for. Once the aetiology of the erosion has been identified, steps must be taken to preserve the remaining tissue, typically via repair with an appropriate material. Repairs may use either composite resin [115,116] or glass-ionomer cement, and these materials give good levels of protection against further damage, as well as sound aesthetic repair. Steps to manage the condition are also essential, for example referring the patient to a gastroenterologist for medical management of their condition, or to a psychologist for behavioural management of an eating disorder [113,114].

1.5 Dental prophylaxis

This book is mainly concerned with repair materials for teeth damaged in a variety of ways. However, clinical dentistry also has to be concerned with the source of much of the damage, namely oral bacteria. Dental prophylaxis is that aspect of dentistry concerned with cleaning of the oral cavity as well as strengthening the teeth against acid attack, and is thus important as a preventive treatment to assist in the maintenance of sound oral health in patients.

Prophylaxis is the term also applied to extensive tooth cleaning, typically carried out by a trained professional such as a dental hygienist. The cleaning involves removing calculus from the surfaces of the teeth above the gum line, usually followed by cleaning between the teeth with dental floss. Cleaning is finished by polishing with pumice paste using a rubber cup on a slow speed hand-piece.

The purpose of this treatment is to clean the teeth and gums thoroughly, so that caries, gingivitis and periodontal disease are prevented from developing and progressing. Periodontal disease in particular is an extremely widespread condition, with recent estimates suggesting that something of the order of 90% of the world's population has at least mild periodontal disease [117]. The incidence is lower in developed countries but despite this, in the United States around 50% of individuals aged 30 or over are estimated to have moderate to severe periodontal disease [118,119]. Effects of periodontal disease vary with its severity, but the condition is characterized by loss of alveolar bone [120–122], resulting in loss of support for the tooth [123] and, eventually, complete loss of the tooth. In fact, periodontal disease is the major cause of tooth loss in adult populations [117].

Periodontal disease is caused by the oral biofilm, known as plaque, which as we have seen is also the cause of dental caries. Plaque accumulates around the teeth and becomes calcified into a form known as calculus. In this form, it also contributes to adverse effects. The current view is that almost all types of periodontal disease are the result of mixed microbial infections involving a variety of pathogenic bacteria [124–126]. Plaque may also grow sub-gingivally in the periodontal pockets around the teeth that have become deepened. Predominant bacterial species associated with moderate to severe periodontal disease are typically Gram-negative [127,128], with the species *Porphyromonas gingivalis* [129] and *Aggregatibacter actinomycetemcomitas* [130,131] being particularly implicated in periodontal disease in adults. There are factors in addition to bacterial plaque that increase the likelihood of periodontal disease occurring, including smoking, stress, cardiovascular disease and diabetes [123].

The progress of periodontal disease follows a distinct and recognized pattern. Colonization of teeth and periodontal pockets by the key pathogenic bacteria leads to tissue inflammation within the periodontal tissue, which with time leads to destruction of adjacent connective tissue and the alveolar bone. Chronic inflammation of this type goes on to cause atherosclerosis and to aggravate conditions such as cardiovascular disease and type 2 diabetes [132,133].

Microbial plaque is the primary cause of both dental caries and periodontal disease [134,135]. In principle, most plaque can be removed using appropriate oral hygiene devices, such as toothbrushes and dental floss, but in practice many patients lack both the skill and the motivation to maintain a reliable plaque-free state [136]. For this reason, professional dental prophylaxis has an important part to play in helping maintain sound oral health in individuals. The primary function of such prophylaxis is removal of plaque, stain and calculus [137] and elimination of the factors that cause plaque to build up and be retained [138]. This may be augmented by the topical application of fluoride in an appropriate form.

Professional prophylaxis is performed using toothbrushing, rubber cup polishing and flossing. Rubber cup polishing is carried out using a fine grit, typically pumice, and this removes extrinsic staining and smoothes rough enamel surfaces following scaling [137]. Following this part of the treatment, application of fluoride is used, to assist remineralization and to enhance the resistance of enamel to acid attack.

Rubber cup prophylaxis with pumice paste removes a small amount of surface enamel, typically corresponding 0.6–4.0 μm of the outer layer [139]. The actual amount removed depends on the speed of the hand-piece, the abrasivity of the paste and the time spent cleaning the teeth [139,140]. The layer removed includes the fluoride-rich layer formed as a result of exposure to fluoridated toothpastes. This level of fluoride can be replaced by applying further fluoride topically after the polishing step [141].

Professional prophylaxis is typically applied at 6-month intervals [142]. However, patients vary in their risk of developing caries and/or periodontal disease so that for some there are clinical advantages in applying prophylactic techniques at shorter time intervals. Ideally, dentists and their teams will develop individualized preventive plans to control those factors leading to destructive dental caries or periodontal disease so that patients can benefit from improved oral health.

1.6 Conclusions

This chapter has outlined the conditions that lead to damage to the teeth, and shows that the effects of dental caries, trauma and periodontal disease can be profound in terms of loss of tooth structure and indeed of the teeth themselves. In the clinic, dentists carry out repairs on these conditions routinely using a variety of artificial materials. These materials have emerged as a result of many years of extensive research carried out internationally by the research community that includes basic scientists with interests in chemistry, materials science and bioengineering, as well as clinicians.

However, it is important from the oral health perspective not to lose sight of the importance of prevention of tooth damage. Trauma, being in its nature unpredictable, is difficult to prevent, though in aggressive contact sports such as boxing or rugby, some preventive methods, such as the wearing of mouth-guards, are recommended. Prevention of dental caries and periodontal disease are more straightforward, in that they are predictable conditions but in neither case is prevention easily achieved. Consequently there remains a widespread need for materials and techniques to repair and replace teeth that have been damaged or lost as a result of these conditions. The preventive methods of dental prophylaxis are discussed towards the end of this chapter, and some key references for further reading are included. This is an extremely importance subject from the clinical point of view, and is included for completeness. However, the focus of the remainder of this book is on the repair of teeth and in particular, the variety of modern materials that are used for this purpose.

References

[1] P.W. Lucas, Dental Functional Morphology: How Teeth Work, Cambridge University Press, Cambridge, 2007.

[2] A.R. ten Cate, Oral Histology: Development, Structure and Function, Mosby, London, 1998.

[3] D.M. Davis, J.M. Fiske, B. Scott, D. Radford, The emotional effects of tooth loss: a preliminary quantitative study, Br. Dent. J. 188 (2000) 503–506.

[4] G.V. Lubarsky, R.A. D'Sa, S. Deb, B.J. Meenan, P. Lemoine, The role of enamel proteins in protecting mature human enamel against acidic environments, Biointerphases 7 (2000) 14, http://dx.doi.org/10.10007/513758-011-0014-6.

[5] H. Slavkin, B.J. Baum, Relationship of dental and oral pathology to systemic illness, J. Am. Med. Assoc. 284 (2000) 1215–1217.

[6] T.S. Fill, R.W. Toogood, P.W. Major, J.P. Carey, Analytically determined mechanical properties of, and models for the periodontal ligament: critical review of literature, J. Biomech. 45 (2012) 9–16.

[7] W.J. Ralph, Tensile behaviour of the periodontal ligament, J. Periodont. Res. 17 (1982) 423–426.

[8] O. Fejerskov, E.A.M. Kidd (Eds.), Dental Caries: The Disease and Its Clinical Management, Blackwell and Munksgaard, Oxford, 2008.

[9] D.T. Zero, M. Fontana, E.A. Martinez-Miller, A. Ferreira-Zandona, A. Ando, C. Gonzalez-Cabezas, S. Bayne, The biology, prevention, diagnosis and treatment of dental caries: scientific advances in the United States, J. Am. Dent. Assoc. 140 (2009) 255.

[10] B.J. Paster, S.K. Boches, J.L. Galvin, R.E. Ericson, C.N. Lau, V.A. Lavanos, A. Sahasrabudhe, F.E. Dewhirst, Bacterial diversity in subgingival plaque, J. Bacteriol. 183 (2001) 3770.
[11] S. Hojo, N. Takahashi, T. Yamada, Acid profile in caries dentin, J. Dent. Res. 70 (1991) 182–186.
[12] J.D.B. Featherstone, The continuum of dental caries – evidence for a dynamic disease process, J. Dent. Res. 83 (Special issue C) (2004) C39–C42.
[13] J.D.B. Featherstone, The science and practice of caries prevention, J. Am. Dent. Assoc. 131 (2000) 887–889.
[14] J.D.B. Featherstone, The science and practice of caries prevention, J. Am. Dent. Assoc. 131 (1983) 887–889.
[15] R.Z. LeGeros, Calcium Phosphates in Oral Biology and Medicine, Karger, Basel, 1991.
[16] E.C. Reynolds, Remineralization of enamel subsurface lesions by casein phosphopeptide-stabilized calcium phosphate solutions, J. Dent. Res. 76 (1997) 1587–1595.
[17] E.C. Reynolds, Anticariogenic complexes of amorphous calcium phosphate stabilized by casein phosphopeptides: a review, Spec. Care Dent. 18 (1998) 8–16.
[18] W.E. Brown, T.M. Gregory, L.C. Chow, Effects of fluoride on enamel solubility and cariostasis, Caries Res. 11 (1977) 118–141.
[19] S.O. Griffin, E. Regnier, P.M. Griffin, V. Huntley, Effectiveness of fluoride in preventing caries in adults, J. Dent. Res. 86 (2007) 410–415.
[20] J.N. ten Cate, J.D. Featherstone, Mechanistic aspects of the interactions between fluoride and dental enamel, Crit. Rev. Oral Biol. Med. 2 (1991) 283–286.
[21] N.H. de Leeuw, Resisting the onset of hydroxyapatite dissolution through the incorporation of fluoride, J. Phys. Chem. B. 108 (2004) 1809–1811.
[22] C.A. Robinson, R.C. Shore, S.J. Brooks, S. Stafford, S.R. Wood, J. Kirkham, The chemistry of enamel caries, Crit. Rev. Oral Biol. Med. 11 (2000) 481–495.
[23] A. Yehia, K. Ezzat, Fluoride uptake by synthetic apatites, Adsorpt. Sci. Technol. 27 (2009) 337–347.
[24] M.J. Larsen, O. Fejerskov, Chemical and structural challenges in remineralization of dental enamel lesions, Scand. J. Dent. Res. 97 (1989) 285–296.
[25] J.A. Cury, L.M.A. Tenuta, Enamel remineralization: controlling the caries disease or treating the early caries lesions? Braz. Oral Res. 23 (Suppl. 1) (2009) 23–30.
[26] R.P. Ellwood, O. Fejerskov, J.A. Cury, B. Clarkson, Fluoride in caries control, in: O. Fejerskow, E.A.M. Kidd (Eds.), Dental Caries: The Disease and Its Clinical Management, Blackwell and Munksgaard, Oxford, 2008.
[27] M.J. Larsen, F.R. von der Fehr, J.M. Birkeland, Effect of fluoride on the saturation of an acetate buffer with respect to hydroxyapatite, Arch. Oral Biol. 21 (1976) 723–728.
[28] J.D.B. Featherstone, Prevention and reversal of dental caries: role of low level fluoride, Comm. Dent. Oral Epid. 27 (1999) 31–40.
[29] W.J. Loesche, Role of *Streptococcus mutans* in human dental decay, Microbiol. Rev. 50 (1986) 353–380.
[30] D.L. Mager, L.A. Ximenez-Fyvie, A.D. Haffajee, S.S. Socransky, Distribution of selected bacterial species on intraoral surfaces, J. Clin. Periodontol. 30 (2003) 644–654.
[31] P.W. Caufield, G.R. Cutler, A.P. Dasanayake, Initial acquisition of mutans streptococcui by infants: evidence for a discrete window of infectivity, J. Dent. Res. 72 (1993) 37–45.
[32] R.H. Selwitz, A.I. Ismail, N.B. Pitts, Dental caries, Lancet 369 (2007) 51–59.
[33] L.E. Bertassoni, S. Habelitz, J.H. Kinney, S.J. Marshall, G.W. Marshall Jr., Biomechanical perspective on the remineralization of dentin, Caries Res. 43 (2000) 70–77.
[34] V. Imbeni, J.L. Kruzic, G.W. Marshall, S.J. Marshall, R.O. Ritchie, The dentin-enamel junction and the fracture of human teeth, Nature Mater. 4 (2005) 229–232.

[35] L. Zheng, J.F. Hilton, S. Habelitz, S.J. Marshall, G.W. Marshall, Dentin caries activity status related to hardness and elasticity, Eur. J. Oral Sci. 111 (2003) 243–252.
[36] M.K. Pugach, J. Strother, C.L. Darling, D. Fried, S.A. Gansky, S.J. Marshall, G.W. Marshall, Dentin caries zones: mineral, structure and properties, J. Dent. Res. 88 (2009) 71–76.
[37] J.H. Kinney, M. Balooch, S.J. Marshall, G.W. Marshall Jr., T.P. Weihs, Hardness and Young's modulus of human peritubular and intertubular dentin, Arch. Oral Biol. 41 (1996) 9–13.
[38] J.H. Kinney, S. Habelitz, S.J. Marshall, G.W. Marshall Jr., The importance of intrafibrillar mineralization of collagen on the mechanical properties of dentin, J. Dent. Res. 82 (2003) 957–961.
[39] M. Balooch, I.C. Wu-Magidi, A. Balaza, A.S. Lunqvist, S.J. Marshall, G.W. Marshall, W.J. Siekhaus, J.H. Kinney, Viscoelastic properties of demineralized human dentin measured in water with atomic force microscope (AFM) based indentation, J. Biomed. Mater. Res. 40 (1998) 539–544.
[40] L. Angkur, N. Nijhof, M.V. Swain, N.M. Kilpatrick, Influence of hydration and mechanical characterization of carious primary dentine using an ultra-micro indentation system (UMIS), Eur. J. Oral Sci. 112 (2004) 231–236.
[41] J.D. Featherstone, Modelling the caries-inhibitory effects of dental materials, Dent. Mater. 12 (1996) 194–197.
[42] J.M. ten Cate, Remineralization of deep enamel dentine caries lesions, Aust. Dent. J. 53 (2008) 281–285.
[43] T.P.N. Bhardwaj, P. Solmon, A. Parameswaran, Tooth restored with composite resin – a comparative analysis, Trends Biomater. Artif. Organs 15 (2002) 57–60.
[44] U. Glendor, Epidemiology of traumatic dental injuries – a 12 year review, Dent. Tramatol. 24 (2008) 603–611.
[45] N. Zerman, G. Cavalliera, Traumatic injuries to permanent teeth, Endodod. Dent. Traumatol. 9 (1993) 61–64.
[46] L.M. Kaste, H.C. Gift, M. Bhat, P.A. Swango, Prevalence of incisor trauma in persons 6 to 50 years of age: United States, 1988–1991, J. Dent. Res. 75 (1996) 696–705.
[47] J.D. Shulman, J. Peterson, The association between incisor trauma and occlusal characteristics in individuals 8–50 years of age, Dent. Traumatol. 20 (2004) 67–74.
[48] D. Locker, Prevalence of traumatic dental injury in grade 8 children in six Ontario communities, Can. J. Public Health 96 (2005) 73–76.
[49] W. Marcenes, S. Murray, Social deprivation and traumatic dental injuries among 14-year-olds in Newham, London, Dent. Traumatol. 17 (2001) 17–21.
[50] W. Marcenes, S. Murray, Changes in prevalence and treatment need for traumatic dental injuries among 14-year-old children in Newham, London: a deprived area, Community Dent. Health 19 (2002) 104–108.
[51] H.D. Sgan-Cohen, G. Megnagi, Y. Jacobi, Dental trauma and its association with anatomic, behavioral and associated variables among fifth and sixth grade schoolchildren in Jerusalem, Community Dent. Oral Epidemiol. 33 (2005) 174–180.
[52] O.D. Otuyemi, I.O. Segun-Ojo, A.A. Adegboye, Traumatic anterior dental injuries in Nigerian preschool children, East Afr. Med. J. 73 (1996) 604–606.
[53] D.J. Burden, An investigation of the association between overjet size, lip coverage, and traumatic injury to maxillary incisors, Eur. J. Orthod. 17 (1995) 513–517.
[54] M.J. Rocha, M. Cardoso, Traumatized permanent teeth in Brazilian children assisted at the Federal University of Santa Caterina, Brazil, Dent. Traumatol. 17 (2001) 245–249.

[55] J. Traebert, M.A. Peres, V. Blank, R.D. Boell, J.A. Pietruza, Prevalence of traumatic dental injury and associated factors among 12-year-old school children in Florianopolis, Brazil, Dent. Traumatol. 19 (2003) 15–18.
[56] U. Glendor, A. Halling, L. Andersson, E. Eilert-Petersson, Incidence of traumatic tooth injuries in children and adolescents in the county of Vastmanland, Sweden, Swed. Dent. J. 20 (1996) 15–28.
[57] J. Traebert, D.D. Bittencourt, K.G. Peres, M.A. Peres, J.T. de Lacerda, W. Marcenes, Aetiology and rates of treatment of traumatic dental injuries among 12-year-old school children in a town in southern Brazil, Dent. Traumatol. 22 (2006) 173–178.
[58] G.T. Davis, S.C. Knott, Dental trauma in Australia, Aust. Dent. J. 29 (1984) 517–521.
[59] T.J. Holland, D.M. O'Mullane, H.P. Whelton, Accidental damage to incisors amongst Irish adults, Endod. Dent. Traumatol. 10 (1994) 191–194.
[60] W.M. Thomson, S. Stephenson, J.A. Kieser, J.D. Langley, Dental and maxillofacial injuries among older New Zealanders during the 1990s, Int. J. Oral Maxillofac. Surg. 32 (2003) 201–205.
[61] L.K. Bakland, J.O. Andreasen, Examination of the dentally traumatized patient, J. Calif. Dent. Assoc. 2 (1996) 35–44.
[62] A. Reis, A. Kraul, C. Francci, T.R.G. Assis, D.D. Crivelli, M. Oda, A.D. Loguercio, Reattachment of anterior fractured teeth: fracture strength using different materials, Oper. dent. 27 (2002) 621–627.
[63] B. Farik, E.C. Munksgaard, S. Kreiborg, J.O. Andreassen, Adhesive bonding of fragmented anterior teeth, Endodod. Dent. Traumatol. 14 (1998) 119–123.
[64] B. Farik, E.C. Munksgaard, J.O. Andreassen, Impact strength of teeth restored by fragment-bonding, Endodod. Dent. Traumatol. 16 (2000) 151–153.
[65] J.A. Dean, D.R. Avery, M.L. Swartz, Attachment of anterior tooth fragments, Pediatr. Dent. 8 (1986) 139–143.
[66] L.N. Baratieri, S. Monteiro Jr., M.A.C. Andrada, Tooth fracture reattachment: case reports, Quintessence Int. 21 (1990) 261–270.
[67] J.O. Grippo, Abfractions: a new classification of hard tissue lesions of teeth, J. Esthet. Dent. 3 (1991) 14–18.
[68] J.O. Grippo, M. Simring, T.A. Coleman, Abfraction, abrasion, biocorrosion and the enigma of noncarious cervical lesions: a 20-year perspective, J. Esthet. Restor. Dent. 24 (2012) 10–23.
[69] G.S. Sarode, S.C. Sarode, Abfraction: a review, J. Oral Maxillofac. Pathol. 17 (2013) 222–227.
[70] L.C. Levitch, J.D. Bader, D.A. Shugars, H.O. Heymann, Non-carious cervical lesions, J. Dent. 22 (1994) 195–207.
[71] G. McCoy, The etiology of gingival erosion, J. Oral Implantol. 10 (1982) 361–362.
[72] D.W. Bartlett, P. Shah, A critical review of non-carious cervical (wear) lesions and the role of abfraction, erosion, and abrasion, J. Dent. Res. 85 (2006) 306–312.
[73] L.A. Litonua, S. Andreana, A.K. Patra, J.S. Cohen, An assessment of stress analysis in the theory of abfraction, Biomed. Mater. Eng. 14 (2004) 311–321.
[74] J.S. Rees, H. Hammadeh, C.C. Jagger, Abfraction lesion formation in maxillary incisors, canines and premolars: a finite element study, Eur. J. Oral Sci. 111 (2003) 149–153.
[75] G. McCoy, On the longevity of teeth, J. Oral Implantol. 11 (1983) 248–267.
[76] J.O. Grippo, Tooth flexure, J. Am. Dent. Assoc. 122 (1991) 13.
[77] W.C. Lee, W.S. Eakle, Possible role of tensile stress in the etiology of cervical erosive lesions of teeth, J. Prosthet. Dent. 52 (1984) 374–380.

[78] H. Spranger, Investigation into the genesis of angular lesions at the cervical region of teeth, Quintessence Int. 26 (1995) 149–154.
[79] J.O. Grippo, M. Simring, S. Schreiner, Attrition, abrasion, corrosion and abfraction revisited: a new perspective on tooth surface lesions, J. Am. Dent. Assoc. 135 (2004) 1109–1118.
[80] J.S. Rees, A review of biomechanics of abfraction, Eur. J. Prosthodont., Restor. Dent. 8 (2000) 139–144.
[81] J.A. Hood, Experimental studies on tooth deformation: stress distribution in class V restorations, NZ Dent. J. 68 (1972) 116–131.
[82] K.F. Leinfelder, Restoration of abfraction lesions, Compendium 159 (1994) 1396–1400.
[83] C.H. Gibbs, P.E. Mahan, H.C. Lundeen, K. Brehnan, E.K. Walsh, W.B. Holbrook, Occlusal forces during chewing and swallowing as measured by sound transmission, J. Prosthet. Dent. 46 (1981) 443–449.
[84] S.R. Suit, C.H. Gibbs, S.T. Benz, Study of gliding contacts during mastication, J. Periodontol. 47 (1976) 331–334.
[85] M. Tanaka, T. Naito, M. Yokata, Finite element analysis of the possible mechanism of cervical lesion formation by occlusal force, J. Oral Rehabil. 30 (2003) 60–67.
[86] G. McCoy, The etiology of gingival erosion, J. Oral Implant. 10 (1982) 361–362.
[87] A. Asundi, A. Kishen, A strain gauge and photoelastic analysis of in vivo strain and in vitro stress distribution in human dental supporting structures, Arch. Oral Biol. 45 (2000) 543–550.
[88] T. Kuree, H. Itoh, A.A. Caputo, H. Nakahara, Potential for load-induced cervical stress concentration as a function of periodontal support, J. Esthet. Dent. 11 (1999) 215–222.
[89] A. Manns, R. Miralles, J. Valdivia, R. Bull, Influence of variation in antereoposterior occlusal contacts on electromyographic activity, J. Prosthet. Dent. 61 (1989) 617–623.
[90] J.S. Rees, The role of cuspal flexure in the development of abfraction lesions: a finite element study, Eur. J. Oral Sci. 106 (1998) 1028–1032.
[91] J.A.A. Hood, Biomechanics of the intact, prepared and restored tooth: some clinical implications, Int. Dent. J. 41 (1991) 25–32.
[92] J.S. Rees, D.C. Jagger, Abfraction lesions: myth or reality? J. Esthet. Restor. Dent. 15 (2003) 263–271.
[93] H.E. Lee, C.L. Lin, C.H. Wang, C.H. Cheng, C.H. Chang, Stresses at the cervical lesion of maxillary premolar – a finite element investigation, J. Dent. 30 (2002) 283–290.
[94] H.O. Heymann, J.R. Sturdevant, S. Bayne, A.D. Wilder, T.B. Sluder, W.D. Brunson, Examining tooth flexure effects on cervical restorations: a two-year clinical study, J. Am. Dent. Assoc. 122 (1991) 41–47.
[95] A.L. Tattram, K.W.J. Wright, H.M. Pickard, Finite element stress analysis of the crown of normal and restored teeth, J. Dent. Res. 55 (1976) 1004–1011.
[96] V.K. Goel, S.C. Khera, J.L. Ralston, J.H. Chang, Stresses at the dentinoenamel junction of human teeth – a finite element investigation, J. Prosthet. Dent. 66 (1991) 451–459.
[97] I. Idhim, Q. Li, J. Lougham, Restoration of non-carious cervical lesions Part 1: modelling of restorative fracture, Dent. Mater. 23 (2007) 1553–1561.
[98] J.S. Rees, M. Hammedeh, D.C. Jagger, Abfraction lesion formation in maxillary incisors, canines and premolars: a finite element study, Eur. J. Oral Sci. 111 (2003) 149–154.
[99] J.S. Rees, A review of the biomechanics of abfraction, Eur. J. Prosthodont. Rest. Dent. 8 (2000) 139–144.
[100] J.S. Rees, P.H. Jacobsen, The effect of cuspal flexure on a buccal Class V restoration: a finite element study, J. Dent. 26 (1998) 361–367.
[101] J.S. Rees, The biomechanics of abfraction, Proc. Inst. Mech. Eng. H 220 (2006) 69–80.

[102] P. Lambrechts, M. Braem, G. Vanherle, Evaluation of clinical performance for posterior composite resins and dentin adhesives, Oper. Dent. 12 (1987) 53–78.
[103] E. Reyes, C. Hildebolt, E. Langenwalter, D. Miley, Abfractions and attachment loss in teeth with premature contacts in centric relation: clinical observations, J. Periodontol. 80 (2009) 1955–1962.
[104] J.O. Grippo, Bioengineering seeds of contemplation: a private practitioner's perspective, Dent. Mater. 12 (1996) 198–202.
[105] M. Aliping-McKenzie, J.W. Nicholson, R.W.A. Linden, The long-term effect of Coca-Cola and fruit juices on the surface hardness of glass-ionomers and compomers, J. Oral Rehabil. 31 (2004) 1046–1052.
[106] K. Lyons, Aetiology of abfraction lesions, NZ Dent. J. 97 (2001) 93–98.
[107] L. Shaw, A. Smith, Erosion in children: an increasing clinical problem? Dent. Update 21 (1994) 103–106.
[108] J.H. Nunn, Prevalence of dental erosion and the implications for oral health, J. Oral Sci. 104 (1996) 156–161.
[109] A. Milosevic, M.A. Lennon, S.C. Fear, Risk factors associated with tooth wear in teenagers: a case control study, Community Dent. Health 14 (1997) 143–147.
[110] B.G. Smith, N.D. Robb, The prevalence of tooth wear in 1007 dental patients, J. Oral Rehabil. 23 (1996) 232–239.
[111] V. Jarvinen, J.H. Meurman, H. Hyvarinen, I. Rytomaa, H. Murtomaa, Dental erosion and upper gastrointestinal disorders, Oral Surg. Oral Med. Pathol. 65 (1988) 298–303.
[112] I. Rytomaa, V. Javinen, R. Kanerva, O.P. Heinonen, Bulimia and tooth erosion, Acta Odontol. Scand. 56 (1998) 36–40.
[113] M.G.D. Kellehe, D.I. Bonfim, R.S. Austin, Biologically based restorative management of tooth wear, Int. J. Dent. 2012 (2012). Article ID 742509.
[114] D. Bartlett, Intrinsic causes of erosion, Monogr. Oral Sci. 20 (2006) 119–139.
[115] N.J. Poyser, P.F.A. Briggs, H.S. Chana, M.G.D. Kelleher, R.W.J. Porter, M.M. Patel, The evaluation of direct composite restorations for the worn mandibular anterior dentition—clinical performance and patient satisfaction, J. Oral Rehabil. 34 (2007) 361–376.
[116] K.W. Hemmings, U.R. Darbar, S. Vaughan, Tooth wear treated with direct composite restorations at an increased vertical dimension: results at 30 months, J. Prosthet. Dent. 83 (2000) 287–293.
[117] B.L. Pihlstrom, B.S. Michalowicz, N.W. Johnson, Periodontal disease, Lancet 366 (2005) 1809–1820.
[118] J.M. Albandar, J.A. Brunelle, A. Kingman, Destructive periodontal disease in adults 30 years of age and older in the United States 1988–1994, J. Periodontol. 70 (1999) 13–29.
[119] J.M. Albandar, Understanding of periodontitis in NHANES surveys, J. Periodontol. 82 (2011) 337–341.
[120] P.E. Petersen, H. Ogawa, Strengthening the prevention of periodontal disease: the WHO approach, J. Periodontol. 76 (2005) 2187–2193.
[121] G.C. Armitage, M.P. Cullinan, Comparison of the clinical features of chronic and aggressive periodontitis, Periodontology 53 (2000) 12–27.
[122] J.G.C. Armitage, Development of a classification system for periodontal diseases and conditions, Ann. Periodontol. 4 (1999) 1–6.
[123] Y.A. Al Jehan, Risk factors of periodontal disease: a review of the literature, Int. J. Dent. 2014 (2014). Article 182513.
[124] G. Blandino, I. Milazzo, D. Fazio, S. Puglisi, M. Pisano, A. Speciale, S. Pappalardo, Antimicrobial susceptibility and ß-lactamase production of anaerobic and aerobic bacteria isolated from pus specimens from orofacial infections, J. Chemother. 19 (2007) 495–499.

[125] P.J. Pussinen, S. Paju, P. Mantyla, T. Sorsa, Serum microbial- and host-derived markers of periodontal disease: a review, Curr. Med. Chem. 14 (2007) 2402–2412.
[126] J. Ruby, J. Barbeau, The buccale puzzle: the symbiotic nature of endogenous infections of the oral cavity, Can. J. Infect. Dis. 13 (2002) 34–41.
[127] A.D. Haffajee, S.S. Socransky, Microbial etiological agents of destructive periodontal diseases, Periodontology 5 (2000) 78–111.
[128] W.E. Moore, L.V. Moore, The bacteria of periodontal diseases, Periodontology 5 (2000) 66–77.
[129] A.L. Griffen, M.R. Becker, S.R. Lyons, M.L. Moeschberger, E.J. Leys, Prevalence of Porphryomonas gingivalis and periodontal health, J. Clin. Microbiol. 36 (1998) 3239–3242.
[130] B. Dogan, A.S. Kipalev, E. Okte, N. Sultan, S.E. Asikainen, Consisent intrafamilial transmission of Actinobacillus actinomycetemcomitans despite clonal diversity, J. Periodontol. 79 (2008) 307–315.
[131] J.M. Lovegrove, Dental plaque revisited: bacteria associated with periodontal disease, J. NZ Soc. Periodontol. 87 (2004) 7–21.
[132] I. Niedzielska, T. Janic, S. Cierpka, E. Swietochowska, The effect of chronic periodontitis on the development of atherosclerosis: review of the literature, Med. Sci. Moni. 14 (2008) RA103–RA106.
[133] J.H. Meurman, M. Sanz, S.J. Janket, Oral health, atherosclerosis and cardiovascular disease, Crit. Rev. Oral Biol. Med. 15 (2004) 403–413.
[134] J.D.B. Featherstone, The science and practice of caries prevention, J. Am. Dent. Assoc. 131 (2000) 887–899.
[135] V. Clerehugh, A. Tugnair, Periodontal diseases in children and adolescents: 1. Aetiology and diagnosis, Dent. Update 28 (2001) 222–230.
[136] American Academy of Periodontology Research Science and Therapy Committee, Treatment of plaque-induced gingivitis, chronic periodontitis and other clinical conditions, J. Periodontol. 72 (2001) 1790–1800.
[137] V. Clerehugh, A. Tugnair, Periodontal diseases in children and adolescents: 2. Management, Dent. Update 28 (2001) 274–281.
[138] M. Quirynen, C.M.L. Bollen, The influence of surface roughness and surface-free energy on supra- and subgingival plaque formation in man. A review of the literature, J. Clin. Periodontol. 22 (1995) 1–14.
[139] G.K. Stookey, In vitro estimates of enamel and dentin abrasion associated with a prophylaxis, J. Dent. Res. 57 (1978) 36.
[140] J.R. Mellberg, The relative abrasivity of dental prophylactic pastes and abrasives on enamel and dentin, Clin. Prev. Dent. 1 (1979) 13–18.
[141] N. Tinanoff, S.H.Y. Wei, F.M. Parkins, Effect of a pumice prophylaxis on fluoride uptake in tooth enamel, J. Am. Dent. Assoc. 88 (1974) 384–389.
[142] Y. Hosoya, J.W. Johnston, Evaluation of various cleaning and polishing methods on primary enamel, J. Pedod. 13 (1989) 253–269.

Classification of restorative materials and clinical indications

2

2.1 Introduction

This chapter is concerned with the essential classification of the materials used to repair teeth and restore their function. As far as direct restoratives are concerned, we follow the classification on Mount et al. [1] and consider that the two basic types of modern tooth-coloured materials are the composite resins and the glass-ionomer cements. They are fundamentally different, and though hybrids have been attempted, combining their advantages is not feasible for sound scientific reasons.

Composite resins consist of blends of large monomer molecules, filled with unreactive reinforcing filler. As such, they are hydrophobic, which means that they are unable to bond to the hydrophilic prepared tooth surface [1]. Glass-ionomer cements, by contrast, consist of aqueous solutions of polymeric acid, typically poly(acrylic acid) and powdered reactive glass. These two components react together in an acid–base reaction, and thus cause the cement to set. These materials are hydrophilic, and therefore capable of wetting the prepared tooth surface and forming true adhesive bonds.

The difference between these materials in terms of their hydrophobic or hydrophilic nature is fundamental, and is the reason that it is difficult to combine their best characteristics into a single hybrid material. Nonetheless, materials exist that are based on modifications of these two basic types, and they will be considered briefly in this chapter, and in much greater detail in individual chapters later in the book.

The essential features of the two basic types of restorative material are given in Table 2.1. From this, it can be seen that each type has its own advantages and disadvantages. In terms of overall properties, modern composite resins appear to be favoured, and there is evidence that these materials are the ones used in the majority of aesthetic repairs in dentistry, particularly in adults. However, as the development of the polyacid-modified composite resins (compomers) shows, these materials are far from perfect, and there is unquestionably scope to enhance their properties. Glass-ionomer cements have properties that would seem to indicate the direction in which improvements could be made, despite the technical difficulties in doing so.

2.2 Basic types of dental restorative material: composite resins and glass-ionomer cements

2.2.1 Composite resins

The term 'composite resin' is applied to a group of dental restoratives that set by an addition polymerization mechanism. Originally these were based on poly(methyl

Materials for the Direct Restoration of Teeth. http://dx.doi.org/10.1016/B978-0-08-100491-3.00002-7

Table 2.1 Essential features of composite resins and glass-ionomer cements

Material	Advantages	Disadvantages
Composite resin	Photo-activated, hence 'command-set' Excellent aesthetics Tough hence durable	Hydrophobic, hence no adhesion to tooth No inherent fluoride release
Glass-ionomer cement	Inherent 'ion-exchange' bonding because hydrophilic Acceptable aesthetics Fluoride release	Sensitive to loss of moisture when newly placed Brittle

Source: G.J. Mount, M.J. Tyas, J.L. Ferracane, J.W. Nicholson, J.H. Berg, R.J. Simonsen, H.C. Ngo, A revised classification for direct tooth-colored restorative materials, Quintessence Int. 40 (2009) 691–697.

methacrylate), filled with finely divided quartz powders [1]. Modern versions of these materials are based on more complex monomers that consist of large molecules containing two alkene functional groups capable of undergoing addition polymerization. Current substances employed are primarily bisphenol glycidyl methacrylate (bis-GMA) or urethane dimethacrylate. Other lower molar mass monomers are also included in the formulations, such as diethylene glycol dimethacrylate (DEGDMA) or triethylene dimethacrylate (TEGDMA). These act as diluents and improve the application viscosity, which would otherwise be unworkably high [2,3].

Modern composite resins are typically cured with photo-initiators and in deep cavities need to be applied layer-by-layer in a technique known as incremental build-up [3]. Their ability to be photo-cured allows them to be presented to the clinician as single pastes, typically in black plastic capsules or syringes to prevent the unset pastes from being exposed to daylight. This is to stop premature polymerization [4]. However, they can also be supplied as two-paste systems, with each paste containing a different component of the polymerization initiator. Mixing the pastes brings the two components, which results in the generation of free radicals, and these free radicals initiate polymerization and cause the composite resin to set. This was the way composite resins were supplied to the profession when they first appeared in the 1960s [1]. Such systems are still available, but are much less widely used in the modern dental clinic than single-paste light-cured composites, and very few manufacturers still make them [5].

In addition to the blend of monomers, composite resins contain fillers. These are typically finely divided quartz or barium silicate glasses, and their function is to provide strength for the fully formulated composite [2]. These fillers are linked to the polymer phase by coupling agents, which are typically silane-based substances [2]. Composite reins are characterized by the absence of a chemical reaction between the filler and the monomer or polymer phase. Also, they show no inherent adhesion to the tooth but instead they have to be bonded to the tooth with bespoke bonding agents. These are discussed in detail in Chapter 5.

2.2.2 *Glass-ionomer cements*

As we have seen, in the classification of tooth-coloured dental restorative materials, the composite resins represent one of the major types [1,6]. The other major type is the glass-ionomer cement.

Within clinical dentistry, there are several types of cement available, including the zinc phosphate and the zinc polycarboxylate. They share with glass-ionomers the feature of being acid–base cements and setting as the result of a neutralization reaction, and consequently they are hydrophilic by nature [7]. These cements differ from each other in that they have different acid and base components, but they resemble each other in that the acid is always an aqueous solution and the base is a water-insoluble solid metal oxide powder. The setting reaction, which begins immediately when the components are mixed, involves acid attack on the solid powdered base, and leads to the release of metal ions into the aqueous phase. In this phase, the metal ions interact with the acid (or its anion) to form metal salts, and these are rigid and insoluble. As these salts form, so the overall cement hardens and becomes insoluble in saliva and other aqueous media [7].

Cements are formulated from minimal amounts of water [7,8]. This has two practical consequences within dentistry, namely (i) that the initial cement consists of a highly viscous paste which has sufficient stiffness to be used and placed in clinical service, and (ii) that the formation of a solid mass on setting is not accompanied by phase separation. Instead water from the initial formulation becomes incorporated within the cement by some means.

The precise structural role of the water molecules in these cements is not always clear, though there are various possibilities. Water is capable of occupying co-ordination sites around the key metal ions used in the bases, such as Ca^{2+}, Zn^{2+} or Al^{3+} [7]. It may occupy sites adjacent to the anions within the cement, such as polyacrylate [9]. Whatever the detail, though, the overall effect is that water becomes bound within the set cement, and the cement hardens with little or no loss of the water with which it was mixed initially.

Historically, two acid–base cements were used in dentistry, their use dating back to the late 19th century. These were the zinc phosphate and dental silicate cements [7]. These two remained in clinical service until at least the 1970s, and zinc phosphate continues to be used today, with its principal application being the luting of crowns [2].

Both types of cement are made from aqueous solutions of phosphoric acid that are typically deactivated slightly by the inclusion of aluminium and zinc. Compositions differ slightly, as shown in Table 2.2.

Table 2.2 **Composition of cement-forming liquids**

Cement	Composition of liquid (%)	References
Zinc phosphate	H_3PO_4 45.3–63.2 Al 1.0–3.1 Zn 0–9.9	[10,11]
Dental silicate	H_3PO_4 48.8–65.9 Al 1.6–2.5 Zn 0–9.1	[12]

The zinc phosphate cement dates back to at least 1879, when Rollins reported a formulation based on syrupy orthophosphoric acid [13]. The first really satisfactory cement of this type was reported by Fleck in 1902 [14]. His report described a paper based on zinc oxide that had been deactivated by heating, together with a solution of phosphoric acid modified by the inclusion of aluminium and zinc. These two approaches to moderating the reaction led to a setting process that took place at a sufficiently slow speed that a smooth paste could be prepared from the components, and there was time to apply it before hardening took place.

The development of the dental silicate cement in its final, satisfactory form occurred slightly later than the development of the zinc phosphate, though it, too, traces its earliest history back to the later 1870s. The pioneering work on this material was reported in 1878 and 1879 by Fletcher [15,16], and involved cements prepared from concentrated solutions of orthophosphoric acid and sintered mixtures of oxides, including silica and alumina, with inclusions of calcium oxide and zinc oxide. One of these cements showed slight translucency when set [16], but overall the cements were not a success clinically [7].

In the early years of the 20th century, a number of individuals made experiments on the composition of the glasses for dental silicate cements. For these studies, which were often published in obscure journals or in the patent literature, forms of glass emerged that were based on alumino-silicate formulations augmented with fluoride [7]. The addition of fluoride was important in that the first aspect of its use was that it acts as a flux in the glass-forming process, ie, it reduces the melting temperature of the molten glass. However, fluoride also makes the resulting cement stronger as well as conferring beneficial therapeutic effects as the fluoride ion can be released slowly from the set cement. By the late 1930s, all of these compositional features were established and the dental silicate cements available to the dental profession were all of this type [17].

Dental silicate cements were used as aesthetic repair materials for anterior teeth [7]. Though they lacked the ability to adhere to the tooth, they did have a reasonable match for the appearance of the natural tooth, both in terms of colour and translucency. Nonetheless, they were not entirely satisfactory in clinical service and in particular were susceptible to acid erosion and staining in the mouth [7].

These drawbacks were sufficiently important that, in the early 1960s, the UK Laboratory of the Government Chemist was commissioned to investigate these materials, partly with a view to determining whether there was scope to improve them [18]. Work was carried out by a small group led by Dr Alan Wilson, with initial studies aimed at elucidating the setting mechanism of the cement. From the 1930s, setting had been attributed to gelation of silicic acid, which was thought to be produced as a result of acid attack on the silicate glass powder [19]. However, this was shown to be untrue in a study of the acid solubility of a number of formulations of dental silicate cement. Their solubility was such that they could not possibly be composed of silica gel, as assumed [20]. Later structural studies of the set cement confirmed that the material was substantially composed of aluminium phosphates and was thus a phosphate-bonded cement rather than a silicate cement [21].

As these studies were in progress, the first report of the novel zinc polycarboxylate appeared [22]. This material was invented in the mid 1960s by Dr (later Professor)

Denis Smith, and the development showed that satisfactory cements could be made by reacting heat-treated zinc oxide of the type used in zinc phosphate dental cements with concentrated solutions of poly(acrylic acid). This demonstrated that an alternative cement-forming acid was available, and one, which offered the prospect that cements formed from it, would adhere to the tooth [22,23].

It was not a straightforward matter to take the next step of making an acceptable cement from dental silicate glass and aqueous poly(acrylic acid) [18]. When it was first tried, the result was a disappointing material that set very slowly and was extremely weak. It was so poor that the result was not reported at the time in a pioneering study of novel cement-forming acids [24]. It was only some years later that Wilson mentioned this experiment and its unfortunate outcome [18].

The problem was that the dental silicate glass was not sufficiently basic to react rapidly with poly(acrylic acid) and thereby form a satisfactory cement. The dental silicate glass had been developed to react with orthophosphoric acid, a strong acid, rather than a weak acid such as poly(acrylic acid). In order to produce an acceptable cement, the basicity of the glass needed to be adjusted. Fortunately, as part of the fundamental studies on the setting of the dental silicate cement, Wilson and his team had showed that basicity of the glass is controlled by its ratio of alumina to silica [25]. Armed with this knowledge, they were able to set out to alter the composition of the glass in an appropriate direction, eventually producing a large number of experimental glasses [26], one of which, known as G200, proved acceptable. Cements based on this glass were first reported in 1971 [27] and the name 'glass-ionomer' applied to them.

These early cements had relatively poor properties compared with modern glass-ionomers. They set relatively slowly, but quickly became unworkable, and were weak when fully hardened [28]. Also, as the glass G200 was relatively high in fluoride, it was opaque, which meant that the set cements lacked translucency [18]. This meant that the early glass-ionomer cements had relatively poor aesthetics.

Nonetheless these early cements exhibited all of the important defining characteristics of glass-ionomers that remain important today [29]. Some of these are shown in Table 2.1, and overall the important characteristics are:

(i) setting by a neutralization (acid–base) reaction;
(ii) no significant setting shrinkage;
(iii) no significant setting exotherm;
(iv) no release of potentially hazardous monomer;
(v) adhesion to the tooth surface;
(vi) release of fluoride, with its potential therapeutic effect;
(vii) a reasonable aesthetic match for the colour and translucency of the natural tooth.

These features are the critical ones of glass-ionomer cements, but not always recognized. For example, certain manufacturers have provided materials consisting of the ionomer glass component dispersed in composite resin monomers, and described the result as a 'light-cured glass-ionomer'. This is clearly misleading, since these products do not set by neutralization. In addition, they have a polymerization contraction and are too hydrophobic to bond to the tooth surface. The defining aspect of glass-ionomers is that they undergo a neutralization reaction, though as we will see later in this chapter, there are the resin-modified glass-ionomers in which this neutralization reaction is supplemented by a true polymerization [6].

2.3 Resin-modified glass-ionomer cements

Two types of hybrid materials became available in the early 1990s that attempted to combine the properties of composite resins and glass-ionomers. The first of these was the group known as resin-modified glass-ionomers, originally described as light-cured glass-ionomers [30,31] and designated for use as liners and bases, rather than full restorations. They contained, in addition to the usual components of a glass-ionomer cement, an amount of water-soluble monomer, plus photo-initiator. The monomer used is usually 2-hydroxyethyl methacrylate, usually referred to as HEMA [7].

The advantage of the resin-modified glass-ionomer over conventional materials is that, with the light-cured versions, there is a significant degree of control over the setting reaction for the clinician. This arises because the polymerization part of the setting reaction does not begin until the cure light is beamed onto the cement. However, this advantage is absent from the self-cured version of the resin-modified glass-ionomer.

Properties of resin-modified glass-ionomer cements vary between brands, but they have been found to lie in the same range as those of conventional glass-ionomer materials. The acid–base part of the setting chemistry is still able to occur, despite the presence of the HEMA. However, HEMA has been shown to inhibit this reaction to an extent [32], probably because the organic monomer causes the poly(acrylic acid) molecules to adopt more tightly coiled configurations than they do in pure water [33]. This is because HEMA is a less good solvent for poly(acrylic acid) in thermodynamic terms than pure water [32,33].

Use of resin-modified glass-ionomers has grown considerably since their introduction in 1991, and versions are available that are suitable for use as full restorations [34]. However, because of limited penetration by light, deep cavities may need to be filled using the incremental build-up technique usually associated with composite resins. Resin-modified glass-ionomers show good adhesion to dentine [31] and also release useful amounts of fluoride [31,35].

In their original paper on the classification of tooth-coloured dental restoratives, McLean et al. argued for these materials to be called resin-modified glass-ionomers [6]. A variety of other terms have been used, including light-cured glass-ionomers [30,31], resin-ionomers [36] and resin-reinforced glass-ionomers [37]. The latter is particularly inexcusable, given that they are no stronger than conventional glass-ionomers and that what limited experimental evidence there it suggests that the presence of the HEMA component not only slows down the setting reaction but also weakens the set cement [32].

Despite these occasional alternative names for these materials, the term 'resin-modified glass-ionomer' seems to have become the most widely used of them all. It is the one that most manufacturers favour in describing their products, and is also the one used most extensively in the scientific and clinical literature. Because of its scientific accuracy [6], it is our preferred term and the one we apply to these materials throughout the current book.

2.4 Polyacid-modified composite resins

The term *polyacid-modified composite resin* was originally proposed for these materials by McLean et al. in 1994 [6], and was felt to be a more accurate description than the term 'compomer' under which they had been first marketed. The latter word was coined as a hybrid of the terms 'composite' and 'glass-ionomer', but lacked any indication that the materials in question more closely resembled conventional composite resins than glass-ionomer cements. In particular, they are formulated without any water present, and are substantially hydrophobic, albeit less so than conventional composite resins. Also, despite early claims, they show no inherent adhesion to the tooth surface, and have to be used in association with bonding agents of the type used with conventional composites [1,6].

Polyacid-modified composite resins were developed in an attempt to make a composite resin with the sort of ion-release capability of glass-ionomer cements, especially of fluoride [38]. They are similar to conventional composites in that they are mainly based on the hydrophobic monomers bis-GMA or urethane dimethacrylate, and their setting is typically initiated by light. In addition, they contain inert fillers of appropriate particle size.

In addition, they contain extra components. Part of the filler phase is made up of particles of fluoroaluminosilicate glass of the type used in glass-ionomer cements. There is also a small quantity of a proprietary acid-functional monomer, the so-called 'acid resin' [1]. This is not sufficient to allow the monomer to be soluble in water, but it does confer a small degree of hydrophilic character on the set matrix. This causes water from the surroundings to be drawn into the structure, and results in ionization of the acid-functional groups and reaction with the ionomer glass component [38]. Any such reaction is limited, but potentially useful in allowing the set material to release fluoride.

Polyacid-modified composite resins have undergone considerable development since they first appeared. The very limited nature of the acid–base reaction means that they have had to have the fluoride-releasing capability augmented, for example, through the inclusion of extra ytterbium fluoride in the formulation [38]. There has also been concern that the ability to draw in water from the environment might also lead to staining and softening, and reformulation has partly been driven by the need to minimize any such moisture uptake, so as to preserve the physical properties of the composite.

Filler loadings are low by comparison with some of the better conventional composites available, and this means that there is a relatively large volumetric shrinkage on polymerization [1]. However, to an extent swelling due to moisture uptake offsets this. Despite this moisture uptake, aesthetics of these materials are reasonable though they are now generally recommended for use in children's dentistry, and are available in a variety of colours (pink, blue, green) so that aesthetics in the sense of a close visual appearance to the natural tooth is less of a concern [38].

Though these materials were designed to combine properties of glass-ionomers with those of composites [39], their handling is entirely that of a typical composite. Through cure limitations, coupled with the need for photo-initiation, means that incremental build-up has to be used for deep cavities. Also, there is no inherent adhesion to the tooth as ion-exchange bonding does not occur.

As mentioned, these materials seem to have found particular application in children's dentistry. The successive reformulations mean that they may have lost their original distinctive characteristic of having a small amount of acid–base reaction following post-cure moisture uptake. There is evidence that modern polyacid-modified composite resins primarily release fluoride as a result of the additional fluoride compound, as with fluoridated conventional composites, and that any acid–base reaction is so slight that it has little, if any, effect on the properties of the material. Overall, these materials do not duplicate the properties of either of the parent materials particularly well, and their current use in clinical dentistry is fairly limited [1].

2.5 Clinical aspects of the tooth-coloured restorative materials

The original classification of dental restorative materials proposed by McLean et al. [6] was based on the setting chemistry of the materials. Specifically, this distinguished the addition polymerization of the monomers in composite resins from the acid–base neutralization in glass-ionomers, and highlighted these as the key differences. However, these chemical differences lead to the two groups having distinctive properties that, in turn, contribute to different outcomes in clinical service. Some of these differences have only emerged since the original classification was published in 1994. This part of the chapter aims to explain these differences in detail, and to highlight those factors that should inform materials selection to ensure optimum clinical outcomes.

Composite resins have continued to undergo improvements, notably through modifications to the filler type and content, and filler particle size and distribution [1,30]. In addition, there have been considerable developments in bonding systems, as discussed in detail in Chapter 5.

A concern with the use of composites in the dental clinic is their polymerization shrinkage. This is unavoidable with polymerizing systems, and arises because the tethered ends of the repeat units in the polymer occupy less free volume than the equivalent ends of the unpolymerized monomers [40]. Shrinkage of modern composites varies between 2% and 5% by volume, depending on the filler loading (usually expressed as volume percent) and on the blend of monomers used [41]. Modern composite resins are generally classified as packable and flowable, with packable composites having higher filler loadings [42,43]. As their name suggests, they are stiff pastes, readily packed into cavities using a reasonable amount of force. As such, when they are cured, they have better physical properties and provide strength to the bulk of the restoration [43]. In addition, their shrinkage is towards the lower end of the quoted range [43].

Flowable composites, by contrast, have lower filler loadings and a higher proportion of low viscosity monomers. They are thus more readily able to flow into surface irregularities on the prepared and bonded tooth surface. Consequently, they complete the restoration in such a way that little if any unoccupied space remains. By comparison with packable composites, however, they shrink more on setting [43].

Both types of composite resin should be applied using the technique of incremental build-up in which layers not exceeding 2 mm are placed and light-cured prior to the placement of the next layer [44]. This allows the layers to be fully cured all the way through, and layers will adhere to each other, so that this technique does not introduce any points of weakness to the material. Occasional claims of 'bulk cure' being acceptable have been made, ie, where layers of 5 mm or so are cured in a single burst of light. However, the scientific evidence does not support such claims, and they should be treated with caution [1].

Currently composite resins are the materials of choice with many clinicians for anterior restorations [45], particularly in adults. Clinical studies of their performance are generally positive, though there have been some concerns about their susceptibility to stain and discolour [45]. Also, where loads are high, the edges of composite resin restorations show a tendency to chip. On the other hand, survival rates have been shown to be excellent, with up to almost 20 years acceptable service being recorded [46] and annual failure rates working out at about 2% [45]. Overall, they are known to be versatile and reliable materials, and their future in restorative dentistry is assured [47].

The alternative tooth-coloured material, the glass-ionomer cement, has also been widely studied, especially in terms of its bioactivity. This arises from its ability to exchange ions with its surroundings when placed in the mouth. Typical conventional glass-ionomers have been shown to release sodium, silicon and phosphorus under neutral conditions, and also calcium and aluminium under acidic conditions [48]. The non-metals are assumed to be released as silicate, SiO_3^{2-}, and phosphate, PO_4^{3-}, respectively. In addition, they release fluoride [49], a process that is capable of continuing for several years [50].

As well as releasing ions, conventional glass-ionomers can take up ions. Fluoride ion uptake has been demonstrated in a number of studies [51–53], and has been claimed to be the basis for fluoride recharge [1]. However, recent studies have cast doubt on this notion, particularly raising the question of the relationship between specimen maturity and fluoride uptake [54].

Studies have also shown that calcium and phosphate can be taken up from saliva [55]. Specimens that were exposed to saliva not only had an altered chemical composition in the surface, but they were also significantly harder than specimens exposed only to pure water. This showed that the calcium phosphate-enriched surfaces were mechanically different from the unmodified ones. In a clinical study of glass-ionomer fissure sealants, residual cement left at the bottom of deep fissures was found to form an enamel-like structure with time, either by ion-exchange with the saliva or ion-exchange with the tooth [56].

Bonding of glass-ionomers has also been found to be altered by the ability to exchange ions. When glass-ionomers are applied to the tooth surface, they are able to wet the substrate and form attachments [7]. With time, ions are exchanged between the tooth surface and the cement, and an interfacial zone is formed that contains intermingled elements that were originally present in either the tooth surface of the cement [57]. This ion-exchange layer appears strong and durable, and may be the reason that glass-ionomers show such good long-term adhesion to the tooth, despite relatively low initial bond strengths [58].

The features that characterize conventional glass-ionomer cements, including ion-exchange bonding, are discussed in much greater detail in Chapter 6. The overall conclusion from this section of the present chapter, though, is that the classification proposed in 1994 by McLean et al. [6] has stood the test of time, and is scientifically sound. It reflects not only the fundamental chemistry of the materials formulations, but also the resulting biological and clinical properties. The two important subgroups of the main two (polyacid-modified composites and resin-modified glass-ionomers) turn out to be much more closely allied to their main parent than was originally hoped.

This means that polyacid-modified composites are essentially composite resins. As such, they must be bonded to the tooth with appropriate bonding agents, applied in increments, and show no ion-exchange properties, though they will release fluoride [38]. Similarly, resin-modified glass-ionomers are very similar to conventional glass-ionomers. They show inherent adhesion to the tooth [30], long-term fluoride release [31] and ion-release under neutral and acidic conditions [59].

Another thing that follows from this is that occasional recent claims from manufacturers of the invention of a completely new type of materials are incorrect. Thus, both 'giomers' and 'ormocers' are types of composite resin, albeit with novel fillers and, in the case of ormocers, novel monomers, though they still set by the same type of chemistry, ie, addition polymerization [45]. They are also fundamentally hydrophobic, and do not form inherent bonds to the tooth surface. These materials are discussed later in the book, in Chapter 3, where their principal features are described and related to their essential chemistry as types of composite.

2.6 Materials for pulp capping

The tooth pulp can become exposed by a variety of processes, including deep caries, trauma or accidentally during cavity preparation in the dental chair [60]. The consequences can be severe, and include pain, infection and necrosis. When the pulp is exposed, steps need to be taken to manage the situation, and these involve either pulp capping with an appropriate material [60,61] or removal of the pulp followed by sealing of the tooth roots. In the present section of the chapter, we consider briefly materials for the first of these options, pulp capping.

Pulp capping is the term given to the procedure of the dressing of an exposed pulp of the tooth, and has the aim of maintaining the pulp in its vital condition [61]. A vital pulp is essential for the long-term well being of a tooth, since it contributes to secondary dentine formation and also to general dentine repair following damage due to biological or pathological assault. The pulp tissue also has the role of maintaining the dentin in its moist state, and this ensures that dentine retains its biomechanical properties of resilience and toughness. All together, these features mean that the pulp contributes to the overall function of the vital tooth.

However, the pulp is a delicate biological system, comprising as it does a collection of fibroblasts, blood vessels and nerves. As such, it can suffer damage when it is exposed, and this damage can threaten its vitality [60,61]. Capping, if successful, allows the tooth to heal and the pulp to retain its biological function.

The main material used in this procedure is calcium hydroxide, $Ca(OH)_2$, which was first introduced to the dental profession in 1921. It is widely considered to be the best material available, since it is easy to use and is bioactive. Its bioactivity is demonstrated in that it stimulates migration, proliferation and differentiation of pulp fibroblast cells in vivo [62]. In this way, calcium hydroxide stimulates dentine formation and causes complete healing of the tooth [63]. It is also usually antibacterial as a result of its high pH and therefore contributes to the disinfection of the pulp, an important aspect of the healing process [43].

In principle, the only substance that needs to be provided to stimulate healing of the tooth following pulp exposure is calcium hydroxide. In practice, supplying this as a simple suspension in water is quite challenging, because the solution is difficult to manipulate and maintain in place [2]. Also, it forms a very friable and unsatisfactory covering to the pulp that is fragile and mechanically weak. Consequently, it needs to be covered with zinc oxide-eugenol cement plus another acid–base cement (zinc phosphate, zinc polycarboxylate or conventional glass-ionomer) to complete the treatment and keep the calcium hydroxide in place. This makes the procedure difficult. However, pure calcium hydroxide slurry placed in this way is well tolerated by the injured pulp.

As an alternative, calcium hydroxide is often supplied as two-paste material that also includes zinc oxide in a suspension of calcium hydroxide in the organic liquid ethyl toluene sulphonamide, mixed with glycol salicylate containing inert fillers, pigments and radiopacifiers. These two organic liquids react together in an acid–base process catalysed by moisture from the surroundings to form a chelate structure bonded together by salicylate units co-ordinated with zinc and calcium ions. This material is more easily handled than the simple calcium hydroxide suspension, and sets to form a weak cohesive cement [2].

In recent years, a light-curable version of the calcium hydroxide cement has become available [64,65]. This is claimed to have superior properties to conventional calcium hydroxide cements, including ease of handling [64]. However, there is evidence that they absorb water [66], which is likely to cause swelling, and they also likely to undergo polymerization shrinkage. This latter point does not seem to have been investigated, and its potential clinical consequences are unclear. A further questionable aspect of these materials is that the calcium hydroxide is effectively sealed away inside the resin system, and this must reduce its ability to provide a high pH in the region surrounding the material. Thus the desirable bioactivity of the calcium hydroxide component is likely to be substantially compromised.

Another chelate cement, zinc oxide-eugenol has been suggested as a treatment for exposed and inflamed pulp [61]. However, its use has been reported to cause adverse biological responses, including chronic inflammation and eventual necrosis of the pulp [67,68]. As a result, its use is no longer recommended for direct application to the pulp. However, its application with a calcium hydroxide system as the means of retaining the calcium hydroxide remains widely used and is recommended.

On the other hand, the new material known commercially as 'Biodentine' is much more promising [61,69]. It is a hydraulic cement manufactured by the French company Septodont and consisting mainly of tricalcium silicate [70]. In this it resembles the endodontic sealer Mineral Trioxide Aggregate, MTA, though it has a different overall composition. Like MTA, it can be used in endodontics as a root canal sealer for teeth from which the pulp has been removed, and also to repair root perforations [70]. It is also advocated for pulp capping.

Biodentine is supplied as a powder and a liquid. The powder contains, in addition to the calcium silicates, calcium carbonate and calcium oxide as fillers, iron oxide for pigmentation, and zirconium oxide as a radiopacifier. The liquid is mainly water and contains calcium chloride as an accelerator, plus a water-soluble polymer [70].

When hardened, Biodentine shows good biocompatibility with the oral tissues and, in particular, exerts minimal influence on cells of the adjacent pulp. Some loss of cell viability has been reported, but this has been attributed to apoptosis and necrosis, rather than the toxicity of the material [71]. In one study of the performance of Biodentine, it was found that the material caused complete dentinal bridge formation in molars while creating no inflammatory response on the cells of the pulp [72]. Both of these features suggest that this material has promise for application in pulp capping. Its ability to promote regeneration of the hard tissue is particularly noteworthy, and will be considered in more detail in Chapter 9.

2.7 Endodontic materials

For a tooth in which the pulp is too damaged by trauma or infection to survive, the usual clinical procedure is extirpation of the pulp, followed by sealing of the root system of the tooth. This procedure is aimed at preserving the structure of the tooth despite its loss of vitality, and typically employs pre-formed gutta percha points to prove the bulk of the obturation. There is also some sort of sealing material employed as well [73].

The root canal is usually a complex shape and filling it to prevent leakage and consequent infection is a skilled task. In the clinic, root canals need preparation to clean them and modify their internal shape. This is followed by irrigation with a series of solutions including sodium hypochlorite solution to sterilize the region ready for sealing.

The main material used for obturation of the cleaned and disinfected root canal in contemporary endodontics is gutta percha. This is used because it is plastic and will take up the shape of the root canal when pressed into place [74]. A sealant is used in association with these gutta percha points, and its function is to fill any gaps between the points and the canal walls. This has the effect of improving the quality of the overall seal at the tooth root [73].

As is described in Chapter 10, several different materials have been considered as sealants. These include zinc oxide-eugenol cements, epoxy resins and glass-ionomer cements [73,74]. In addition, calcium hydroxide paste has been used, though this material appears to be susceptible to leakage and may not be entirely satisfactory in forming a durable seal. However, its bioactivity is able to promote the physiological closure of the apex with dentine and cementum via stimulation of the odontoblast and cementoblast cells present [75].

Table 2.3 **Components of MTA**

Component	Nominal formula
Tricalcium silicate	$(CaO)_3 \cdot SiO_2$
Dicalcium silicate	$(CaO)_2 \cdot SiO_2$
Tricalcium aluminate	$(CaO)_3 \cdot Al_2O_3$
Tetracalcium aluminoferrate	$(CaO)_4 \cdot Al_2O_3 \cdot Fe_2O_3$
Gypsum	$CaSO_4 \cdot 2H_2O$
Bismuth oxide	Bi_2O_3

Mineral trioxide aggregate has also been widely used [73] and appears to be an exceptionally good material for repairing interfaces between the root canal system and the external surface of the tooth. It was originally developed as a material for root-end filling [74] but has since been shown to give good results when used to repair perforations. It will also induce apical closure in immature tooth roots [73].

MTA has the composition shown in Table 2.3. Essentially, it sets by reaction of the calcium silicate and calcium aluminate components with water and, like Biodentine, is classified as a hydraulic cement [76]. It has been suggested for use in pulp capping, though this is not its major application. MTA has good biocompatibility when used to seal tooth roots and is also bioactive, due to its high pH. This stimulates osteoblasts and cementoblasts resulting in regeneration of osseous and dental tissues [77]. These biological properties and the clinical applications of MTA are discussed fully in Chapter 10.

References

[1] G.J. Mount, M.J. Tyas, J.L. Ferracane, J.W. Nicholson, J.H. Berg, R.J. Simonsen, H.C. Ngo, A revised classification for direct tooth-colored restorative materials, Quintessence Int. 40 (2009) 691–697.

[2] J.F. McCabe, A.W.G. Walls, Applied Dental Materials, Ninth ed., Blackwell Munsgaard, Oxford, 2008.

[3] S. Pamela, J.S. Stein, J.E. Haubenreich, P.B. Osborne, Composite resin in medicine and dentistry, J. Long Term Eff. Med. Implants 15 (2005) 641–654.

[4] J.W. Stansbury, Curing dental resins and composites by photopolymerisation, J. Esthet. Dent. 12 (2000) 300–308.

[5] J.L. Ferracane, Current trends in dental composite resins, Crit. Rev. Oral Biol. Med. 6 (1995) 302–318.

[6] J.W. McLean, J.W. Nicholson, A.D. Wilson, Proposed nomenclature for glass-ionomer dental cements and related materials, Quintessence Int. 25 (1994) 587–589.

[7] A.D. Wilson, J.W. Nicholson, Acid–Base Cements, Cambridge University Press, Cambridge, 1993.

[8] A.D. Wilson, J.W. McLean, Glass-Ionomer Cement, Quintessence Publishing, Chicago, 1988.

[9] A. Ikegami, Hydration of polyacids, Biopolymers 6 (1968) 431–440.

[10] B. Axelsson, Kemisk analys av dentala zinkfosfatcement, Odont. Revy 16 (1965) 126–130.

[11] A.D. Wilson, G. Abel, B.G. Lewis, The solubility and disintegration test for zinc phosphate dental cements, Br. Dent. J. 137 (1974) 313–317.
[12] A.D. Wilson, B.E. Kent, D. Clinton, R.P. Miller, The formation and microstructure of the dental silicate cement, J. Mater. Sci. 7 (1972) 220–238.
[13] W.H. Rollins, A contribution to the knowledge of cements, Dental Cosmos 21 (1879) 574–576. Quoted in Reference [7].
[14] H. Fleck, The chemistry of oxyphosphates, Dent. Items Interest 24 (1902) 906–935. Quoted in Reference [7].
[15] T. Fletcher, Compound for filling decayed teeth etc, Brit. Pat. 3028 (1878). Quoted in Reference [7].
[16] T. Fletcher, New filling, Br. J. Dent. Sci. 22 (1879) 74. Quoted in Reference [7].
[17] G.C. Paffenbarger, I.C. Schoonover, W. Souder, Dental silicate cements: physical and chemical properties and a specification, J. Am. Dent. Assoc. 25 (1939) 32–87.
[18] A.D. Wilson, A hard decade's work: the invention of glass-ionomer cement, J. Dent. Res. 75 (1997) 1723–1727.
[19] K.W. Ray, The behaviour of siliceous cements, J. Am. Dent. Assoc. 21 (1934) 237–251.
[20] A.D. Wilson, R.F. Batchelor, Dental silicate cements. III. Environment and durability, J. Dent. Res. 47 (1968) 115–120.
[21] A.D. Wilson, B.E. Kent, R.F. Mesley, R.P. Miller, D. Clinton, K.E. Fletcher, Formation of dental silicate cement, Nature 225 (1970) 272–273.
[22] D.C. Smith, A new dental cement, Br. Dent. J. 125 (1968) 381–384.
[23] D.C. Smith, Development of glass ionomer cement systems, Biomaterials 19 (1998) 467–478.
[24] A.D. Wilson, Dental silicate cements. VII. Alternative liquid cement formers, J. Dent. Res. 47 (1968) 1133–1136.
[25] B.E. Kent, B.G. Lewis, A.D. Wilson, Glass ionomer cement formulations. I. The preparation of novel fluoroaluminosilicate glasses high in fluorine, J. Dent. Res. 58 (1979) 1607–1619.
[26] A.D. Wilson, S. Crisp, H.J. Prosser, B.G. Lewis, S.A. Merson, Aluminosilicate glasses for polyelectrolyte cements, Ind. Eng. Chem. Prod. Res. Dev. 19 (1980) 263–270.
[27] A.D. Wilson, B.E. Kent, The glass-ionomer cement, a new translucent cement for dentistry, J. Appl. Chem. Biotechnol. 21 (1971) 313.
[28] J.W. Nicholson, Adhesive dental materials – a review, Int. J. Adhes. Adhes. 18 (1998) 229–236.
[29] G.J. Mount, Color Atlas of Glass Ionomer Cement, third ed., Dunitz, London, 2002.
[30] S.B. Mitra, Adhesion to dentin and physical properties of a light-cured glass-ionomer liner/base, J. Dent. Res. 70 (1991) 72–74.
[31] S.B. Mitra, In vitro fluoride release from a light-cured glass-ionomer liner/base, J. Dent. Res. 70 (1991) 75–78.
[32] H.M. Anstice, J.W. Nicholson, Studies on the structure of light-cured glass-ionomer cements, J. Mater. Sci. Mater. Med. 3 (1992) 447–451.
[33] J.W. Nicholson, H.M. Anstice, The physical chemistry of light-curable glass-ionomer cements, J. Mater. Sci. Mater. Med. 5 (1994) 119–124.
[34] S.K. Sidhu, Clinical evaluations of resin-modified glass-ionomer restorations, Dent. Mater. 26 (2010) 7–12.
[35] O.T. Al-Naimi, T. Itota, R.S. Hobson, J.F. McCabe, Fluoride release from restorative materials and its effect on biofilm formation in natural saliva, J. Mater. Sci. Mater. Med. 19 (2008) 1243–1248.

[36] K.M.Y. Hse, S.K. Leung, S.H.Y. Wei, Resin-ionomer restoration materials for children – a review, Aust. Dent. J. 44 (1999) 1–11.
[37] W. Zhang, S.I. Masumi, X.M. Song, Bonding property of two resin-reinforced glass-ionomer cements to zirconia ceramic, Quintessence Int. 41 (2010) e132–e140.
[38] J.W. Nicholson, Polyacid-modified composite resins ('compomers') and their use in clinical dentistry, Dent. Mater. 23 (2007) 615–622.
[39] A.U.J. Yap, C.H. Tan, S.M. Chung, Wear behaviour of new composite restoratives, Oper. Dent. 29 (2004) 277–282.
[40] C.J. Kleverlaan, A.J. Feilzer, Polymerization shrinkage and contraction stress of dental resin composites, Dent. Mater. 21 (2005) 1150–1157.
[41] C.L. Davidson, A.J. Feilzer, Polymerization shrinkage and polymerization shrinkage stress in polymer-based restoratives, J. Dent. 25 (1997) 435–440.
[42] M. Helvatjoglu-Antoniades, Y. Papadogiannis, R.S. Lakes, P. Dionysopoulos, D. Papadogiannis, Dynamic and static elastic moduli of packable and flowable composite resins and their development after initial photo curing, Dent. Mater. 22 (2006) 450–459.
[43] K.K. Choi, J.L. Ferracane, T.J. Hilton, D. Charlton, Properties of packable dental composites, J. Esthet. Dent. 12 (2000) 216–226.
[44] F. Lutz, I. Krejci, T.R. Oldenburg, Elimination of polymerization stresses at the margins of posterior composite resin restorations: a new restorative technique, Quintessence Int. 17 (1986) 777–784.
[45] J.L. Ferracane, Resin composite – state of the art, Dent. Mater. 27 (2011) 29–38.
[46] P.A. DaRosa Rodolpho, M.S. Cenci, T.A. Donassollo, A.D. Loguercio, F.F. Demarco, A clinical evaluation of posterior composite restorations: 17-year findings, J. Dent. 34 (2006) 427–435.
[47] N. Moszner, U. Salz, New developments of polymer dental composites, Prog. Polym. Sci. 28 (2002) 535–576.
[48] B. Czarnecka, H. Limanowska-Shaw, J.W. Nicholson, Buffering and ion release by a glass-ionomer cement under near-neutral and acidic conditions, Biomaterials 23 (2002) 2783–2788.
[49] L. Forsten, Fluoride release and uptake by glass-ionomers and related materials and its clinical effect, Biomaterials 19 (1998) 503–508.
[50] L. Forsten, Fluoride release from a glass ionomer cement, Scand. J. Dent. Res. 85 (1977) 503–504.
[51] M.G. Gandolfi, S. Chersoni, G.L. Acquaviva, G. Piana, C. Prati, R. Mongiorgi, Fluoride release and absorption at different pH from glass-ionomer cements, Dent. Mater. 22 (2006) 441–449.
[52] S.L. Creanor, L.H.C. Carruther, W.P. Saunders, R. Strang, R.H. Foye, Fluoride uptake and release characteristics of glass ionomer cements, Caries Res. 28 (1994) 322–328.
[53] A.J. Preston, S.M. Higham, E.A. Agalamanyi, L.H. Mair, Fluoride recharge of aesthetic dental materials, J. Oral Rehabil. 26 (1999) 936–940.
[54] B. Czarnecka, J.W. Nicholson, Maturation affects fluoride uptake by glass-ionomer dental cements, Dent. Mater. 28 (2012) e1–e5.
[55] K. Okada, S. Tosaki, K. Hirota, W.R. Hume, Surface hardness change of restorative filling materials stored in saliva, Dent. Mater. 17 (2001) 34–39.
[56] R.N. van Duined, C.L. Davidson, A.J. de Gee, A.J. Feilzer, In situ transformation of glass-ionomer into an enamel-like material, Am. J. Dent. 17 (2004) 223–227.
[57] H. Ngo, G.J. Mount, M.C.R.B. Peters, A study of glass-ionomer cement and its interface with enamel and dentin using a low-temperature, high-resolution scanning electron microscope technique, Quintessence Int. 28 (1997) 63–69.

[58] H. Ngo, G.J. Mount, J. McIntyre, J. Tuisuva, J. von Doussa, Chemical exchange between glass-ionomer restorations and residual carious dentine in permanent molars: an in vivo study, J. Dent. 34 (2006) 608–613.

[59] H. Forss, Release of fluoride and other elements from light-cured glass ionomers in neutral and acidic conditions, J. Dent. Res. 72 (1993) 1257–1262.

[60] T.J. Hilton, Keys to clinical success with pulp capping: a review of the literature, Oper. Dent. 34 (2009) 615–625.

[61] L.W. Stockton, Vital pulp capping: a worthwhile procedure, J. Can. Dent. Assoc. 65 (1999) 328–331.

[62] U. Schröder, Effects of calcium hydroxide-containing pulp-capping agents on pulp cell migration, proliferation, and differentiation, J. Dent. Res. 64 (1985) 541–548.

[63] P. Hörsted-Bindslev, V. Vilkinis, A. Sidlauskas, Direct capping of human pulps with a dentin bonding system or with calcium hydroxide cement, Oral Surg. Oral Med. Oral Pathol. Oral Radiol. Endod. 96 (2003) 591–600.

[64] T.R. Pitt Ford, G.J. Roberts, Immediate and delayed direct pulp capping with the use of a new visible light cured calcium hydroxide preparation, Oral Surg. Oral Med. Oral Pathol. 71 (1991) 338–342.

[65] Y. Kitasak, S. Shibat, J. Tagami, Migration and particle clearance from hard-setting $Ca(OH)_2$ and self-etching adhesive resin following direct pulp capping, Am. J. Dent. 19 (2006) 370–375.

[66] L.F. Francisconi, A.P. de Freitas, P.M.C. Scaffa, R.F.L. Mondelli, P.A.S. Francisconi, Water sorption and solubility of different calcium hydroxide cements, J. Appl. Oral Sci. 17 (2009) 427–431.

[67] Y. Chang, K. Tai, F. Huang, M. Huang, Cytotoxic and nongenotoxic effects of phenolic compounds in human pulp, J. Endod. 26 (2000) 440–443.

[68] Y. Ho, F. Huang, Y. Chang, Mechanisms of cytotoxicity of eugenol in human osteoblastic cells in vitro, Int. Endod. J. 39 (2006) 389–393.

[69] P. Laurent, J. Camps, M. de Meo, J. Dejou, I. About, Induction of specific cell responses to a Ca_3SiO_5-based posterior restorative material, Dent. Mater. 24 (2008) 1486–1494.

[70] O. Malkondu, M.K. Kazandag, E. Kazazglu, A review of Biodentine, a contemporary dentine replacement and repair material, BioMed. Res. Int. 2014 (2014) 160951.

[71] H.-M. Zhou, Y. Shen, Z.-J. Wang, L. Li, Y.F. Zheng, L. Häkkinen, M. Haapasalo, In vitro cytotoxicity evaluation of a novel root repair material, J. Endod. 39 (2013) 478–483.

[72] A. Nowicka, M. Lipska, M. Parafiniuk, D. Lichota, J. Buczkowska-Radlinska, Response of human dental pulp capped with biodentine and mineral trioxide aggregate, J. Endod. 39 (2013) 743–747.

[73] P. Carotte, Endodontics: Part 5. Basic instruments and materials for root canal treatment, Br. Dent. J. 197 (2004) 455–464.

[74] M. Torabinejad, C.U. Hong, F. McDonald, T.R. Pitt Ford, Physical and chemical properties of a new root-end filling material, J. Endod. 21 (1995) 349–353.

[75] L. Tronstad, F. Barnett, M. Flax, Solubility and biocompatibility of calcium hydroxide-containing root canal sealers, Endod. Dent. Traumatol. 4 (1988) 152–159.

[76] J. Camilleri, The chemical composition of mineral trioxide aggregate, J. Conserv. Dent. 11 (2008) 141–143.

[77] M. Parirokh, M. Torabinejad, Mineral trioxide aggregate: a comprehensive literature review – Part I: chemical, physical, and antibacterial properties, J. Endod. 36 (2010) 16–27.

Composite resins

3

3.1 Introduction

Within the field of materials science, the term 'composite' is applied to a material that consists of a combination of phases. Typically, there are two phases, a continuous one, known as the matrix, and a discontinuous one, dispersed within the matrix phase [1]. The majority of composites consist of an inorganic filler, either particles or fibres, dispersed in a matrix of organic polymer. However, other technically useful composites exist, including all-ceramic composites [2] and metal matrix composites [3].

In the case of polymer-based materials, composites are often preferred because the mechanical properties of the pure polymer phase are inadequate for the proposed application [4]. To overcome this problem, polymeric materials are reinforced in some way, typically by incorporating a substantial amount of rigid filler. For some polymers, the problem may be that they lack the toughness required for a particular application, and for these materials, elastomeric fillers are used. These fillers have the effect of increasing toughness and the concomitant effect of reducing brittleness. However, this approach is not used for restorative dental materials.

The reason that fabricating composites lead to improved properties is that the overall properties are broadly a reflection of the properties of the individual components. These become combined to give some sort of weighted mean of the properties of the components in what is known as the 'Rule of Mixtures' [1]. For any mechanical property, the value obtained for the composite must lie somewhere between the value of the matrix polymer and the value for the inorganic filler. In other words, the uppermost and lowermost possible values are defined by the properties of the individual components and the resulting value for the composite lies somewhere in between.

As an example, we can consider the elastic modulus of a composite that consists of a polymer matrix and a filler phase only. Taking the volume fraction of filler as V_f, and the individual elastic moduli as E_p and E_f for polymer and filler respectively, the overall predicted modulus of the composite is given by [5]:

$$E_c = (1 - V_f)E_p + V_f E_f$$

In fact, this equation is not particularly useful for accurate modelling studies. It provides a simple approach to determining the baseline value of the elastic modulus, but it is not used in detailed modelling studies because it is only an approximation of the way properties combine in real composite materials [6]. Nonetheless, it is useful in demonstrating that the properties of arise from the interplay between properties of the individual components and the amount of those components present in the composite material, as measured by volume fraction. Similar effects are known for other mechanical properties, and also for physical properties such as electrical and thermal conductivity.

Materials for the Direct Restoration of Teeth. http://dx.doi.org/10.1016/B978-0-08-100491-3.00003-9

Various other equations have been proposed that attempt to combine the properties of components in such a way that the properties of the resulting composites can be predicted [5]. In real systems, however, complications arise from the size, shape, orientation and state of adhesion between the filler and the matrix [5]. Real systems also suffer from imperfect dispersion of the filler within the matrix, and the entrapment of air in the composite during the mixing process. Both have profound effects on the mechanical properties of the resulting composite. Nonetheless, the principle remains that composite materials are used because they have improved properties compared to those of the polymer phase alone.

Composite materials are widely used in dentistry, mainly for tooth repair, but also for bonding orthodontic brackets. The range of components that can be used is restricted by a number of considerations, including the need to match the appearance (colour and translucency) of the natural tooth, and the need to restrict the substances used to those which are non-toxic. It is also important to use materials having appropriate mechanical properties. Current materials are described in this chapter, with information on their clinical applications and performance. Some information is also included on recent developments in these materials and these may affect their clinical use in the future.

3.2 Composites in dentistry

In dentistry, the term 'composite' has a more restricted meaning than the one we have just described. It is applied to a limited group of materials only, namely those that comprise a polymeric matrix with an inert filler, and where setting occurs by free radical addition polymerization [6]. We need to note in passing, though, that dental cements (glass-ionomers, zinc phosphates, etc.) are also composites according to the strict scientific definition. In their set state, they also consist of a matrix phase that is filled with a particulate reinforcing phase [7]. However, for convenience in dentistry, we restrict the term composite to those materials that consist of an organic polymer and an inert filler only, and typically describe them as 'composite resins' (or 'resin composites' in the American usage).

Although the details of the composition of individual brands vary, modern composite resins are all broadly similar. They consist of the following components [8]:

(i) A matrix phase generally made from a dimethacrylate monomer or blend of monomers.
(ii) Reinforcing fillers made of finely divided silicate or glass particles, possibly with added radio-opacifying agent, such as barium oxide.
(iii) A silane coupling agent to attach the filler to the matrix.
(iv) An initiator system to promote the setting polymerization reaction.

The main monomer used is the substance generally known as bisGMA, but whose systematic chemical name is 2,2-bis[4-(2-hydroxy-3-methacrylyloxypropoxy)phenyl] propane (Fig. 3.1). Composites based on this substance were developed originally by Bowen in the early 1960s in an attempt to combine the chemistry of epoxy and methacrylate systems [9]. This monomer is a liquid of high viscosity and to prepare composite

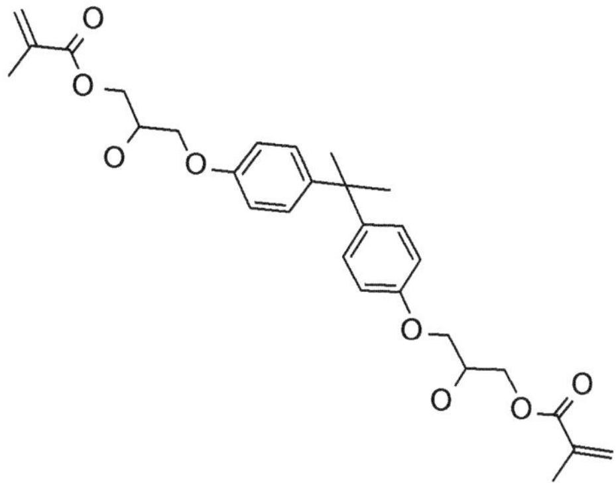

Fig. 3.1 BisGMA.

formulations of clinically acceptable viscosity, bisGMA is blended with other lower viscosity dimethacrylates, such as triethylene glycol dimethacrylate, TEDGMA (Fig. 3.2). Alternatively, the monomer urethane dimethacrylate (Fig. 3.3) may be used. It has a lower viscosity than bisGMA and may be used as either the base monomer in its own right in a composite formulation, or as a diluent to lower the viscosity of a formulation based on bisGMA [10].

The most widely used approach to polymerization of modern composites is photoinitiation [8]. However, earlier formulations were supplied as two-paste systems, where mixing two components, one of which would be present in each of the pastes, formed the initiator. A typical initiator system for this approach is benzoyl peroxide, present in a base paste at about 1% by volume [11], with tertiary amine activator, present in the other catalyst paste at 0.5%. The most widely used activator in these two-component initiators is *N,N*-dihydroxyethyl-*p*-toluidine [12].

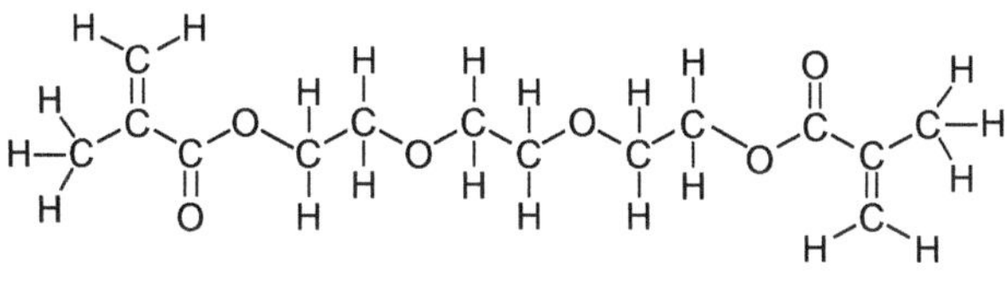

Fig. 3.2 TEGDMA.

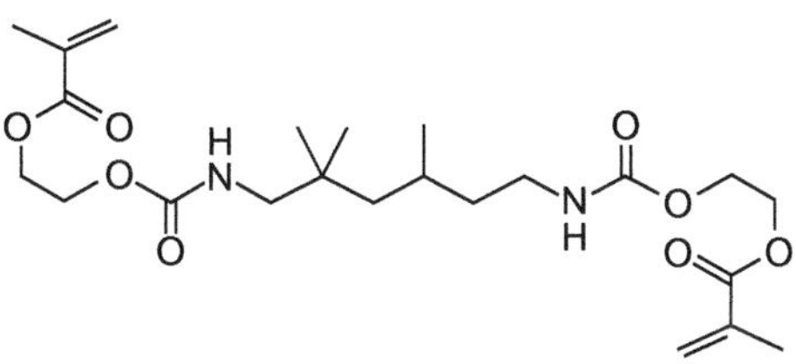

Fig. 3.3 Urethane dimethacrylate.

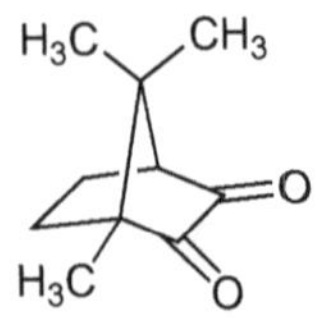

Fig. 3.4 Camphorquinone.

The concept behind this approach is that when equal volumes of pastes are mixed, benzoyl peroxide is introduced to the tertiary amine and free radicals are generated. These free radicals promote polymerization of dimethacrylate monomers and cause the composite to harden. There are still a few commercial composite resins supplied as two-paste systems, but their number is dwindling and this technology is fast becoming obsolete in developed countries [8].

By contrast, most modern composites cure by a light-activated process. The typical photoinitiator system used is based on camphorquinone (Fig. 3.4) with an aromatic tertiary amine as accelerator [13]. These are sensitive to blue light at 468 nm, and irradiation causes homolytic decomposition of the camphorquinone to form free radicals, which then initiate the polymerization and associated hardening of the composite resin.

Other initiator systems have been used, such as PPD (1-phenyl-1,2-propanedione) [14] and bis-acylphosphine oxide [15]. They have the advantage of being less intensely coloured than camphorquinone, and consequently there is a much closer colour match between the composite in its cured and uncured states. This makes choosing the correct shade of composite to match the tooth more straightforward [8]. Despite the differences in the chemistry of these substances, their essential mode of action is the same in all cases. They become excited by light of a specific wavelength, as a result of which they fragment into free radicals, and the free radicals then go on to promote polymerization of the monomers.

Light-curable composites show variations in cure with depth into the materials [11,16]. This is partly because light is attenuated at greater depths, some of it as the light passes through the polymer phase and some of it due to reflection of the light from the filler particles. Attenuation of light is also partly due to absorption by the initiator molecules in the upper layers, which means that there is a lower intensity of light at the critical wavelength available to excite initiator molecules at deeper inside the composite.

In clinical use, the standard approach for dealing with this problem is to place the composite in layers of a maximum thickness of 2 mm within the cavity [8]. This is generally considered sufficient to ensure that there is adequate cure all the way through the layer. It is also helpful in mitigating problems caused by contraction of the material as a result of polymerization (for further information on this, see Section 3.3). Various techniques have been proposed for exactly how this incremental build-up should be done in clinical practice, involving different patterns of overlaying and variations in orientation with respect to the floor of the cavity [17,18]. However, no one method appears to be ideal and there is no clinical evidence that any particular method is superior to any other [8].

Depth of cure is tested in the laboratory by curing a sample of composite typically in a metal mould, removing it and scraping away the bottom with a plastic spatula [17]. This technique is widely used, and it is certainly able to establish whether or not there is uncured composite paste at the lower end of the specimen. However, it is somewhat crude test. It also suffers from questionable clinical relevance, as the optical properties of a metal or even a plastic mould differ substantially from those of the natural tooth. Consequently, light transmission is likely to be different, resulting in a different pattern of curing.

The alternative approach used in published studies has been to determine the micro-hardness at varying depths [18,19], an approach that assumes the existence of a correlation between micro-hardness and degree of conversion (DC) of monomer to polymer. Studies using this approach have shown that depth of cure does not correlate well with measurements made using a proper hardness measurement technique, in this case Vicker's hardness [20]. In particular, for the so-called 'bulk fill' materials the ISO 4049 method, which involves scarping away unset material from the base of a cylinder of composite that has been exposed to light from the top, was found to overestimate the depth of cure compared to that determined from Vickers hardness number.

Depth of cure has also been shown to vary significantly with the shade of the formulation and that for some shades a 2 mm layer may be too thick for adequate through-cure [15]. Given the variety of materials available on the market, this is a serious finding. It has been suggested that, as clinicians lack the means to monitor extent of reaction within a composite restoration, manufacturers could helpfully provide quantitative data about the cure of their particular materials. This would include information about how cure varies with time of exposure to light, its intensity and the shade of the product. This would be important to guide clinicians on how to approach the question of placement technique and cure regime for materials placed in specific cavities [15]. This would help to counteract the unfortunate clinical tendency of increasing the thickness of the layers and reducing the cure times in order to reduce the overall time needed to place a composite restoration.

3.3 Curing of composite resins

Composite resin pastes generally set by free radical polymerization, a process which is a chain reaction that involves opening of the terminal carbon–carbon double bonds in the dimethacrylate monomers [21]. There are three steps in the overall process, beginning with initiation, followed by propagation and termination.

In the initiation step, the initiator is typically irradiated with light at the appropriate wavelength, and this causes it to fracture into free radicals. This fracture involves the formation of two reactive species containing an unpaired electron, and splitting of a chemical bond. Breaking a chemical bond in this way is termed *homolytic fission.* The high reactivity of the resulting free radicals means that they will react readily with nearby monomer molecules, forming an enlarged radical as a complete molecule of monomer becomes incorporated. This process is repeated many times in rapid succession, causing the polymer to grow quickly. This rapid sequence of additions of

$$R\text{-}CH_2CH_2\cdot \ + \ \cdot CH_2CH_2\text{-}R \rightarrow R\text{-}CH_2CH_3 + \ H_2C{=}CH\text{-}R$$

Fig. 3.5 Termination of polymerization by disproportionation.

monomer molecules is known as propagation, and is characterized by retention of the unpaired electron, with consequent high reactivity [22].

Eventually, there are so many growing polymer molecules in the system that the possibility of two unpaired electron radical centres coming together increases. When this happens, the result is that the radical centres are extinguished. This can occur either by combination, in which the individual unpaired electrons of the free radicals pair up to form a covalent bond, or by disproportionation. In the latter case, one free radical removes a hydrogen atom from the other free radical, leading to the formation of two molecules, each with different end groups. One is terminated in a methyl group (CH_3–), and the other in a double bond (>C=CH_2) [4]. These two possibilities are shown in Fig. 3.5.

The extent of polymerization can be quantified by comparing the proportion of double bonds in the set material with those in the composite paste as formulated initially [21]. This is typically expressed as a percentage, and called the degree of polymerization (DP), or DC. Values vary widely in practical dental composites, ranging from 35% to 77% [23].

The majority of the polymerization of a dental composite resin occurs very quickly, typically during the 20–40 s or so of light irradiation from the dental cure lamp. However, free radicals within the material do not terminate immediately the lamp switches off. Hence they are able to continue their propagation steps for some time after this initial cure, as growing polymer molecules containing free radical centres continue to incorporate extra monomer molecules [24]. Shrinkage, which is associated with polymerization, has been shown to continue for up to 24 h after initial setting [25] in a process known as 'post-polymerization' [26].

Because dimethacrylate monomers have at least two double bond sites capable of undergoing polymerization, their reaction leads to the formation of a highly crosslinked network [21]. Immediately after light irradiation begins, there is a rapid reaction that causes the DC to rise quickly, and the crosslink density to develop with similar speed. This brings about a rapid increase in the viscosity of the system leading to gelation of the viscous liquid composite [17]. At gelation, there is a substantial reduction in the mobility of the molecules in the system, though this affects the higher molar mass species more than the lower mass one. Since the higher molar mass species are the polymer chains containing several monomer molecules and retaining the free radical centre, whereas the low molar mass species are unreacted monomer molecules, it follows that the polymer chains become almost completely immobile. This prevents the termination reactions from occurring, while leaving both initiation and propagation processes to continue. Hence the rate of reaction takes off dramatically, causing the phenomenon of autoacceleration to occur [27]. As it does so, the viscosity becomes so high that even the monomer molecules become unable to move through the network. When this stage is reached, there is another change of state, this time from rubbery polymer to a glassy one [28]. This vitrification prevents further reaction and traps unreacted monomer molecules and partly polymerized free radicals in the structure [22]. This explains why the maximum DC is limited to about 75–80% in these systems. It also explains why there are still radical centres in existence at the end of the setting process. Their presence explains the post-polymerization phase of setting, which probably occurs due to slight molecular motion within the vitrified structure that allows further polymerization to take place at a very slow rate [25]. Free radicals may continue to be detected for several weeks after vitrification [29,30], though there is little further polymerization beyond 24 h.

3.3.1 Degree of conversion

The DC achieved within a composite is important because it controls several properties of the cured material, including mechanical strength [31,32], polymerization shrinkage [33], wear behaviour [34] and monomer release [35]. It is most commonly determined by fourier transform infrared spectroscopy (FTIR) [36] since the double bond in the monomer molecules gives rise to a sharp and distinct peak at $1640\,cm^{-1}$. DC can be determined by measuring the reduction in the intensity of this peak relative to a reference peak that is known to be unaffected by polymerization. The peak usually chosen as the reference peak is the one at $1608\,cm^{-1}$, which arises from absorption by the aromatic rings in bisGMA [36].

FTIR may be complicated because there are several functional groups capable of absorbing infrared radiation in the region of interest for carbon–carbon double bonds. These peaks may reduce the signal-to-noise ratio at $1640\,cm^{-1}$, and thereby interfere with the quantification process. There is also a problem caused by the presence of double bonds in the silane coupling agent at the filler–matrix interface. These may also complicate the determination of the DC [37].

An alternative spectroscopic technique that has been used in studies of DC is Raman spectroscopy [38]. Raman bands appear at the same wavelength as those used in FTIR, as they are active in both infrared and Raman absorption modes. No particular advantages arise from the use of Raman spectroscopy over FTIR, and as a technique it has not been used quite as much for studies of this type [39].

In addition to spectroscopic techniques, DC has been studied indirectly using micro-hardness methods, either Vicker's or Knoop hardness. There is a good relationship between the DC and micro-hardness [37,40], though the relationship is complicated because micro-hardness is affected not only by DC but also be extent of crosslinking [41]. It can also be affected by accidentally placing the micro-hardness indenter directly on a filler particle. A further disadvantage of the use of micro-hardness is that measurements cannot provide quantitative information on the fraction of double bonds that have undergone polymerization.

3.3.2 Crosslinking

DC is not the only feature of the polymerization process that affects mechanical properties [42]. Another important aspect is the degree of crosslinking between the molecules. This not only affects mechanical strength and hardness of the cured composite, it also affects stability and appearance because materials with lower crosslink density can take up moisture and hence swell more easily. This can lead to hydrolytic degradation [29,43]. Swelling may also alter the appearance of the composite, either because coloured substances are taken up and the shade changes, or because uptake of saliva causes the translucency to change.

Crosslinking cannot be measured directly, because it arises from the same reaction as the polymerization of the monomers, namely conversion of the C=C double bonds to single bonds. However, an indirect technique can be used instead. One possibility is to determine the extent of softening of the composite when immersed in ethanol. This technique involves comparing values for the surface hardness before and after storage in ethanol [29,44].

An alternative possibility is to measure the glass transition temperature, T_g. This property can be determined either by differential scanning calorimetry or by dynamic mechanical analysis [45]. The glass transition temperature is the temperature at which vitrification occurs during the cure reaction, and above this temperature the polymer is rubbery, while below this temperature, the polymer is glassy. As with other means of studying crosslinking, T_g gives only an indication of the crosslink density, because its value depends not only on degree of crosslinking but also on DC and other factors, such as the viscosity of the monomer phase [45].

3.3.3 Depth of cure

Depth of cure is influenced by the way light is transmitted through the composite resin [21]. The interaction of light with the material is complicated and affected by several factors. Some of the light may be reflected from the surface and not enter the composite at all [46,47]. Some light may be absorbed by the filler and especially by the pigments [48], which is the reason that darker shades have lower depths of cure than lighter ones [49]. Filler particles can reduce the transmission of light by scattering, an effect that depends on both the particle size of the filler and the wavelength of the light. This effect is most pronounced with filler particles of the order of half the wavelength of the light, ie, in the region of 200–250 nm [50–52].

Fillers also interfere with the transmission of light because of the difference in refractive index between them and the matrix phase. This causes refraction at the interface between the filler and the polymer [53,54], which results in altered light intensity and thus recued conversion of monomer to polymer. This effect is particularly severe in the so-called flowable formulations which contain relatively high levels of diluent molecules because the mismatch in the refractive index between these substances and the fillers is greater than that with bisGMA or UDMA [55].

3.3.4 Oxygen inhibition

When composite resins undergo polymerization, a thin layer exposed to the air fails to react. This is due to the presence of oxygen. The oxygen molecule is a di-radical, that is, it has two unpaired electrons. This makes it reactive towards the free radicals within the setting composite, and it reacts readily with these free radicals to form unreactive electron pair bonds. This quenches the radical centre and inhibits the polymerization process. Studies have shown that this layer is of the order of 13–20 μm thick in commercial methacrylate-based composite resins [56].

When restorations are placed in increments, the thin oxygen-inhibited layer of one increment is covered by the next increment. This shields it from ingress of further oxygen, so that it cures when irradiated through the next increment. Because the oxygen-inhibition layer is unpolymerized, in principle there can be some limited mixing when a new layer of uncured paste is placed over it. This has been considered to be important in bonding the increment layers together [57].

However, recent studies have shown this not to be the case. In one study, for example, shear bond strength was determined for specimens prepared in increments both in the presence of air and in an inert atmosphere [57]. No significant differences in shear bond strength were found, a result that was taken to show that the free radical polymerization reactions were able to proceed equally in both conditions. This, in turn, meant that oxygen inhibition was not significant in these systems.

In another study, the interfacial bond strength between the increments was determined at various times in air and in a nitrogen atmosphere, and again no significant differences were found [56]. From these findings, it must be concluded that, though a thin oxygen-inhibition layer undoubtedly occurs in these materials, it is too thin to influence the eventual properties of the cured composite resin, and its presence is not responsible for the layers bonding together.

3.3.5 Polymerization shrinkage and shrinkage stress

When composite resins undergo polymerization they shrink slightly [21,58]. This is because, in an addition polymerization, the free volume occupied by the double bonded end of a monomer molecule is greater than that occupied by the equivalent single bond in the polymer molecule. This effect classically allows addition polymerization to be studied by the technique of dilatometry, whereby the reduction in volume of a substance such as methyl methacrylate is followed by observing the contraction in a narrow-bore tube of a device known as a dilatometer [59].

For a filled system such as dental composite resin, contraction does not correlate simply with DP, because only the polymer matrix phase undergoes contraction, not the filler. However, there is a link between contraction and DP [33]. Shrinkage has important clinical consequences for these materials, and can result in either interfacial gap formation at the margins of the restoration or cuspal movement in repaired teeth [60,61]. As composites undergo cure, so stresses develop within the material. These are the result of a complex interplay between the forces due to polymerization shrinkage, polymerization rate, onset of gelation and elastic modulus of the set composite [21]. Another important factor is the shape of the cavity being restored, since it imposes restrictions on the possible volumetric change of the composite. Also, compliance of the walls of the cavity towards flexure has an influence on the resulting stresses [62,63].

The phenomenon of polymerization shrinkage in composite resins based on either bisGMA or UDMA is considered to be their most important deficiency

[21,64]. For many years now, a substantial effort has been devoted to the search for alternative monomer systems that show lower or even no contraction when they polymerize. These efforts have led to some successes, as demonstrated in research publications. For example, a series of monomers, such as spiro-orthocarbonates, have been employed which undergo expansion on polymerization due to differences in configuration between the tightly coiled monomer and the less tightly coiled polymer [65]. In addition, epoxy-polyol molecules have been studied, and these cure by a ring-opening reaction that shows up to 50% less shrinkage than the polymerization of monomers used in conventional composites [66]. Despite these findings, the current dental composites remain mainly formulated from bisGMA and/or UDMA systems. Moreover, the clinical technique of incremental build-up is able to mitigate partly against the problems caused by polymerization shrinkage, since by placing the composite in thin layers and curing them individually, contraction takes place in that part of the restoration, and the next layer is placed so as to fill some of the space vacated by the contraction. In this way, correct clinical handling of the material ensures that problems arising from polymerization shrinkage are minimized.

3.3.6 Soft-start polymerization

The technique of the so-called soft-start polymerization was developed in the late 1990s in order to reduce the rate of initial shrinkage [67,68] and potentially maintain the integrity of the bond to the tooth. It employs a cure lamp that either emits only low irradiance for the first 10 s, after which it switches to maximum output for the remaining duration of the light exposure; or emits a progressively increasing irradiance in the early stages, after which it, too, emits maximum output for a brief period [67,69].

At the molecular level, the effect of soft-start polymerization is to extend the gelation time of the composite [67]. By reducing the rate of early polymerization, the rate of shrinkage is also reduced. This helps to maintain the seal at the margins of the restoration, and may allow relaxation processes to take place, so that stresses do not build up to the same extent as in conventional cure regimes.

Laboratory studies have suggested that soft-start polymerization may be beneficial [70–74]. In particular, marginal adaptation appears to be improved [75–77], with a corresponding reduction in marginal leakage [78]. However, these findings do not seem to translate to measurable improvements in clinical performance. Though soft-start polymerization undoubtedly improves the marginal seal, as well as increasing the micro-hardness of the set composite [79], it did not reduce sensitivity to a cold stimulus in patient evaluations [67]. Two cure regimes were employed on composites in Class I and Class II restorations, one a soft-start technique, and the other a conventional steady irradiation technique. Sensitivity to a cold stimulus was evaluated using a standardized approach at 2 weeks, 3, 12 and 24 months, and no differences were found between the two cure techniques. Patients reported equal discomfort with both approaches to the cure of their composite restorations. This suggests that soft-start polymerization does not offer any advantages, and that it is not necessary with these materials.

3.3.7 Photoinitiators

When composite resins were first introduced, their polymerization involved free radical initiation by a combination of benzoyl peroxide with tertiary amine activator, delivered in two different pastes, known respectively as base and catalyst. Contemporary composites are visible light-activated one-paste systems and the principal photoinitiator used is camphorquinone [70,80]. It is used in conjunction with a co-initiator, typically an amine [81]. This latter compound does not absorb light, but is necessary to react with the light-activated camphorquinone molecule to generate free radicals and hence initiate the chain polymerization.

When camphorquinone is irradiated by light of the appropriate wavelength, the carbonyl groups react as shown in Scheme 3.1. For camphorquinone there are two carbonyl groups, both of which can undergo the processes illustrated in Scheme 3.1 to generate radical centres. This means that a total of four radical centres are produced from one camphorquinone molecule. It is also the reason that the optimum ratio of camphorquinone to amine is 1:2, and this is the ratio typically included in a composite formulation [81–83].

Camphorquinone has an absorbance range between 400 and 500 nm wavelength, with a maximum at 468 nm [84]. This is in the blue region of the visible spectrum, and is the reason that camphorquinone appears yellow in white light [85,86]. Inclusion of camphorquinone in a composite formulation introduces a yellow colour, some of which remains after curing. Because this affects the overall aesthetics, it is considered undesirable and alternative photoinitiators have been sought. The most widely studied of these is PPD [81].

PPD absorbs in a slightly different region of the spectrum from camphorquinone, since the molecule mainly absorbs in the near UV region, with a maximum absorption at 398 nm, and absorption extends only slightly into the visible region [83]. It thus appears less yellow than camphorquinone. It generates free radicals by the homolytic fission process illustrated in Scheme 3.2.

This process yields a total of two free radicals per PPD molecule. An advantage of this is that the radical fragments are smaller and more independent than those produced by camphorquinone, where two of the radical centres are on the same molecular

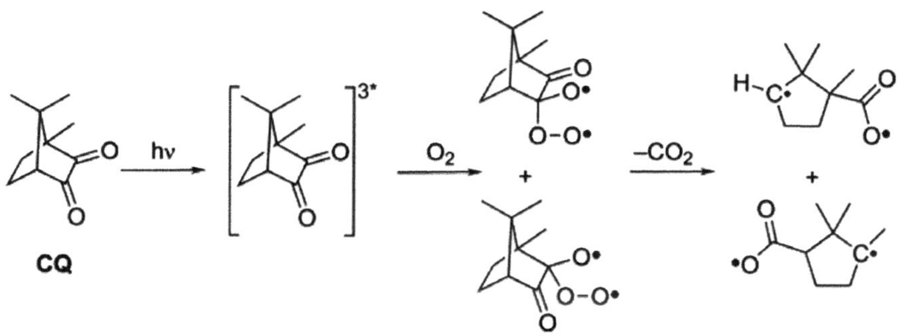

Scheme 3.1 Free radical generation by camphorquinone.

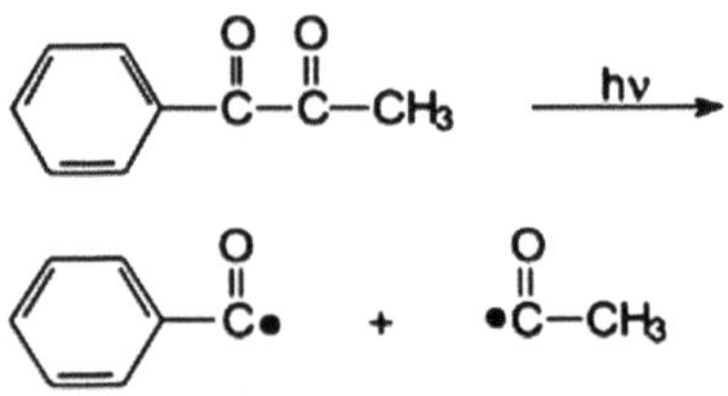

Scheme 3.2 Free radical generation by PPD.

species and the molecular fragments relatively large [87]. This means that diffusion apart of the radicals is more difficult, so that there is a greater likelihood of radical recombination in the camphorquinone system than in the PPD one. This, in turn, implies that PPD would have a greater efficiency than the camphorquinone system. Against that, the rate of formation of free radicals from camphorquinone is higher than that from PPD [81].

The effectiveness of these photoinitiators is dependent on the lamp used to bring about cure with them. Initially, cure lamps employed quartz-tungsten-halogen (QTH) bulbs, which emit blue light with a maximum emission around 470 nm and a wide spectral output. These favour the camphorquinone system and give effective degrees of conversion in composites that contain this system. More recently, cure lamps using light-emitting diodes (LEDs) for their light emission have been used. These have a narrower spectral output than QTH bulbs and a slight shift in the maximum output into the region 450–460 nm [81]. In principle, this may make them marginally more effective with PPD than with camphorquinone. In practice, however, experimental studies have shown no significant differences in DC for different cure lamps applied to formulations containing either of these two initiator systems [81]. Experiments of this type can thus be seen to confirm the effectiveness of the camphorquinone-amine initiator and explain its continuing pre-eminence as the initiator system in visible light-cured composite resins [21].

3.4 Cure lamps

As the majority of composites used in contemporary dentistry are light-cured, it follows that the nature and effectiveness of the cure lamp is critical to the performance of the composite in clinical practice. As previously mentioned, the original cure lamps used QTH bulbs [88]. These emit light of wavelength around 430–500 nm, ie, at the blue end of the visible spectrum, and hence they are well suited for compositions containing the camphorquinone-amine initiator system [89]. However, the wavelength of maximum absorption for camphorquinone (468 nm) represents only a fraction of the spectral output of such lamps, so that much of the energy is outside the range useful for promoting cure, and hence wasted [90]. On the other hand, QTH lamps also emit heat [91,92], which may help to increase the degree of cure, particularly within the material [93]. This may be a useful adjunct to the cure induced by the light itself.

More recently there have been moves to replace QTH lamps with LEDs [93]. These have very narrow emission ranges and their output is concentrated in the blue wavelength region of the spectrum, ie, in the range 440–480 nm [94,95]. They are therefore able to cure composites at least as well as QTH lamps [96], while generating much less heat [97,98]. Composites cured using LEDs appear at least as well polymerized as those cured with QTH lamps [94] and to have similar mechanical properties [99].

Wavelength of emitted light is not the only criterion when considering the effectiveness of dental cure lamps. The power output is also important. This is because high power emission results in the generation of more free radicals per unit time than lower power emission. On the other hand, higher concentrations of free radicals in a polymerizing system result in lower molar mass polymers [4]. This is because each free radical generated by an initiator molecule begins a chain reaction involving the available monomer molecules. If there are more such free radicals, each has fewer monomer molecules available from which to build its polymer.

High power versions of both QTH and LED are available, and offer the prospect of shorter cure times with improvements in the speed with which a restoration can be completed [100]. Despite the anticipated change in the detailed structure of the polymerized composite resin, physical properties of materials cured with these high power systems are comparable with those of composites cured with lower power units [93,100].

It is difficult to draw hard and fast conclusions concerning the relative merits of the various types of cure lamp on the market. All types seem capable of producing an acceptable degree of cure, and differences found in scientific studies probably do not translate into significant differences in clinical performance. In practice, the performance of all cure lamps appears to give acceptable degrees of cure of commercial composite resins, and so any type of commercial dental cure lamp can safely be used for activating the cure of composites.

3.5 Fillers

The role of the fillers in composite resins is to reinforce their mechanical properties and provide a blended material whose overall properties make it suitable for the clinical repair of teeth. A limited range of materials has been used, with greater emphasis on variations in the particle size and size distribution than on chemical composition. Early materials were filed with powdered quartz, whereas modern composites are more likely to be filled with finely divided barium silicate or a radio-opaque silicate glass [8]. Filler loadings are typically of the order of 55% by volume, as they were in Bowen's original formulation [9].

In addition to the filler, a coupling agent is employed. This is typically a silicon-based substance that contains two types of functionality in the same molecule, an alkoxy end which binds to the filler particle surface, and a vinyl end which undergoes an addition reaction to become incorporated into the resin matrix [101]. The most commonly

Table 3.1 **Particle size and size distribution of fillers in composites**

Type	Size distribution
Macrofill	10–50 μm
Microfill	40–50 nm
Hybrid	10–50 μm + 40 nm
Minifill	1–10 μm + 40 nm
Nanofill	5–100 nm

used substance for this purpose is γ-methacryloxy-propyl tri-methoxysilane [11]. This substance not only promotes bonding between the filler particles and the resin matrix, thereby proving mechanical reinforcement, it also resists ingress of water at the interface. Water would otherwise migrate to the inorganic surface, attacking the interface and destroying the bond between the filler and the resin. Silanes provide a water-resistant bond at the interface between the inorganic and the organic components, and this makes the resulting composite durably in clinical service [101].

The size range of the filler particles was the basis of an early classification of composite resins [102]. Though the range of particle sizes has now been extended to include nano-particles [103], this is still a useful approach to classifying these materials. Table 3.1 shows the order of development of composite resins based on the particle size of their fillers.

The earliest commercial composites for use in dentistry had particle sizes in the range 10–50 μm and would now be considered 'macrofill' materials [8]. They were strong mechanically but difficult to polish. In addition, wear caused the surfaces to roughen readily, resulting on poor long-term aesthetics. To overcome these problems, composites were blended with much smaller particles to create 'microfill' materials. However, because these particles are harder to blend into the monomer mixture due to adsorption of monomer molecules on their much larger relative surface areas, the total volume fraction of filler that could be achieved was lower than for macrofills. Consequently, the mechanical properties were inferior. This led rapidly to the approach of blending the large and the small filler particles to create the so-called 'hybrid' composites. These had good mechanical properties, mainly because of the higher filler loadings that could be achieved with the lager particles, and were less susceptible to wear due to the influence of the smaller particles [8].

Since these developments, there have been further refinements in filler technology, which have mainly involved the use of still finer filler particles (typically in the μm range), often in conjunction with slightly larger particle sizes [104]. As shown in Table 3.1, one version is the minifill [105], also known as microhybrid composites. They are considered to be universal composites because they can be used for most anterior and posterior repairs, due to their combination of mechanical strength, polishability and long-term aesthetic properties.

Nanofilled materials are the most recent of the composite types, and these are based on fillers of nanoparticle dimensions [106]. Full details of their composition are typically confidential because of commercial considerations, but one approach to problems

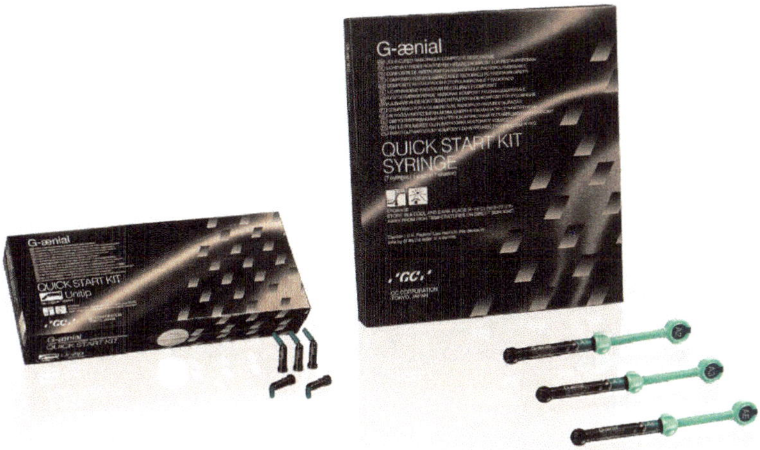

Fig. 3.6 Example of composite resin (G-aenial Composite, GC, Japan).
Used with permission.

caused by incorporating such fine particles has been to incorporate them first into composite that is pre-polymerized, then fractured and dispersed in further amounts of resin monomer, usually with slightly larger filler particles [107].

Physical properties of these materials are generally very good [104,108] and their volumetric shrinkage and water sorption properties also compare favourably with composites containing larger particle size fillers [104]. Studies have shown them to combine the mechanical strength of hybrid composites [109,110] with the polishability of the microfills [109,110]. They also have good wear resistance [111,112] and good optical properties [109]. An example of a modern commercial brand of composite resin is shown in Fig. 3.6.

As well as classifying composite resins by their particle size and size distribution, modern composites are distinguished by their consistency. The two broad groups are termed 'packable' (sometimes referred to as 'condensable') and 'flowable', and they differ in their viscosity. Packable composites are more viscous as a result of modifications to the filler particle size distribution, though they generally do not have higher overall levels of filler than universal composites [113]. Flowable composites, by contrast, are of lower viscosity. As a result, they can be dispensed from syringes with very fine bore needles into small spaces, thereby enhancing the adaptation of the composite restoration. Their lower viscosity is achieved by a slight reduction in the filler content and also by adding other compounds such as surfactants to enhance their flow properties [114]. Though the details of these alterations to composite formulations are not made public by manufacturers, it is known that they do not compromise the mechanical strength properties of the set cement [8].

The different consistencies influence the ways in which these types of composite are used in the clinic. While a universal restorative may have either a stiff consistency or a more fluid one, depending on the details of its composition [8], they are

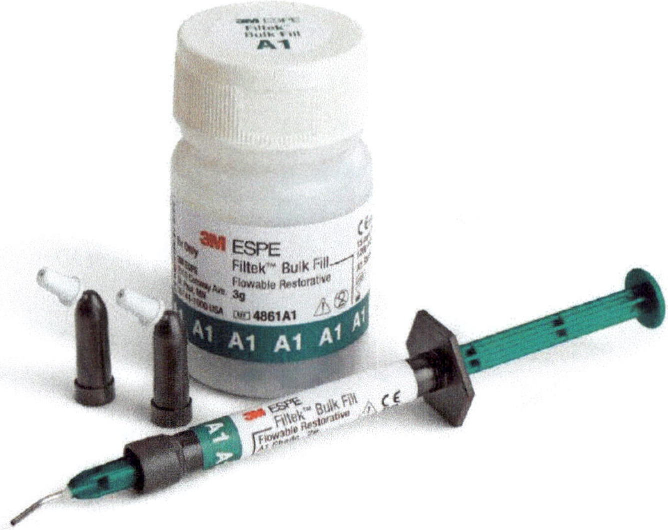

Fig. 3.7 Filtek™ Bulk Fill Flowable Restorative from 3M, as an example of bulk fill composite. Used with Permission.

designed to be capable of use both for fine margins of restorations and for bulk (incremental) filling. By contrast, packable and flowable composites are designed for different purposes, and usually are used together for different parts of a single cavity restoration.

Packable composites are designed to be placed with the aid of an amalgam condenser or other instrument and, when cured, they have good mechanical and wear properties [115]. Their high viscosity prevents them from slumping and enhances the ability to obtain tight interproximal contacts in practical use [8,116]. Flowable composites (Fig. 3.7), because of their lower viscosity, are able to penetrate into irregularities, thereby ensuring a good seal at the margins of restorations. It is claimed that they can be used to prepare thin layers of cured material that do not entrap air and also that, when set, they are flexible enough to be able to survive in regions of high stress, such as the margins of Class I or Class II cavities and in Class V cavities. However, this seems somewhat questionable and is not supported by any scientific evidence.

3.6 Clinical applications of composite resins

The main application of composite resins in contemporary dentistry is as direct repair materials in a variety of cavities teeth [117] and it is estimated that 95% of all anterior restorations and 50% of all posterior restorations are now made with composite resin [118]. In addition, they are also being increasingly used as indirect repair materials for a number of uses, including as onlays and inlays [119], and as fissure sealants.

The main material used for many years for the direct repair of teeth was silver amalgam [120]. This combined ease of placement with adequate physical properties, and so was the material of choice. However, there are increasing concerns about its use, and direct composites are replacing it in clinical practice in many parts of the world [21]. Composites have the considerable advantage of superior aesthetics, being fully capable of matching the natural tooth in terms of shade and translucency. For amalgams, there is also growing concern with environmental issues of waste disposal and the misplaced perception of their toxicity, due to the mercury that they contain [121]. Modern direct composites survive well in the mouth and numerous clinical studies attest to their ability to remain functional for extended periods of time, ie, 10–15 years or more [21,122]. There is a problem with claims of longevity, however, and that is that, by the time long-term studies have been completed, the brands in question are obsolete and have been replaced on the market. As far as durability is concerned, we can assume that the newer formulations do not differ significantly from the earlier brands, though this is not what the manufacturers claim.

The mechanical properties of composites vary widely, as shown in Table 3.2. As we have seen, this is a function mainly of their filler particle size and size distribution, and also the specific application for which the composite has been formulated. Overall, though, these properties give rise to their highly satisfactory clinical performance.

In addition to their good mechanical properties, composites typically show low thermal conductivities and minimal water absorption [21]. This allows them to protect the tooth from thermal damage when hot foodstuffs or beverages are consumed. Also, colour and appearance remain stable over extended periods of time.

In addition to their use to repair teeth damaged by caries, direct composites can be used to repair teeth damaged by trauma [123]. This application also exploits their good aesthetics, while also making use of their toughness and durability. Composites can also be used in children's teeth as pit and fissure sealants, where they have good survival rates and are clinically effective in reducing the onset of caries [124].

In general in direct applications, composite resins are built up in increments [8,21]. They can also be used in deep cavities in the so-called sandwich technique, in which glass-ionomer (either conventional or resin-modified) is placed first in bulk to ensure bonding to dentine and also a good marginal seal, with composite resin being placed on top to finish the restoration [123]. In principle, conventional glass-ionomers are preferred in this application, because they do not leach harmful monomers in a position close to the pulp.

Table 3.2 Properties of contemporary composite resins

Property	Range of values
Compressive strength	260–300 MPa
Tensile strength	40–50 MPa
Flexural strength	80–150 MPa
Young's modulus	6–14 GPa

The building of composite increments has been studied in a variety of possible orientations (horizontal, oblique and vertical) but none appears particularly advantageous, and all give good results in anterior teeth [125–127]. The clinical outcomes for the resulting restorations have been widely studied, and results are generally good [121,128–130], though there is some concern that the use of these materials is more technique-sensitive than the use of amalgams [131]. Also, they are more expensive [21].

Following placement and incremental cure, the composite restoration needs to be finished. This can involve correcting of contours and smoothing of margins by abrasion in order to remove excess material and adjust occlusion [132]. Polishing in order to provide a smooth surface completes the restoration. This prevents plaque retention [133] and eliminates problems of further caries development and potential periodontitis [132]. These finishing steps may be carried out with a variety of devices, including diamond rotary cutting instruments, carbide burs, abrasive discs and rubber cups, the latter in association with polishing pastes [134,135]. Once these finishing steps have been performed, occlusion is verified and any final corrections made [136].

Composite resins may also be used for indirect repairs [119]. In this, a variety of polymerization techniques combining irradiation with light and application of heat, vacuum or pressure is used. This results in higher degrees of conversion than are generally achieved for direct composites [136–138] and gives them better aesthetics and long-term colour stability than direct composites [139]. They also give rise to less postoperative sensitivity than direct composites [139]. These materials are used for onlays and inlays, and can also be used to modify existing prostheses or to replace metal-ceramic restorations [118]. They are being used increasingly as alternatives to porcelain, including as crowns, in which application they show good survival rates [140]. They can also be used to make veneers [141] and anterior bridges [142]. This aspect has been explored less than the use of composites for direct tooth repair, but there is every likelihood that this application will grow in importance in the coming years.

3.7 Fluoride-releasing composite resins

Composite resins are not inherently capable of releasing fluoride, but if appropriate fluoride compounds are added, they may become so. Suitable compounds include inorganic salts such as sodium fluoride or stannous fluoride, fluoridated glasses or organic fluoride compounds. Longer-term sustained release requires only sparingly soluble fluoride salts, such as SrF_2 or YbF_3, or leachable glass fillers [143]. Fluoride release from these substances requires water to diffuse into the composite resin, a process that is slow, because the resin polymer system is quite hydrophobic [144]. However, the presence of hydrophilic or ionic additives can accelerate the process [145], allowing water uptake to occur at a sufficient rate to promote the release of fluoride from the composite restoration.

The amount of fluoride released by composites tends to be much lower than that released by either conventional or resin-modified glass-ionomer. It is also lower than the level released by polyacid-modified composite resins. The reason for this is not clear. It may be because the simple water uptake/dissolution process is less effective at providing fluoride than the mechanisms in glass-ionomers or polyacid-modified composites; or it may be a reflection of the lower fluoride loadings in the composite formulations [146,147].

Fluoride release from composite resins does not show the 'early burst' that glass-ionomers display and also there appears to be no ability for fluoride to recharge in most systems. However, recharge has been demonstrated for an experimental composite system [148]. On the other hand, fluoride release has been shown to continue over long periods of time, at least a year having been reported in a number of studies [149,150].

The kinetics of fluoride release from composite resins vary widely, and are straightforward than those of glass-ionomers. Various types of behaviour have been observed, including fluoride release being directly proportional to time and fluoride release being approximately proportional to either the logarithm of time or to the inverse square root of time, $t^{-1/2}$ [150,151]. The clinical significance of these differences is not clear.

3.8 Modern alternative composite resins

As well as conventional composites of the type based on bisGMA and/or UDMA and filled with silicate-based filler, there are now materials available that are essentially composites in that they comprise a polymeric matrix reinforced with finely divided filler. However, either the polymer system or the filler phase is of a different chemical composition from that of conventional composite resins. Three such materials are currently available, and these are the ormocers, the siloranes and the giomers. Their details are given in Table 3.3, and their characteristics are described in the following subsections.

3.8.1 Ormocers

The term 'ormocer' derives from 'organically modified ceramic' and these materials were developed at the Fraunhofer Institute, Würzburg, Germany. Their original use was as speciality coatings for various technical applications, such as protective coatings,

Table 3.3 Modern modified composite resins used in dentistry

Type	Polymer system	Filler	Setting reaction
Ormocer	Polysiloxane functionalized with organic groups terminated in double bonds	Conventional silicate glass filler	Additional polymerization
Silorane	Oxirane (epoxy) polymers attached to silane centre	Conventional silicate glass filler	Ring-opening polymerization
Giomer	Conventional composite matrix based on bisGMA chemistry	Crushed pre-reacted glass-ionomer cement	Addition polymerization

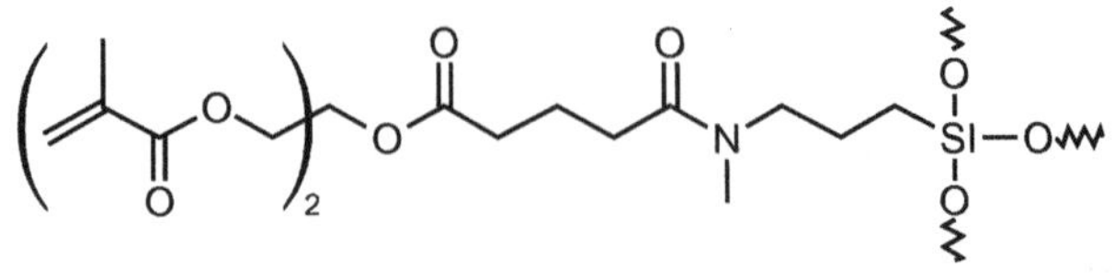

Fig. 3.8 Example of ormocer monomer.

non-stick surfaces and anti-static coatings [152]. They have now been pioneered as composite dental restorative materials, with commercial materials based on these new systems being available for clinical use.

The principal novelty of ormocers compared with conventional composites is that their polymer systems are prepared from alkoxysilanes, ie, molecules of the type $R_nSi(OR')_{(4-n)}$. This gives them an inorganic centre containing silicon and oxygen atoms, which are inorganic and the atoms that occur in glasses and other clay-derived ceramics. The organic parts (R or R′) are multifunctional urethane and thioether(meth) acrylate groups which contain carbon–carbon double bonds, through which the ormocer is cured by addition polymerization [153] (see Fig. 3.8). Because the starting material is essentially a pre-polymer of reasonable molar mass, polymerization (cross-linking) results in minimal shrinkage compared with conventional composites, even though the reaction is an addition polymer of carbon–carbon double bonds [154]. Ormocers contain virtually no residual monomer [153], which is advantageous, and they also have very good appearance. These features make them highly suitable for use in dentistry.

Ormocers have been developed for clinical use in the repair of teeth and a number of commercial materials are now available. Experiments have confirmed that they have reduced setting shrinkage compared with conventional composites, and also they have very good aesthetics and good wear properties [155]. Clinical studies have shown ormocers to perform well in the mouth and findings show that their overall clinical performance is reported to be at least as good as that of conventional composites [156–158]. Nonetheless, they are difficult to handle because their pastes have a high viscosity, and that makes them difficult to condense and to achieve good marginal adaptation.

3.8.2 Siloranes

The term ‘silorane’ is derived from the words ‘siloxane’ and ‘oxirane’, indicating that the molecules involved are both siloxanes and oxiranes, ie, they consist of Si(OR) species, where the R groups are terminated in oxirane (epoxy) rings:

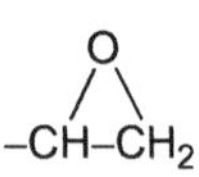

The constituent molecules of siloranes are large, as shown in Fig. 3.9, and have a reasonable viscosity, though less so that bisGMA.

Setting of materials based on this chemistry set by ring-opening polymerization initiated by a three-component photoinitiator system consisting of camphorquinone,

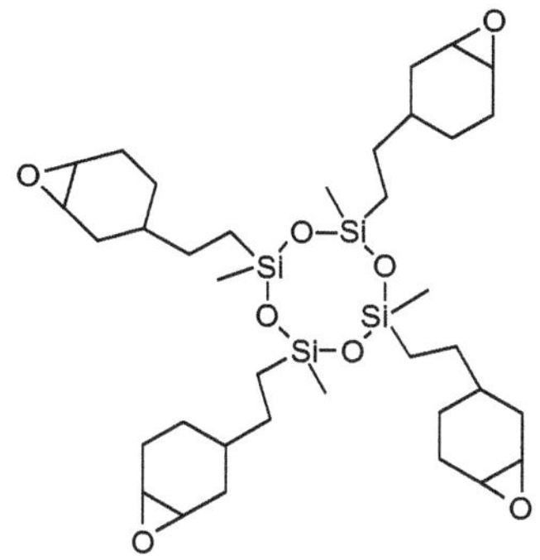

Fig. 3.9 Silorane monomer, showing terminal oxirane (epoxy) rings.

an amine and an iodonium salt, such as those based on diphenyliodonium cations [159]. In this system, camphorquinone absorbs light at 468 nm and in the excited state reacts with the amine, an electron donor. This causes the amine to form a cation, which further reacts with the diphenyl iodonium salt to generate an acidic cation. This cation then reacts to open the oxirane ring, according to Scheme 3.3.

The loss of free volume associated with the ring-opening reaction is less than that associated with the polymerization of double bonds. This means that the fully formulated composite shows less shrinkage on setting than conventional composites [160]. This, in turn, lowers shrinkage stress to under 1% by volume, compared with 2–3% for conventional methacrylate-based composites [161]. Unfortunately, this reduced shrinkage does not appear significant under clinical conditions, and margins of restorations do not appear any better than those of conventional composites [162].

Siloranes are filled with finely ground quartz particles in size the range 0.1–2.0 µm (100–2000 nm), and are described in the literature as nanofilled materials. They also include the compound ytterbium fluoride as a source of soluble fluoride to provide some anti-caries activity. Only one company, 3M in the America, manufactures these materials, for which they use the generic brand name Filtek™. A number of different specific versions of Filtek™ are available.

$$\underset{R^2\text{-}CH—CH_2}{\overset{O}{/\backslash}} + RR^1NCH_2^+ \rightarrow RR^1NCH_2—O—CH_2\overset{+}{C}HR^2—$$

Then:

$$RR'NCH_2—O—CH_2\overset{+}{C}HR^2 + \underset{CH_2CH—}{\overset{O}{/\backslash}} \rightarrow RR^1NCH_2—O—CH_2CHR^2—O—CH_2\overset{+}{C}HR^2$$

Scheme 3.3 Ring-opening polymerization of epoxy resins.

Studies have shown these siloranes to have good stability when stored in various media [163], a consequence of their relatively hydrophobic nature that also results in low water absorption and low water solubility [164]. They have been used in all of the applications of conventional composites, including Class I and Class II cavities, Class V restorations and as posterior filling materials. Results have generally been good [165–168], mainly as a result of the very fine filler employed, which gives good wear properties and hence clinical durability.

3.8.3 Giomers

Giomers are a type of conventional composite resin that is generally formulated with a 'flowable' consistency. Their distinctive feature is that they are filled, in part, with pre-reacted glass-ionomer cement that has been finely crushed [169]. This makes giomers moderately fluoride-releasing [170], due to the pre-reaction at the glass surface of the filler particles, but their overall properties are those of conventional composite resins. There is some evidence that they release sufficient fluoride to be considered anti-bacterial [171]. Their remaining filler has been little discussed in the literature, but from reports of their clinical performance [172,173], it is likely that they are also filled with nano-particle fillers, which give them sound clinical durability and the ability to retain their aesthetics for at least 2 years.

Clinical summary

- Composite resins are tough aesthetic materials for repairing teeth.
- They are typically one-paste light-cured systems, but two-paste self-cured brands are still available.
- They set by polymerization, which inevitably causes shrinkage.
- To overcome the effects of setting shrinkage and also to ensure thorough cure, composite resin restorations should be built up in increments.
- Composites are not adhesive and must be used with bonding agents.
- They are available as packable (high viscosity), flowable (lower viscosity) or universal grades. The majority of a restoration should be built up from packable or universal material.
- Some authorities advocate soft-start polymerization, but this practice is not supported by the evidence.
- Various types of cure lamp are available for use with composite resins, and all of them seem to give clinically acceptable degrees of cure.
- A wide range of repairs is possible with composite resins.
- Some brands are available that release fluoride, but levels released are low.
- Most composites are methacrylate-based, but other types are available (ormocers, siloranes, giomers). Each is claimed to offer some advantages over methacrylate systems, but is not yet clear whether these improvements make a significant difference to their clinical performance.

Clinical use of composite resins

(a) Step-by-step guide to using light-cured composite resins

  (i) Prepare the cavity — remove plaque and pellicle from the surface using a non-fluoridated cleaning paste and a rotary brush. Then remove all caries and cut the enamel.

  (ii) In the case of deep caries, cover the pulpal wall with calcium hydroxide cement, followed by either zinc polycarboxylate or glass-ionomer cement. Do not use zinc

oxide-eugenol, as eugenol is released from this material and it inhibits the polymerization of the composite resin.
(iii) Prepare cut surface and apply appropriate bonding agent, preferably a four-step one (see Chapter 5).
(iv) Apply first composite layer approximately 1 mm thick and light-cure for 40 s.
(v) Apply subsequent layers, curing each for 40 s.
(vi) Remove excess material (use diamond bur, finishing bur or Arkansas stone). Polish with fluoride-containing paste and silicone discs.
(vii) The patient can eat and drink immediately this procedure is completed.

(b) Step-by-step guide to using two-paste composite resins
(i) Prepare the cavity in the same way as above.
(ii) Condition the surface and apply bonding agent.
(iii) Mix one drop of resin with one drop of catalyst and apply to the cavity surface with an applicator or micro-brush.
(iv) Mix equal portions of base and catalyst pastes, and completely fill the cavity with one portion of this mixture. Wait until the material sets.
(v) Remove excess material (use diamond bur, finishing bur or Arkansas stone). Polish with fluoride-containing paste and silicone discs.
(vi) The patient can eat and drink immediately this procedure is completed.

References

[1] M.S.M. Alger, Polymer Science Dictionary, second ed., Springer Publishing, New York, 1997.
[2] F. Riley, Structural Ceramics, The University Press, Cambridge, 2009.
[3] A. Mortensen, J. Llorca, Metal matrix composites, Annu. Rev. Mater. Res. 40 (2010) 243–270.
[4] J.W. Nicholson, The Chemistry of Polymers, fourth ed., RSC, Cambridge, 2012.
[5] T.S. Chow, The effect of particle shape on the mechanical properties of filled polymers, J. Mater. Sci. 15 (1980) 1873–1888.
[6] R.J. Magya, S. Root, T.R. Mattsson, Equations of state for mixtures: results from density functional (DFT) simulations compared to high accuracy validation experiments on Z, J. Phys. Conf. Ser. 500 (2014). Article 162004.
[7] A.D. Wilson, J.W. Nicholson, Acid–Base Cements, The University Press, Cambridge, 1993.
[8] J.L. Ferracane, Resin composite – state of the art, Dent. Mater. 27 (2011) 29–38.
[9] R.L. Bowen, Properties of a silica-reinforced polymer for dental restorations, J. Am. Dent. Assoc. 66 (1963) 57–64.
[10] A. Peutzfeldt, Resin composites in dentistry: the monomer systems, Eur. J. Oral Sci. 105 (1997) 97–116.
[11] J.F. McCabe, A.W.G. Walls, Applied Dental Materials, ninth ed., Blackwell Munksgaard, Oxford, 2008.
[12] E.C. Combe, Notes on Dental Materials, Churchill Livingstone, Edinburgh, 1992.
[13] J.W. Stansbury, Curing dental resins and composites by photopolymerization, J. Esthet. Dent. 12 (2000) 300–308.
[14] Y.J. Park, K.H. Chai, H.R. Rawls, Development of a new photoinitiation system for dental light-cure composite resins, Dent. Mater. 15 (1999) 120–127.
[15] B.K. Moore, J.A. Platt, G. Borges, T.M. Chu, I. Katsilieri, Depth of cure of dental resin composites: ISO 4049 depth and microhardness of types of materials and shades, Oper. Dent. 33 (2008) 408–412.

[16] H. Matsumoto, J.E. Gres, V.A. Marker, T. Okabe, J.L. Ferracane, G.A. Harvey, Depth of cure of visible light-cure resin: clinical simulation, J. Prosthet. Dent. 55 (1986) 574–578.
[17] International Organisation for Standardisation, Dentistry: Polymer-Based Restorative Materials, ISO 4029, ISO, Geneva, Switzerland, 2009.
[18] J.L. Ferracane, Correlation between hardness and degree of conversion during the setting reaction of unfilled dental restorative resins, Dent. Mater. 1 (1985) 11–14.
[19] F.A. Rueggeberg, R.G. Craig, Correlation parameters used to estimate monomer conversion in a light-cure composite, J. Dent. Res. 67 (1988) 932–937.
[20] S. Flury, S. Hayoz, A. Peutzfeldt, J. HÜsler, A. Lussi, Depth of cure of resin composites: is the ISO 4049 method suitable for bulk fill materials? Dent. Mater. 28 (2012) 521–528.
[21] J.G. Leprince, W.M. Palin, M.A. Hadis, J. Devaux, G. Lehoup, Progress in dimethacrylate-based dental composite technology and curing efficiency, Dent. Mater. 29 (2013) 139–156.
[22] E. Andrzejewska, Photopolymerization kinetics of multifunctional monomers, Prog. Polym. Sci. 26 (2002) 605–665.
[23] G. Schmalz, Resin-based composites, in: G. Schmalz, D. Arenholt-Bindslev (Eds.), Biocompatibility of Dental Materials, Springer-Verlag, Berlin/Heidelberg, Germany, 2009, pp. 99–137.
[24] N. Scott, A. Venturello, F.A.C. Borga, D. Pasqualini, D.S. Paolino, F. Geobaldo, E. Berutti, Post-curing conversion kinetics as functions of the irradiation time and increment thickness, J. Appl. Oral Sci. 21 (2013) 190–195.
[25] D. Truffier-Boutry, S. Demoustier-Champagne, J. Devaux, J.J. Biebuyck, M. Mestdagh, P. Larbanois, G. Lehoup, A physico-chemical explanation of the post-polymerization shrinkage in dental resins, Dent. Mater. 22 (2006) 405–412.
[26] R.L. Leung, P.L. Fan, W.M. Johnston, Post-irradiation polymerization of visible light-activated composite resin, J. Dent. Res. 62 (1983) 363–365.
[27] K. Anseth, S.M. Newman, C.N. Bowman, Polymeric dental composites: properties and reaction behaviour of multimethacrylate dental restorations, Adv. Polym. Sci. 122 (1995) 177–217.
[28] L.G. Lovell, J.W. Stansbury, D.C. Stypes, C.N. Bowman, Effects of composition and reactivity on the reaction kinetics of dimethacrylate/dimethacrylate copolymerizations, Macromolecules 32 (1999) 3913–3921.
[29] E. Asmussen, A. Peutzfeldt, Influence of selected components on crosslink density in polymer structures, Eur. J. Oral Sci. 109 (2001) 282–285.
[30] J.G. Leprince, G. Lamblin, J. Devaux, M. Dewaele, M. Mestdagh, W.M. Palin, B. Gallez, G. Lehoup, Irradiation modes' impact on radical entrapment in photoactive resins, J. Dent. Res. 89 (2010) 1494–1498.
[31] J.L. Ferracane, E.H. Greener, The effect of resin formulation on the degree of conversion and mechanical properties of dental restorative resins, J. Biomed. Mater. Res. 20 (1986) 121–131.
[32] J. Li, H. Li, A.S.L. Fok, D.C. Watts, Multiple correlations of material parameters of light-cured dental composites, Dent. Mater. 25 (2009) 829–836.
[33] M. Dewaele, D. Truffier-Boutry, J. Devaux, G. Lehoup, Volume contraction in photocured dental resins; the shrinkage-conversion relationship revisited, Dent. Mater. 22 (2006) 359–365.
[34] J.L. Ferracane, J.C. Mitchem, J.R. Condon, R. Tod, Wear and marginal breakdown of composites with various degrees of cure, J. Dent. Res. 76 (1997) 1508–1516.

[35] J.L. Ferracane, Elution of leachable components from composites, J. Oral Rehabil. 21 (1994) 441–452.
[36] J.L. Ferracane, E.H. Greener, Fourier transform infrared analysis of degree of polymerization in unfilled resins – methods comparison, J. Dent. Res. 63 (1984) 1093–1095.
[37] R.H. Halvorson, R.L. Erickson, C.L. Davidson, The effect of filler and silane content on conversion of resin-based composite, Dent. Mater. 19 (2003) 327–333.
[38] C. Pianelli, J. Devaux, S. Bebelman, G. Lehoup, The micro-Raman spectroscopy, a useful tool to determine the degree of conversion of light-activated composite resins, J. Biomed. Mater. Res. 48 (1999) 675–681.
[39] L.C.P. Moraes, R.S.F. Rocha, L.M. Menegazzo, E.B. de Aranjo, K. Yukimito, J.C.S. Moraes, Infrared spectroscopy: a tool for determination of the degree of conversion in dental composites, J. Appl. Oral Sci. 16 (2008) 145–149.
[40] J.G. Leprince, P. Leveque, B. Nysten, B. Gallez, J. Devaux, G. Lehoup, New insight into the 'depth of cure' of dimethacrylate-based dental composites, Dent. Mater. 28 (2012) 512–520.
[41] K. Musanje, B.W. Darvell, Curing-light attenuation in filled-resin restorative materials, Dent. Mater. 22 (2006) 804–817.
[42] K. Tamareselvy, F.A. Rueggeberg, Dynamic mechanical analysis of two crosslinked systems, Dent. Mater. 10 (1994) 290–297.
[43] A.R. Benetti, E. Asmussen, E.C. Munkesgaard, M. Dewaele, A. Peutzfeldt, G. Lehoup, J. Devaux, Softening and elution of monomers in ethanol, Dent. Mater. 25 (2009) 282–285.
[44] E. Asmussen, A. Peutzfeldt, Two-step curing: influence on conversion and softening of a dental polymer, Dent. Mater. 19 (2003) 466–470.
[45] M. Dewaele, E. Asmussen, A. Peutzfeldt, E.C. Munkesgaard, A.R. Benetti, G. Finné, Influence of curing protocol on selected properties of light-curing polymers: degree of conversion, volume contraction, elastic modulus and glass transition temperature, Dent. Mater. 25 (2009) 1576–1584.
[46] A.C. Shorthall, H.J. Wilson, E. Harrington, Depth of cure of radiation-activated composite restoratives – influence of shade and opacity, J. Oral Rehabil. 22 (1995) 337–342.
[47] D.C. Watts, A.J. Cash, Analysis of optical transmission by 400–500 nm visible light into aesthetic dental biomaterials, J. Dent. 22 (1994) 112–117.
[48] F. Goncalves, L.C. Boaro, J.L. Ferracane, R.R. Braga, A comparative evaluation of polymerization stress data obtained with four different mechanical testing systems, Dent. Mater. 28 (2012) 680–686.
[49] A.C. Shorthall, How light source and product shade influence cure depth for a contemporary composite, J. Oral Rehabil. 32 (2005) 906–911.
[50] N. Emami, M. Sjodahl, K.J. Soderholm, How filler properties, filler fraction, sample thickness and light source affect light attenuation in particulate filled resin composites, Dent. Mater. 21 (2005) 721–730.
[51] G.B. dos Santos, R.V. Alto, H.R. Filho, E.M. da Silva, C.E. Fellows, Light transmission on dental resin composites, Dent. Mater. 24 (2008) 571–576.
[52] K. Fujita, T. Ikemi, N. Nishiyama, Effects of particle size of silica filler on polymerization conversion in a light-curing resin composite, Dent. Mater. 27 (2011) 1079–1085.
[53] A.C. Shorthall, W.M. Palin, P. Burtscher, Refractive index mismatch and monomer reactivity influence composite curing depth, J. Dent. Res. 87 (2008) 84–88.

[54] B. Howard, N.D. Wilson, S.M. Newman, C.S. Pfeifer, J.W. Stansbury, Relationships between conversion, temperature and optical properties during composite photopolymerization, Acta Biomater. 6 (2010) 2053–2059.
[55] M.A. Hadis, P.H. Tomlins, A.C. Shorthall, W.M. Palin, Dynamic monitoring of refractive index change through photoactive resins, Dent. Mater. 26 (2010) 1106–1112.
[56] E.S. Shawkat, A.C. Shortall, O. Addison, W.M. Palin, Oxygen inhibition and incremental layer bond strength of resin composites, Dent. Mater. 25 (2009) 1338–1346.
[57] S. Ghivari, M. Chandak, N. Manvar, Role of oxygen inhibition layer on shear bond strength of composites, J. Conserv. Dent. 13 (2010) 39–41.
[58] D. Leung, C.N. Bowman, Reducing shrinkage stress of dimethacrylate networks by reversible addition-fragmentation chain transfer, Macromol. Chem. Phys. 213 (2012) 198–204.
[59] P. Ghosh, P.S. Mitra, Photopolymerization of methyl methacrylate by use of a quinoline-bromine charge transfer complex as the photoinitiator, J. Polym. Sci., Polym. Chem. Ed. 13 (1975) 921–930.
[60] K. Arakawa, Shrinkage forces due to polymerization of light-cured dental composite resin in cavities, Polym. Test. 29 (2010) 1052–1056.
[61] G. Abbass, G.J. Fleming, E. Harrington, A.C. Shorthall, F.J. Burke, Cuspal movement and microleakage in premolar teeth restored with a packable composite cured in bulk or in increments, J. Dent. 31 (2003) 437–444.
[62] R.R. Braga, R.Y. Ballester, J.L. Ferracane, Factors involved in the development of polymerization shrinkage stress in resin-composites: a systematic review, Dent. Mater. 21 (2005) 962–970.
[63] J. Durner, W. Spahl, J. Zaspel, H. Schweikl, R. Hickel, F.X. Reichl, Eluted substances from unpolymerized dental restorative materials and their Nernst partition coefficient, Dent. Mater. 26 (2010) 91–99.
[64] A.H. Garcia, M.A.M. Lozano, J.C. Vila, A.B. Escribano, P.F. Galve, Composite resins. A review of the materials and clinical indications, Med. Oral Patol. Oral Cir. Bucal 11 (2006) E215–E220.
[65] F. Millich, I. Jeang, J.D. Eick, C.C. Chappelow, C.S. Pinzino, Elements of light-cured epoxy-based dental polymer systems, J. Dent. Res. 77 (1998) 603–608.
[66] D.A. Tilbrook, R.L. Clarke, N.E. Howle, M. Braden, Photocurable epoxy-polyol matrices for use in dental composites I, Biomaterials 21 (2000) 1743–1753.
[67] D.C.N. Chan, W.D. Browning, K.B. Frazier, M.G. Brackett, Clinical evaluation of the soft-start (pulse-delay) polymerization technique in Class I and Class II composite restorations, Oper. Dent. 33 (2008) 265–271.
[68] C.M. Amaral, A.K. de Castro, L.A. Pimenta, G.M.B. Ambrosano, Influence of resin composite polymerization technique on microleakage and microhardness, Quintessence Int. 33 (2002) 685–689.
[69] J.O. Burgess, R.S. Walker, C.J. Porche, A.J. Rappold, Light curing – an update, Compend. Contin. Educ. Dent. 23 (2012) 889–896.
[70] A. Mehl, R. Hickel, K.H. Kunzelmann, Physical properties and gap formation of light-cured composites with and without 'softstart-polymerization', J. Dent. 25 (1997) 321–330.
[71] D.C. Watts, A. al Hindi, Intrinsic 'soft-start' polymerization shrinkage-kinetics in an acrylate-based resin-composite, Dent. Mater. 15 (1999) 39–45.
[72] J.O. Burgess, M. DeGoes, R. Walker, A.H. Ripps, An evaluation of four light-curing units comparing soft and hard curing, Pract. Periodontics Aesthet. Dent. 11 (1999) 125–132.

[73] G.K.P. Barros, F.H.B. Aguiar, A.J. Santos, J.R. Lovadine, Effect of different intensity light curing modes on microleakage to two resin composite restorations, Oper. Dent. 28 (2003) 642–646.
[74] C.H. Chye, A.U. Yap, Y.C. Laim, M.S. Soh, Post-gel polymerization shrinkage associated with different light-curing regimes, Oper. Dent. 30 (2005) 474–480.
[75] A. Sahafi, A. Peutzfeldt, E. Asmussen, Soft-start polymerization and marginal gap formation in vitro, Am. J. Dent. 14 (2001) 145–147.
[76] R.C. Alonso, L. Cunha, G.M. Correr, M.F. De Goes, L. Correr-Sobrinho, R.M. Puppin-Rontani, M.A. Ceolho Sinhoreti, Association of photoactivation methods and low modulus liners on marginal adaptation of composite restorations, Acta Odontol. Scand. 62 (2004) 298–304.
[77] N. Hofmann, C. Siebrecht, B. Hugo, B. Klaiber, Influence of curing methods and materials on the marginal seal of Class V composite restorations in vitro, Oper. Dent. 28 (2003) 410–415.
[78] F.H. Aguiar, K.F. Ajudarte, J.R. Lovadino, Effect of light curing modes and filling techniques on microleakage of posterior composite restorations, Oper. Dent. 27 (2002) 557–562.
[79] L.M.A. Cavalcante, A.R. Peris, C.M. Amaral, G.M.B. Ambrosano, A.F. Pimenta, Influence of polymerization technique on microleakage and microhardness of resin composite restorations, Oper. Dent. 28 (2003) 200–206.
[80] Y.Z. Bayindir, M. Yildis, F. Bayindir, The effect of 'soft-start polymerization' on surface hardness of two packable composites, Dent. Mater. J. 22 (2003) 610–616.
[81] W.C. Brandt, L.F.J. Scheider, E. Frollini, L. Correr-Sobrinho, M.A.C. Sinhoret, Effect of different photo-initiators and light curing units on degree of conversion of composites, Braz. Oral Res. 24 (2010) 263–270.
[82] C.M. Amaral, A.R. Peris, G.M. Ambrosano, E.J. Swift Jr., L.A. Pimenta, The effect of light-curing source and mode on microtensile bond strength to bovine dentin, J. Adhes. Dent. 8 (2006) 41–45.
[83] B. Micali, R.T. Basting, Effectiveness of composite resin polymerization using light-emitting diodes (LEDs) or halogen-based light-curing units, Braz. Oral Res. 18 (2004) 266–270.
[84] H.S. Chan, Y. May, H. Kim, K.C.T. Tong, D. Ng, J.C.M. Hsiao, Review: resin composite filling, Materials 3 (2010) 1228–1243.
[85] H.H. Alvim, A.C. Alecio, W.A. Vasconcellos, M. Furlan, J.E. de Oliviera, J.R.C. Saad, Analysis of camphorquinone in composite resin as a function of shade, Dent. Mater. 23 (2007) 1245–1249.
[86] W.D. Cook, M.P. Chong, Colour stability and visual perception of dimethacrylate based dental composite resins, Biomaterials 6 (1985) 257–264.
[87] W. Teshima, Y. Nomura, N. Tanaka, H. Urabe, M. Okazaki, Y. Nahara, ESR study of camphorquinone/amine photoinitiator systems using blue light-emitting diodes, Biomaterials 24 (2003) 2097–2103.
[88] W.J. Dunn, A.C. Bush, A comparison of polymerization by light-emitting diode and halogen-based light-curing units, J. Am. Dent. Assoc. 133 (2002) 335–341.
[89] W.D. Cook, Spectral distributions of dental photopolymerization sources, J. Dent. Res. 61 (1982) 1436–1438.
[90] R.W. Mills, K.D. Jandt, S.H. Ashworth, Dental composite depth of cure with halogen and blue light emitting diode technology, Br. Dent. J. 186 (1999) 388–391.
[91] S. Bouillaguet, G. Caillot, J. Forchelet, M. Cattini-Lorente, J.C. Wataha, I. Krejci, Thermal risks from LED- and high-intensity QTH-curing units during polymerization of dental resins, J. Biomed. Mater. Res. B Appl. Biomater. 72 (2005) 260–267.

[92] D.A. Stewardson, A.C. Shorthall, E. Harrington, P.J. Lumley, Thermal changes and cure depths associated with a high intensity light activation unit, J. Dent. 32 (2004) 643–651.
[93] S.M. Mousavinasab, I. Meters, Comparison of depth of cure, hardness and heat generation of LED and high intensity QTH light sources, Eur. J. Dent. 5 (2011) 299–304.
[94] R.W. Mills, A. Uhl, G.B. Blackwell, K.D. Jandt, High power light emitting diode (LED) arrays versus halogen light polymerization of oral biomaterials: Barcol hardness, compressive strength and radiometric properties, Biomaterials 23 (2002) 2955–2963.
[95] K.M. Wiggins, M. Hartung, O. Althoff, C. Wastian, S.B. Mitra, Curing performance of a new-generation light-emitting diode dental curing unit, J. Am. Dent. Assoc. 135 (2004) 1471–1479.
[96] C. Hasler, B. Zimmerli, A. Lussi, Curing capability of halogen and LED light curing units in deep class II cavities in extracted human molars, Oper. Dent. 31 (2006) 354–363.
[97] B. Ozturk, A.N. Ozturk, A. Usumez, S. Usumez, F. Omer, Temperature rise during adhesive and resin composite photopolymerization with various light curing systems, Oper. Dent. 29 (2004) 325–332.
[98] E. Asmussen, E. Peutzfeldt, Temperature rise induced by some light emitting diode and quartz-tungsten-halogen curing units, Eur. J. Oral Sci. 113 (2005) 96–98.
[99] A. Uhl, R.W. Mills, A.F. Rzanny, K.D. Jandt, Time dependence of composite shrinkage using halogen and LED light curing, Dent. Mater. 21 (2005) 278–286.
[100] C.A. Felix, R.B. Price, P. Andreou, Effect of reduced exposure times on the microhardness of 10 resin composites cured by high-power LED and QTH curing units, J. Can. Dent. Assoc. 72 (2006) 147.
[101] C.Y.K. Lung, J.P. Matinlinna, Aspects of silane coupling agents and surface conditioning in dentistry: an overview, Dent. Mater. 28 (2012) 467–477.
[102] F. Lutz, R.W. Phillips, A classification and evaluation of composite resin systems, J. Prosthet. Dent. 50 (1983) 480–488.
[103] I.D. Siderou, M.M. Karabela, E.Ch. Vouvoudi, Physical properties of current dental nanohybrid and nanofill light-cured resin composites, Dent. Mater. 27 (2011) 598–607.
[104] N. Moszner, U. Salz, New developments of polymeric dental composites, Prog. Polym. Sci. 26 (2001) 535–576.
[105] S.C. Bayne, H.O. Heymann, E.J. Swift Jr., Update on dental composite restorations, J. Am. Dent. Assoc. 125 (1994) 687–701.
[106] A.R. Curtis, W.M. Palin, G.J.P. Fleming, A.C.C. Shorthall, P.M. Marquis, The mechanical properties of nanofilled resin-based composites; the impact of dry and wet cyclic pre-loading on bi-axial flexure strength, Dent. Mater. 25 (2009) 188–197.
[107] J.T. Blackham, K.S. Vanderwalle, W. Lein, Properties of hybrid resin composite systems containing prepolymerized filler particles, Oper. Dent. 34 (2009) 697–702.
[108] N. Ilie, R. Hickel, Investigations on mechanical behaviour of dental composites, Clin. Oral Invest. 13 (2009) 427–438.
[109] S.B. Mitra, D. Wu, B.N. Holmes, An application of nanotechnology in advanced dental materials, J. Am. Dent. Assoc. 134 (2003) 1382–1390.
[110] N. Moszner, S. Klapdohr, Nanotechnology for dental composites, Int. J. Nanotechnol. 2 (2004) 130–156.
[111] A.U. Yap, C.H. Tan, S.M. Chung, Wear behaviour of new composite restoratives, Oper. Dent. 29 (2004) 269–274.
[112] C.P. Turssi, J.L. Ferracane, M.C. Serra, Abrasive wear of resin composites as related to finishing and polishing procedures, Dent. Mater. 21 (2005) 641–648.
[113] K.K. Choi, J.L. Ferracane, T.J. Hilton, D. Charlton, Properties of packable dental composites, J. Esthet. Dent. 12 (2000) 216–226.

[114] S.C. Bayne, J.Y. Thompson, E.J. Swift Jr., P. Stamatiades, M.A. Wilkerson, A characterization of first-generation flowable composites, J. Am. Dent. Assoc. 129 (1998) 567–577.
[115] J. Manhaart, K.-H. Kunzelmann, H.Y. Chen, R. Hickel, Mechanical properties and wear behaviour of light-cured packable composite resins, Dent. Mater. 16 (2000) 33–40.
[116] F.B. de Souza, R.P. Guimaraes, C.H. Silva, A clinical evaluation of packable and microhybrid resin composite restorations: one-year report, Quintessence Int. 36 (2005) 41–48.
[117] P.S. Stein, J. Sullivan, J.E. Hanbereich, P.B. Osborne, Composite resin in medicine and dentistry, J. Long Term Eff. Med. Implants 15 (2005) 641–654.
[118] A. Petropolis, F. Pantzari, N. Nomikos, V. Chronopoulos, S. Kourtis, The use of indirect resin composites in clinical practice: a case series, Dentistry 3 (3) (2013), http://dx.doi.org/10.1111/clr. 2012.23.
[119] I. Gainsford, S. Dunne, Silver Amalgam in Clinical Practice, third ed., Butterworth-Heinemann, Oxford, 1992.
[120] A.M. Brownawell, S. Berent, R.L. Brett, J.V. Bruckner, J. Doull, E.M. Gershwin, R.D. Hood, G.M. Matanoski, R. Rueben, E. Weiss, M.H. Karol, The potential adverse health effects of dental amalgam, Toxicol. Rev. 24 (2005) 1–10.
[121] P.A. DaRosa Rudolpho, M.S. Cenci, T.A. Donassollo, A.D. Loguercio, F.F. Demarco, A clinical evaluation of posterior composite restorations: 17-year findings, J. Dent. 34 (2006) 427–435.
[122] D.C. Sarrett, Clinical challenges and the relevance of materials testing for posterior composite restorations, Dent. Mater. 21 (2005) 9–20.
[123] F. Lutz, I. Krejei, T.R. Oldenburg, Elimination of polymerization stress of the margins of posterior composite restorations: a new restorative technique, Quintessence Int. 17 (1986) 777–784.
[124] K.J. Donly, F. Garcia-Godoy, The use of resin-based composite in children, Pediatr. Dent. 24 (2002) 480–488.
[125] R.E. Kovarik, J.W. Ergle, Fracture toughness of posterior resin composites fabricated by incremental layering, J. Prosthet. Dent. 69 (1993) 557–560.
[126] E.G. Wilson, M. Mandradjieff, T. Brindock, Controversies in posterior resin composite restorations, Dent. Clin. North Am. 34 (1990) 27–44.
[127] D. Stewardson, P. Thornley, T. Bigg, C. Bromage, A. Browne, D. Cottam, D. Dalby, J. Gilmour, J. Horton, E. Roberts, L. Westoby, T. Burke, The survival of Class V restorations in general dental practice: Part 1, baseline data, Br. Dent. J. 208 (2010) 1–5.
[128] P. Gaengler, I. Hoyer, R. Montag, Clinical evaluation of posterior composite restorations: 10-year report, J. Adhes. Dent. 3 (2001) 185–194.
[129] U. Pallesen, V. Qvist, Composite resin fillings and inlays. An 11-year evaluation, Clin. Oral Invest. 34 (2003) 427–435.
[130] M. Bernardo, H. Luis, M.D. Martin, B.G. Leroux, T. Rue, J. Leitao, T.A. DeRouen, Survival and reasons for failure of amalgam versus composite posterior restorations placed in a random clinical trial, J. Am. Dent. Assoc. 138 (2007) 775–783.
[131] J.M. Powers, R.L. Sakaguchi, Craig's Restorative Dental Materials, Mosby, London, 2006.
[132] K.G. Schiebe, K.G. Almeida, I.S. Medeiros, J.F. Costa, C.M. Alves, Effect of different polishing systems on the surface roughness of microhybrid composites, J. Appl. Oral Sci. 17 (2009) 21–26.
[133] A.U. Guler, E. Guler, A.C. Yucel, E. Ertas, Effect of different polishing procedures on color stability of resin composites, J. Appl. Oral Sci. 17 (2009) 108–112.
[134] S.R. Jefferies, Abrasive finishing and polishing in restorative dentistry: a state-of-the-art review, Dent. Clin. N. Am. 51 (2007) 379–397.

[135] B. Lesage, F. Milnar, J. Wohlberg, Achieving the epitome of composite art: creating natural tooth esthetics, texture and anatomy using appropriate preparation and layering techniques, J. Cosmet. Dent. 24 (2008) 42–51.
[136] S. Nandini, Indirect resin composites, J. Conserv. Dent. 10 (2010) 423–431.
[137] M. Nishimaki, Depth of cure and hardness of indirect composite resin materials polymerized with two metal halide laboratory curing units, J. Oral Sci. 54 (2012) 121–125.
[138] R.O. Souza, M. Ozcan, S.M. Michida, R.M. de Melo, C.A. Pavanelli, M.A. Bottino, L.E. Soares, A.A. Martin, Conversion degree of indirect resin composites and effect of thermocycling on their physical properties, J. Prosthodont. 19 (2010) 218–225.
[139] B. Touati, The evolution of aesthetic restorative materials for inlays and onlays: a review, Pract. Periodontics Aesthet. Dent. 8 (1996) 657–666.
[140] L.A. Jongsma, C.J. Kleverlaan, A.J. Feilzer, Clinical success and survival of indirect resin composite crowns: results of a 3-year prospective study, Dent. Mater. 28 (2012) 952–960.
[141] T. Papadopolulos, A. Sarafianou, A. Hatzikyriakos, Colour stability of veneering composites after accelerated aging, Eur. J. Dent. 4 (2010) 137–142.
[142] P. Kharade, S. Sharma, A. Banerjee, T. Gupta, Indirect resin-bonded fibre-reinforced composite anterior bridge: a case report, Gen. Dent. 60 (2012) e170–e172.
[143] X. Xu, J.O. Burgess, Compressive strength, fluoride release and recharge of fluoride-releasing materials, Biomaterials 24 (2003) 2451–2461.
[144] M. Braden, B.E. Causton, R.L. Clarke, Diffusion of water in composite resins, J. Dent. Res. 55 (1976) 730–732.
[145] G.O. Adusei, S. Deb, J.W. Nicholson, The role of the ionomer glass component in polyacid-modified composite resin dental restorative materials, J. Mater. Sci. Mater. Med. 15 (2004) 751–754.
[146] P. Karantakis, M. Helvatjoglou-Antoniades, S. Theodoridou-Pahini, Fluoride release from three glass ionomers, a compomer and a composite resin in water, artificial saliva and lactic acid, Oper. Dent. 25 (2000) 20–25.
[147] A.J. Preston, L.H. Mair, E.A. Agalamanyi, S.M. Higham, Fluoride release from aesthetic dental materials, J. Oral Rehabil. 26 (1999) 123–129.
[148] L. Ling, X. Xu, G.-Y. Choi, D. Bilodeaux, G. Guo, R.M. Diwan, Novel F-releasing composite with improved mechanical properties, J. Dent. Res. 88 (2009) 83–88.
[149] B.J. Cohen, A.S. Deutsch, B.L. Musiant, Fluoride release from four reinforced composite resins: a one year study, Oral Health 85 (1995) 7–8.
[150] G.E.H.M. Djkman, J. de Vries, A. Loding, J. Arends, Long-term fluoride release of visible light-activated composites in vitro: a correlation with in situ demineralisation data, Caries Res. 27 (1993) 117–123.
[151] E.A. Glasspoole, R.L. Erickson, C.L. Davidson, A fluoride-releasing composite for dental applications, Dent. Mater. 17 (2001) 127–133.
[152] A. Sivakumar, A. Valiathan, Dental ceramics and ormocer technology – navigating the future! Trends Biomater. Artif. Organs 20 (2006) 40–43.
[153] S. Kalra, A. Singh, M. Gupta, V. Chadha, Ormocer: an aesthetic direct restorative material, Contemp. Clin. Dent. 3 (2012) 48–53.
[154] A.U. Yap, M.S. Soh, Post-gel polymerization contraction of ‘low shrinkage’ composite restoratives, Oper. Dent. 29 (2004) 182–187.
[155] D. Tagtekin, F.C. Yanikoglu, F.O. Bozkurt, B. Kologlu, H. Sur, Selected characteristics of an Ormocer and a conventional hybrid composite resin, Dent. Mater. 20 (2004) 487–497.
[156] P. Bottenberg, W. Jacquet, K. Alaerts, F. Keulemans, A prospective randomized clinical trial of one bis-GMA-based and two ormocer-based composite restorative systems in class II cavities: five-year results, J. Dent. 37 (2009) 198–203.

[157] S.H. Mahmoud, A.E. El-Embaby, A.M. Abdallah, H.H. Hamama, Two-year clinical evaluation of ormocer, nanohybrid and nanofill composite restorative systems in posterior teeth, J. Adhes. Dent. 10 (2008) 315–322.
[158] C.P. Ernst, M. Brandenbusch, G. Meyer, K. Canbek, F. Gottschalk, B. Willershausen, Two-year clinical performance of a nanofiller vs a fine particle hybrid resin composite, Clin. Oral Invest. 10 (2006) 119–125.
[159] W. Schroeder, S.V. Asmussen, M. Sangermano, C.I. Vallo, Visible light polymerization of epoxy monomers using iodonium salt with camphorquinone/ethyl-4-dimethyl aminobenzoate, Poym. Int. 62 (2013) 1368–1376.
[160] W. Weinmann, C. Thalacker, R. Guggenberger, Siloranes in dental composites, Dent. Mater. 21 (2005) 68–74.
[161] N. Ilie, E. Jelen, T. Clementino-Luedemann, R. Hickel, Low-shrinkage composite for dental application, Dent. Mater. J. 26 (2007) 789–795.
[162] M. Schmidt, L.-L. Kirkevarg, P. Horsted-Bindsler, S. Poulsen, Marginal adaptation of a low-shrinkage silorane-based composite: 1 year randomized clinical trial, Clin. Oral Invest. 15 (2011) 291–295.
[163] N. Ilie, R. Hickel, Macro-, micro- and nano-mechanical investigations on silorane and methacrylate-based composites, Dent. Mater. 25 (2009) 810–819.
[164] W.M. Palin, G.J. Fleming, F.J. Burke, P.M. Marquis, R.C. Randall, The influence of short and medium-term water immersion on the hydrolytic stability of novel low-shrink dental composites, Dent. Mater. 21 (2005) 852–863.
[165] S. Palaniappin, D. Bharadwaj, D.L. Mattar, M. Peumans, B. van Meerbeek, P. Lambrechts, Three-year randomized clinical trial to evaluate clinical performance and wear of a nanocomposite versus hybrid composite, Dent. Mater. 25 (2009) 1302–1314.
[166] L.S. Türkün, E.U. Celik, Noncarious class V lesions with a polyacid modified resin composite and a nanocomposite: a two-year clinical trial, J. Adhes. Dent. 10 (2008) 399–405.
[167] W. Dresch, S. Volpato, J.C. Gomes, N.R. Ribeiro, A. Reis, A.D. Loguercio, Clinical evaluation of a nanofilled composite in posterior teeth: 12-month results, Oper. Dent. 31 (2006) 409–4127.
[168] Z. Ergücü, L.S. Türkün, Clinical performance of novel resin composites in posterior teeth: 18-month results, J. Adhes. Dent. 9 (2007) 209–216.
[169] V. Arora, P. Bogra, Giomer: a new hybrid aesthetic restorative material, J. Conserv. Dent. 5 (2002) 149–155.
[170] N. Nakamura, A. Yamada, T. Iwamoto, M. Arakai, K. Tanaka, S. Aizawa, K. Nonaka, S. Fukumoto, Two-year clinical evaluation of flowable composite resin containing pre-reacted glass-ionomer, Pediatr. Dent. J. 19 (2009) 89–97.
[171] S. Saku, H. Kotake, R.J. Scongall-Vilchis, S. Ohashi, M. Hotta, S. Horuichi, K. Hamada, K. Asoaka, E. Tanaka, K. Yamamoto, Antibacterial activity of composite resins with glass-ionomer filler particles, Dent. Mater. J. 29 (2010) 193–198.
[172] M.C. Sunico, K. Shinkai, Y. Katoh, Two-year clinical performance of occlusal and cervical giomer restorations, Oper. Dent. 30 (2005) 282–289.
[173] U.M. Abdel-Karim, M. El-Eraky, W.M. Etman, Three-year clinical evaluation of two nano-hybrid giomer restorative composites, Tanta Dent. J. 11 (2014) 213–222.

Polyacid-modified composite resins (compomers)

4

4.1 Introduction

Polyacid-modified composite resins are a class of composite material used in dental repair [1]. Like conventional composite materials, they consist of two distinct phases that differ in form and chemical composition and are mutually insoluble in each other. They are combined to form a mixture that has superior mechanical properties to those of the individual phases.

Polyacid-modified composites were introduced into clinical use in about 1992, and aimed to combine the benefits of traditional dental composite resins with those of glass-ionomer cements [2]. Details of the latter materials are found in Chapter 6. The trivial name 'compomer' was applied to these modified composite materials, the term being derived from the words composite ('comp-') and glass-ionomer ('-omer').

However, despite the attempt to combine properties of both types of material, the polyacid-modified composites are, in fact, primarily composite resins [1,3]. They consist mainly of dimethacrylate macromonomers blended with diluents and filled with inert filler, bonded in with silane coupling agent. In addition, they also contain some extra components, including an acid-functional monomer, such as the substance known as TCB resin (which is based on the product of reaction of butane tetra-carboxylic acid with 2-hydroxyethyl methacrylate) plus an ion-leachable glass powder of the type used in glass-ionomer cements. On the other hand, they contain no water, as a result of which there is no reaction between the acid groups and the basic glass during the setting reaction [3].

Rather, the setting reaction is entirely an addition polymerization process, generally photo-initiated, and involving free radicals. Once the material is set, it is able to absorb trace amounts of moisture, and this allows the acid-functional groups to manifest their acidity by dissociating after which they attack the basic glass to form a small amount of salt matrix [1–4]. The effect of this moisture-initiated reaction is discussed in later sections of this chapter.

One of the key features of polyacid-modified composite resins is their lack of adhesion to tooth tissues [5]. This is a feature that they share with conventional dental composite resins, and the contrasts with the behaviour of the glass-ionomer cement. It is further evidence that these materials are essentially composite resins, and have very little of the anticipated 'hybrid character' of composites and glass-ionomers. Bonding therefore requires the type of bespoke bonding agents used for conventional composite resins, together with the appropriate preparation of the freshly cut tooth surface [6].

Materials for the Direct Restoration of Teeth. http://dx.doi.org/10.1016/B978-0-08-100491-3.00004-0

4.2 Curing of polyacid-modified composite resins

Polyacid-modified composite resins resemble traditional composite resins in their setting chemistry, which is based on free radical additional polymerization [1–3]. The usual initiation process is photolysis, using a conventional dental curing light emitting with maximum intensity at a wavelength of 470 nm [1]. Alternatively, there is also the possibility of using two-part free radical initiators, which are brought together when two pastes are mixed [7]. This type of polyacid-modified composite resin has been used as a luting material in the attachment of crowns to prepared teeth [7]. The set material resulting from this process does not differ significantly in its structure or properties from photo-chemically cured polyacid-modified composite [1].

The majority of polyacid-modified composite resin brands are photo-cured, and their principle initiator system is camphorquinone, typically with amine co-initiator, as in conventional composite resins [8]. It is important to ensure adequate cure throughout the material, and depth of cure is an issue for consideration with light-cured polyacid-modified composite resins. The attenuation of light as it passes through the matrix, together with its reflection by the particulate filler, means that deep within the material there is less light available to initiate the polymerization reaction. This leads to the upper layers being better cured than the lower ones [9], and there is some evidence that polyacid-modified composites do not transmit light as well as conventional composites, and hence are more susceptible to inadequate cure at greater depths [10]. Colour also affects this, because darker shades attenuate light to a greater extent than lighter ones [10]. These problems are overcome in clinical practice by the technique of incremental build-up, whereby the material is placed in layers not exceeding 2 mm in thickness, light-cured, followed by the next layer being placed on top and cured in turn. In this way, polyacid-modified composite resins strongly resemble conventional composites.

Polymerization in light-cured polyacid-modified composite resins has been studied in detail using the technique of fourier transform infrared spectroscopy (FTIR) [11]. The disappearance of three peaks that arise from the C=C double bonds was followed, the peaks in question being those at 1700–1730, 1630 and 1230–1320 cm^{-1}. These peaks all reduce in intensity rapidly when the material is irradiated at 470 nm, reaching about 50% after 150 s [11]. After removal of the light, the polymerization reaction was shown to continue for up to 60 h, though at a much reduced rate [11].

Depth of cure in polyacid-modified composites has been studied and compared with that in conventional composites [12]. Two techniques were used to inspect the behaviour of the specimens that had been prepared in split metal mould and cured from one end for 40 s. Depth of cure was then measured either using a penetrometer or by scraping away the inadequately cured material from the end furthest away from the curing lamp using a plastic spatula. These two techniques gave very similar results for all materials. Overall the study showed that clinical materials are able to cure to a variety of depths, depending on the brand and the shade [12].

Like conventional composites, the polymerization reaction in polyacid-modified composite resins is associated with a contraction in the overall volume of the material and a corresponding contraction stress [13]. Experiments showed that the values of this contraction stress varied widely for commercial polyacid-modified composite resins materials, and ranged from 1.27 to 3.41 MPa. This stress developed rapidly, and led to the suggestion that, particularly for the higher values, it could be sufficient to lead to failure of the bond with the tooth [13].

The volume fraction of filler and its effect on properties has been studied in experimental polyacid-modified composite resin systems [14]. As expected, the viscosity of the uncured paste was increased by the inclusion of filler, as were both the compressive and diametral strengths. However, these changes reached their limit at filler volumes of 20–30%, and above this range there were no significant differences in any of the properties. These findings are similar to those of conventional composite resin systems, and demonstrate that polyacid-modified composites have entirely conventional behaviour in this regard.

As part of their formulation, polyacid-modified composite resins also contain a small fraction of basic glass filler of the type used in glass-ionomer cements [1]. Such glasses are typically calcium (or strontium) alumino-fluorosilicates, and react with acids in the presence of water to release ions. The ions released, particularly calcium (or strontium) and aluminium react with the acid to form salts, which in the case of glass-ionomers, are insoluble because they form ionic crosslinks with the polymeric acid. The ions effectively insolubilize the acid-functional polymer chains by this reaction, as well as stiffening the material due to coil expansion and ion-binding. This type of chemistry is available to polyacid-modified composite resins once moisture is present, and these materials are designed for this reaction to occur in the early part of their existence.

4.3 Moisture uptake by polyacid-modified composite resins

As already mentioned, the distinctive property of polyacid-modified composite resins is that, once the polymerization reaction has occurred, the set material is able to take up traces of moisture. This activates the acidic character of the carboxylic functional monomer and triggers an acid–base reaction with the glass [1,2]. The water uptake behaviour of these materials has been studied in detail [15], along with the corresponding water desorption processes. Three commercial polyacid-modified composite resins were used in a study of water uptake and loss, and cured samples were prepared as small discs of size 6 mm diameter × 2 mm thickness. Water uptake was allowed to take place in a controlled humidity environment at 93% relative humidity. Following the initial water uptake, there was an intervening desorption cycle in which specimens were stored in a dry atmosphere over concentrated sulfuric acid.

In one study, it was found that the three brands of polyacid-modified composite gained and lost water in a diffusion process that obeyed Fick's second law of diffusion. Diffusion coefficients were different for the first and second uptake cycles, being greater for the first cycle. Values ranged from $2.37 \times 10^{-9}\,cm^2\,s^{-1}$ to $4.53 \times 10^{-9}\,cm^2\,s^{-1}$

for the first cycle and from $0.85 \times 10^{-9}\,cm^2\,s^{-1}$ to $2.72 \times 10^{-9}\,cm^2\,s^{-1}$ for the second [15]. Equilibration times were longer for the first absorption than the second. Desorption kinetics gave similar results to the second cycle for each material, with comparable diffusion coefficients in all three cases. The results obtained were similar to the behaviour of conventional composite resins stored in water [16], and this led to the conclusion that the presence of the more hydrophilic components of the polyacid-modified composite resin did not increase the rate of water movement through the material. However, there were differences between the first and second cycle sorption rates, suggesting that the presence of free acid functional groups and unreacted basic glass has a greater effect on water transport than the presence of the neutralized acid groups and corresponding trace of polysalt product formed in the specimens following the initial water uptake.

Overall water uptake in polyacid-modified composite resins following immersion in water was found to be similar to that found on storage in a high humidity atmosphere, and represented a gain in mass in the range 1–3.5% [1]. FTIR has been used to study the effect of this water uptake [11]. The bands of interest in the spectrum were those at $1705\,cm^{-1}$, which is due to the free carboxylic acid functional group, and $1555\,cm^{-1}$, which is associated with carboxylate salts, in particular calcium carboxylate. The band at $1705\,cm^{-1}$ was shown to reduce in intensity with time as water was taken up, though it remained visible even when water uptake had equilibrated [11]. The band at $1555\,cm^{-1}$, by contrast, gradually increased with increasing time of exposure to water. It has thus been confirmed that polyacid-modified composite resins undergo a neutralization process when water is taken up. Moreover, it has been shown that the rate of this neutralization is fairly slow, because it is controlled by the rate of water diffusion into the material, itself a slow process [11].

There have been suggestions that the water taken up may have positive effects other than promoting the acid–base reaction between the carboxylic acid functional groups and the basic glass filler [17]. One possibility is that it might act as a plasticizer, thus altering the failure mode from predominantly brittle to tough. This would appear to be supported by the finding that storage in completely dry conditions leads to increased strength in polyacid-modified composite resins [18]. Water sorption may also cause slight swelling, and this may be useful in compensating for the polymerization contraction on setting. This suggestion has been made for conventional composites [19,20] where there are no comparably hydrophilic components and the amount of water taken up might be expected to be more modest.

In fact, studies of water uptake with a direct comparison of water uptake in compomers and conventional composite resins do not show particularly large differences between the two different types of composite material. For example, when the polyacid-modified composite resin brands Dyract® and Compoglass® were compared with the conventional composite resin Pekafill®, there were only minor differences in equilibrium water uptake in both pure water and in 0.9% saline solution (Table 4.1) [18]. Pekafill® showed lowest equilibrium water uptakes in both storage media, but only by a very small amount, and one that was not statistically significant in the case of pure water.

Table 4.1 Variation in equilibrium water content (%) of polyacid-modified and conventional composites resin stored at 37°C (specimens cured for 40 s)

Material	In water	In 0.9% NaCl
Dyract	0.92	1.16
Compoglass	1.20	1.28
Pekafill	0.89	0.88

The effect of this water uptake and ensuing neutralization is complicated, and leads to either no significant changes in mechanical properties, or a reduction in them. Studies have covered compressive strength [18], flexural strength [21] and biaxial flexure strength [17]. All agree that neutralization, at best, causes no reduction in physical properties and, more importantly, leads to no significant improvement.

4.4 The glass component

Selection of the glass component of the filler blend in polyacid-modified composite resins appears straightforward. It needs to have a basic character, as in conventional glass-ionomers, and to be capable of reacting with the acid-functional monomer once sufficient water has been drawn into the set composite structure [21]. However, there are also complications that need to be considered, from which it can be seen that the nature and incorporation of the ionomer glass component into polyacid-modified composite is not as straightforward as it appears at first sight.

The important complication is that the material that is formulated seeks to be a hybrid of hydrophobic and hydrophilic components. In terms of physical chemistry, these are frequently incompatible, and attempting to blend them requires the addition of components that compromise the two contributing types of system [22].

To formulate a successful composite material, and in particular to ensure that there is adequate stress transfer from matrix to filler phase, a coupling agent is deployed at the matrix–filler interface. The type of silane used for conventional dental composite resins effectively forms a mono-molecular hydrophobic layer on the surface of the inorganic filler particles. In silanating the reactive ionomer glass in this way, the chemical reactivity of the glass is affected. It is no longer quite so hydrophilic, and hence is less susceptible to acid attack in the presence of moisture.

This was studied in detail in a series of experiments in which an ionomer glass of known composition, the so-called G338, was reacted with the polymeric acid of the commercial glass-ionomer cement Ketac-Molar [22]. This acid comprises an aqueous solution of acrylic acid–maleic acid copolymer (mole ratio of monomers = 2:1) at a concentration of 47.5% mass/mass [22]. Experimental cements were prepared from both silanted and untreated G338 glass at the powder:liquid ratio of 2.25:1. Setting was studied using both an oscillating rheometer and also FTIR spectroscopy. Biaxial flexure strength was determined after 24 h and net water uptake was also determined after this time. Results are shown in Table 4.2.

These results show that the use of silanated glass resulted in longer setting times and also in significantly weaker set cements. It resulted in apparently higher net water uptake, but this result was not statistically significant. FTIR results were consistent with the reduced rate of setting, as the time to the appearance of a carboxylate peak was longer with the silanated glass than with the untreated glass.

The conclusion from this part of the study was that silanation of the glass powder did, indeed, inhibit the acid–base reaction. As is typical for cements of this type, the slower setting reaction that resulted from silanation yielded significantly weaker cements. Silanation, though necessary to secure a good bond between the glass and the matrix, was found to reduce the effectiveness of the post-cure acid–base reaction that is designed to occur following the uptake of moisture [22].

The other part of this study involved the incorporation of reactive glass (both untreated and silanated) into an experimental composite blend. The formulation of this blend is shown in Table 4.3.

The conventional filler, Raysorb T-4000, is a commercial unreactive particulate glass that is widely used in conventional composite resins, and was also incorporated either untreated or silanated. In all cases, discs of material of dimensions 13 mm diameter × 1 mm thickness were prepared and cured from each side with a conventional dental curing lamp through a glass microscope slide for 40 s. They were stored in water for 24 h, after which they were tested for net water uptake and biaxial flexure strength [23]. Results are shown in Table 4.4.

The first thing that is apparent from these data is that the use of Raysorb T-4000 as filler gave significantly stronger materials, whether or not the filler had been silanated. Secondly, the water uptake was significantly greater when the ionomer glass G338 was used, regardless of whether or not it was silanated. However, the silanted

Table 4.2 Properties of experimental glass-ionomer cements with untreated and silanated glass [22]

	Untreated glass	Silanated glass
Setting time (min)	5	9
Biaxial flexure strength (MPa)	32.1 (SD 2.2)	4.9 (SD 1.0)
Net water uptake (%)	2.6 (SD 0.5)	4.1 (SD 1.8)

Table 4.3 Experimental composite formulation [22]

Component	Composition (%)
bisGMA	14.6
TEGDMA	4.9
Camphorquinone (initiator)	0.3
DMAEM (accelerator)	0.2
Filler (G338 or Raysorb T-4000)	80.0

Table 4.4 Properties of experimental composites to show the effect of silanation [22]

Property	Untreated	Silanated
Filler: Raysorb T-4000		
Biaxial flexure strength (MPa)	104.8 (SD 11.0)	152.0 (SD 6.1)
Net water uptake (%)	0.4 (SD 0.0)	0.1 (SD 0.0)
Filler: G338		
Biaxial flexure strength (MPa)	38.4 (SD 4.7)	68.0 (SD 6.0)
Net water uptake (%)	1.0 (SD 0.1)	0.7 (SD 0.1)

G338 sample had a slightly lower net water uptake as well as much greater biaxial flexure strength than the one with the untreated filler. This demonstrates the importance of silanation of the filler in order to obtain the greatest stress transfer from matrix to filler, and hence the maximum possible strength.

These findings show that the presence of the ionomer glasses, whether silanated or not, leads to a composite material with inferior properties. The ionomer glass is sufficiently hydrophilic to increase water uptake by a composite resin system, even in the absence of an acid-functional monomer, and this appears to cause the resulting material to be much weaker than an equivalent composite resin filled with a conventional particulate filler. Polyacid-modified composite resins are formulated with only comparatively minor amounts of ionomer glass, but nonetheless, as these results show, this results in a material with inferior properties. The need to silanate this ionomer component in order to bind it to the matrix properly inhibits the acid–base reaction. Hence the changes that occur upon taking up moisture are also damaging.

4.5 Physical properties of polyacid-modified composites

The first two polyacid-modified composite resins to be available commercially were Dyract (Dentsply) and Compoglass (Ivoclar Vivadent), followed very soon afterwards by Hytac (ESPE). Several early studies were carried out using these materials to determine their properties. One early study considered a variety of their mechanical properties (compressive strength, flexural strength, microhardness and surface roughness) and these were compared with other tooth-coloured restorative materials, including the commercial composite resin Z100 (3M) [24]. Compressive strength was significantly lower for all three polyacid-modified composite resins than for the conventional composite as prepared, ie, without soaking in water. In the case of Dyract and Compoglass, their strengths did not differ significantly from each other, but were significantly lower than for Hytac [24]. Interestingly, the polyacid-modified composite resins all showed significantly greater yield than the conventional composite resin. Flexural strength properties were similar, with Z100 being the strongest to an extent that was statistically significant. All three polyacid-modified composite resins also showed significantly lower microhardness values than Z100 [24]. Only in surface roughness did they show comparable values to the conventional composite.

As a result of these early findings, the manufacturers quickly re-formulated both of the initial materials. The changes were considered substantial, so that the re-formulated materials were given new brand names, being relaunched as Dyract AP and Compoglass F, respectively. Since then, several additional brands have been brought to the market, in addition to Hytac, including Ana Compomer (Nordiska) and F2000 (3M-ESPE).

As already mentioned, water uptake has been shown to make matters worse in terms of physical properties. Generally, polyacid-modified composite resins have been found to be inferior to conventional composites following this maturation treatment, even those which have been re-formulated. Their compressive strength [25,26] and flexural strength [24,27] are typically lower than those of conventional composite resins, as are their fracture toughness and hardness values [28]. They also have inferior wear properties compared with conventional with conventional composites [27]. These results have led to the conclusion that polyacid-modified composite resins should not be used in load-bearing areas. Reduced physical properties also lead to them having significantly higher wear rates. In one early study, using a three-body wear tester employing toothpaste as the abrasive [29] showed the initial formulation of Dyract to wear at almost three times the rate of conventional composites [29], a particularly disappointing result.

In a typical study of the early brands of polyacid-modified composite resin, Abu-bakr et al. [30] studied selected mechanical properties (compressive strength and Vicker's hardness) of Dyract and Compoglass, as well as the compomer Xeno (Sankin, Tochigi, Japan), following immersion for 3h a day in a variety of liquids for up to 60 days, and compared the findings with those from a resin-modified glass-ionomer (Fuji II LC, GC, Japan) and a conventional composite resin (Clearfil AP X, Kuraray, Japan). Unfortunately, it is clear from their discussion that they regard polyacid-modified composite resins as a type of glass-ionomer and make more of the superiority of the properties of Dyract, Compoglass and Xeno to Fuji II LC than they do of these materials' inferiority to Clearfil AP X. However, the properties of the polyacid-modified composite resins were inferior to those of the conventional composite and in general declined between 1 day and 60 days soaking, indicating beyond all doubt that their water uptake is a damaging property, despite being necessary to promote the post-hardening acid–base reaction. Selected results from this study are shown in Table 4.5.

Table 4.5 Effect of water on the properties of polyacid-modified composite resins [30]

Material	Storage time	Test	Value
Dyract	1 day	VHN	55 kg mm^{-2}
	60 days	VHN	50 kg mm^{-2}
	1 day	Compressive strength	230 MPa
	60 days	Compressive strength	220 MPa
Compoglass	1 day	VHN	50 kg mm^{-2}
	60 days	VHN	50 kg mm^{-2}
	1 day	Compressive strength	265 MPa
	60 days	Compressive strength	230 MPa

The study showed that water affected the properties of the conventional composite resin to slight but statistically significant extents, a finding which is consistent with them taking up small amounts of water under these conditions [31]. Despite the possibility of the water uptake in polyacid-modified composite resins triggering the secondary acid–base reaction, they showed similar behaviour to the conventional composites, with a reduction in both properties on taking up water. This was a greater problem for these materials, as they had lower values to start with.

Re-formulated polyacid-modified composite resins have also been found to have properties that decline following water uptake and secondary acid–base reaction (Table 4.6). In one study that demonstrated this, Dyract AP was shown to have lower compressive and biaxial flexure strength values following soaking in water for 4 weeks than they did at 24 h [32] (Table 4.6). By contrast, when stored in dry conditions, strengths were not significantly different between 24 h and 4 weeks.

In a similar study using re-formulated polyacid-modified composite resins, the effect of specifically acidic storage media on properties was considered [17]. In addition to Dyract AP and Compoglass F, it used F2000, and compared the results with those from the conventional composite resin, Herculite (Kerr), and also a conventional glass-ionomer cement (AquaCem, Dentsply). All materials were found to buffer acidic storage media (ie, dilute solutions of phosphoric, citric or lactic acids) to an extent, shifting the pH some way towards neutral. The glass-ionomer cement was the most effective at this, followed by the polyacid-modified composite resins. Herculite showed no statistically significant changes in pH, suggesting that it possesses no buffering capacity, unlike the polyacid-modified composite resins or the glass-ionomer cement [17]. This study also examined the effect of these acidic storage media, plus water, on the biaxial flexure strengths of the materials. However, results showed no clear trends with either time or storage medium, suggesting that this property in these materials is not affected by either water uptake or secondary acid–base reaction [33].

The effects of aqueous storage on the surface have also received attention. In low pH beverages, such as orange juice, surfaces became visibly rougher when examined by scanning electron microscopy (SEM) [30,33]. The surface developed a pitted appearance with voids present and glass particles protruding from it. These results suggest that polyacid-modified composite resins are particularly susceptible to changes in their surface in clinical condition, and with degradation leading to a surface of rougher texture and duller appearance than when newly placed [30,33].

Table 4.6 Properties of the polyacid-modified composite resin Dyract AP stored in wet and dry conditions [32]

Property	Time	Value (dry) (MPa)	Value (wet) (MPa)
Compressive strength	24 h	213.1 (19.3)	208.7 (19.7)
	4 weeks	206.0 (18.1)	125.1 (32.5)
Biaxial flexure strength	24 h	166.3 (18.7)	166.8 (18.5)
	4 weeks	188.6 (18.3)	137.0 (3.8)

Fracture toughness of polyacid-modified composites has been studied and compared with values obtained for conventional composite resins [27]. Fracture toughness is considered an especially useful laboratory test, because the results can be used to estimate in vivo wear, and also both marginal and bulk fracture strengths of composite resin restorations [34]. Three brands of polyacid-modified composite resin (Dyract Posterior, Compoglass F and F2000) were compared with three brands of conventional composite resin, using single-edged notched specimens to determine fracture toughness following storage in water for 1 week [27]. Results showed that, following this storage treatment, conventional composites had significantly higher fracture toughness values (1.75–1.92 $MPa\,m^{1/2}$) than polyacid-modified composite resins (0.97–1.23 $MPa\,m^{1/2}$). This led the authors to conclude that polyacid-modified composite resins had reduced resistance to crack propagation, so should not be used in stress-bearing situations.

4.6 Fluoride release from polyacid-modified composites

One of the properties of glass-ionomer cements that polyacid-modified composite resins are designed to possess is the ability to release fluoride. The reactive glass filler is an ionomer-type glass, and as such contains fluoride. This becomes available for release following its incorporation into the polysalt phase as a result of the moisture driven acid–base reaction with the acid-functional monomer component [1].

The early brands of polyacid-modified composite resin showed very low values of fluoride release [23,35], so to augment this, additional fluoride species have been incorporated into the re-formulated materials. These include strontium fluoride and ytterbium fluoride [1,25].

As with glass-ionomer cements, fluoride release from polyacid-modified composite resins is sustained for long periods of time [23] and is enhanced by placing the polyacid-modified composite resin in acidic storage media [25,36]. This property has been suggested to be beneficial in the case of resin-modified glass-ionomers [37], since it would lead to enhanced release of protective fluoride ion under the very conditions that promote dental caries. A similar argument can be advanced for polyacid-modified composite resins, and it may be that this ability to release extra fluoride under conditions of low pH is beneficial clinically.

The kinetics of fluoride release under neutral conditions have been shown to follow a different mathematical form from fluoride release from glass-ionomer cements, ie,

$$[F]_C = [F]_I / (t_{1/2} + t) + \alpha t$$

where $[F]_C$ is the total cumulative fluoride release, $t_{1/2}$ is the time for release half its initial value, t is time and α is a constant [25]. By contrast, the second term in the equation for fluoride release from glass-ionomers is in $t^{1/2}$, which indicates a diffusion-based release mechanism [38].

A diffusion-based mechanism has been found when polyacid-modified composite specimens were stored in a lactate buffer [36], and to apply for up to 169 h. Scanning electron microscopy examination of the specimens at the end of the fluoride release experiments showed them to have substantially roughened surfaces, thus confirming previous observations [32,33] and suggesting that attack by the acidic storage medium assists the overall fluoride release from these materials [36].

Like glass-ionomers, polyacid-modified composites have been shown to be capable of taking up fluoride from the surrounding medium where additional fluoride is included [25]. Several brands were studied, and recharge capacity was found to vary between the brands. Polyacid-modified composite resins that showed a high inherent fluoride release were found to have a greater recharge capacity than those with only a low inherent release [25].

In measuring fluoride release, it is conventional to determine total fluoride, which is done by adding TISAB (total ionic strength adjustment buffer) to the solution being analysed [39]. This decomposes any complexes (eg, AlF_4^-) or un-dissociated hydrogen fluoride both of which contain fluoride in a form that would otherwise not be detected by the ion-selective electrode. However, one study was carried out where determinations were also made without the addition of TISAB, thus allowing the unbound and bound fluoride to be distinguished when released from polyacid-modified composite resins stored in neutral or acidic conditions [40]. Results are shown in Table 4.7, and show that there is a disparity between total and free fluoride, in that total fluoride release was generally greater in acidic conditions, but the amount of free fluoride was less (though for Dyract AP it was identical). The clinical significance of this observation is not clear.

The authors concluded that the observed complexation was caused because there were also increased amounts of aluminium released at low pH conditions. For Compoglass F, for example, the aluminium level increased from 4.68 ppm in neutral water to 104 ppm in lactic acid solution, so this interpretation was consistent with all of the observations. There is the alternative possibility, that at low pH, molecules of hydrofluoric acid (HF) formed which are predominantly un-dissociated, but the pH of the lactic acid solution was such that only very small amounts of HF could have been present, which again points to aluminium is the cause of fluoride complexation.

Table 4.7 Fluoride concentrations in storage solutions of polyacid-modified composite resins [40]

Material/conditions	Free fluoride (ppm)	Total fluoride (ppm)	Free fluoride (%)
Compoglass F			
Neutral	2.8	4.5	62.2
Acidic	0.5	15.5	3.2
Dyract AP			
Neutral	19.1	21.3	89.7
Acidic	0.3	21.3	1.4
F2000			
Neutral	2.2	6.2	35.5
Acidic	0.2	15.5	1.3

There is debate about whether the relatively low level of fluoride is effective in preventing caries. It has been shown to be effective in vitro [41], but in the most detailed study, the conclusion was that it was not, and that there was no advantage in using polyacid-modified composite resins over amalgam in terms of any observable anti-caries effect of the fluoride release [42].

4.7 Ion-release and buffering by polyacid-modified composite resins

The release of ions other than fluoride and the ability to buffer organic acids by shifting pH towards neutral is a property of glass-ionomer cements that has been known for some years [43]. Similar properties have been observed in polyacid-modified composite resins.

Storage under both neutral and acidic conditions causes ions such as Ca^{2+}, Al^{3+}, Na^{+} and PO_4^{3-} to be released into solution [36,40]. Like fluoride, greater amounts of all of these species are released under acidic conditions [40]. For polyacid-modified composite resins, too, storage in acidic solutions, such as lactic acid, is associated with substantial shifts in pH towards neutral [43], showing that the capability of buffering storage media is conferred by the acid–base component of the polyacid-modified composite resin.

This ability to buffer external solutions in contact with the polyacid-modified composite resin may be a useful one under clinical conditions. The potential reduction in acidity of caries-generating acids, the main one being lactic acid, would be expected to reduce the rate of caries development in patients [44], and this would give them a useful clinical advantage over conventional composite resins.

4.8 Clinical applications and outcomes

Polyacid-modified composite resins are aimed to be used in similar applications to conventional composites, such as Class II [44] and Class V cavities [45,46], and fissure sealants [47]. They have also been used as bonding agents in orthodontics [48].

Like conventional composites, polyacid-modified composites are not adhesive to the prepared tooth surface [6,49], though this has not always been recognized in the literature. Consequently, they need to been bonded with bonding agents of the type used with conventional composites, following similar surface pre-treatments [49].

Polyacid-modified composite resins are favoured by many clinicians over conventional composites to repair primary teeth [50]. This is on account of their fluoride release [1,50]. To emphasize their application in primary teeth, certain brands have been specifically produced for this purpose and are highly coloured. For example, in America, there is a dual-cure compomer called MagicFil (Zenith Dental, Englewood, New Jersey) which is produced in four colours (pink, green, blue and yellow) with glitter inclusions, and a similar material, Twinky Star (Voco, Germany) is available in Europe [51].

Clinical studies of polyacid-modified composite resins have generally been favourable, though they almost always show that conventional composites have superior performance [52,53]. Typically materials are evaluated against the Ryge criteria [54], a standardized set of criteria including such features as colour stability, marginal integrity and anatomic form after differing lengths of service in patients. These criteria are ranked from alpha (the best) through Bravo to Charlie (the worst) [55]. In a typical study of this sort, Dyract AP was found to score mainly alpha after 2 years of service, though there was some minor discoloration and marginal damage, which both scored bravo [52]. Wear was found to be better than for the original polyacid-modified composite resin Dyract [56], and to be consistent with the results of in vitro wear tests [57].

Colour stability has not always scored so highly, and in certain studies the colour of Dyract AP has been shown to change significantly over 3 years in adults [45]. This has been confirmed in a 5-year study of the same material [58] and shows that components of the typical adult diet, such as coffee and red wine, have a particular influence on the colour stability of these materials. This seems likely to be a consequence of the moisture uptake behaviour of polyacid-modified composite resins which under appropriate circumstances also leads to uptake of natural dyestuffs from food and beverages [1].

Compomers have been found to perform well in Class V cavities [56,59], though it is essential to use an appropriate bonding agent in order to ensure adequate retention [60]. In one study, results were reported for a 2-year trial of Dyract AP, Compoglass F and F2000 [56], and all performed well, scoring predominantly alpha in all criteria. By contrast, in a 1-year study [45], the brand Freedom (SDI, Australia) scored only Bravo or Charlie for all criteria, showing that properties can vary widely between brands. Retention in Class V cavities with bonding agents has been shown to be good for polyacid-modified composites, with one study reporting a 96% survival over a 2-year period. However, this was inferior to a conventional nano-filled composite, which had a 100% survival over the same period [61]. Although retention is good, polyacid-modified composite resins have been shown to discolour with time, especially at the margins [62] and this may limit their use clinically.

In Class I [51] and Class II restorations [63], polyacid-modified composite resins have been found to perform extremely well. Using modern brands, performance over several years (up to 7 in the latter study) showed polyacid-modified composite resins to be indistinguishable from conventional composite resins. The use of polyacid-modified composites in 'open-sandwich' restorations has been reported [64,65], with fairly successful results, and an annual failure rate of only 1.1% [65]. However, using conventional composites for the bulk of the restoration and completing them with either polyacid-modified or conventional composite suggested that the polyacid-modified composite resins were inferior [64], since they showed greater occlusal wear and inferior marginal integrity compared with the composite resin. This result is more consistent with the results of in vitro testing [57] and suggests that care should be taken in selecting polyacid-modified composites for use in clinical applications with perhaps Class V [66] and Class III restorations [59] being more judicious choices.

Polyacid-modified composite resins have been evaluated for other clinical applications. For example, they have been found to perform well as sealants for pits and fissures over a 2-year period [67]. Retention was good and their appearance remained good, though because their level of fluoride release was lower, it was suggested that they were inferior in some respects to glass-ionomer cements for this application [67]. Finally, polyacid-modified composite resins have been used to bond orthodontic brackets to the tooth to secure bands [55]. This is an application for which conventional bonded composite resins are used, and polyacid-modified composites have been found to give satisfactory clinical outcomes, with little or no occurrence of white spot lesions around the brackets.

Clinical summary

- Polyacid-modified composite resins (compomers) are essentially a type of composite, despite having some glass-ionomer cement chemistry.
- They are typically one-paste light-cured systems, but two-paste self-cured brands are also available.
- Like conventional composites, they set by polymerization, which inevitably causes shrinkage. To overcome this they, too, are used in increments.
- Despite the presence of glass-ionomer components, compomers are not adhesive to tooth tissue and must be used with bonding agents.
- Compomers release fluoride.
- They are particularly useful in children's dentistry.

Clinical use

Compomers are used in exactly the same way as conventional composites, and so the steps for clinical use described in Chapter 3 can be applied to them.

References

[1] J.W. Nicholson, Polyacid-modified composite resins ('compomers') and their use in clinical dentistry, Dent. Mater. 23 (2007) 615–622.
[2] N.D. Ruse, What is a compomer? J. Can. Dent. Assoc. 65 (1999) 500–504.
[3] J.W. Nicholson, J.W. McLean, A.D. Wilson, Proposed nomenclature for glass-ionomer dental cements and related materials, Quintessence Int. 25 (1994) 587–589.
[4] J.M. Meyer, M.A. Cattani-Lorente, V. Dupuis, Compomers: between glass-ionomer cements and composites, Biomaterials 19 (1998) 529–539.
[5] J.W. Nicholson, Adhesive dental materials – a review, Int. J. Adhes. Adhes. 18 (1998) 229–236.
[6] R. Martin, S.J. Paul, H. Luthy, P. Scharer, Dentin bond strength of Dyract Cem, Am. J. Dent. 10 (1997) 27–31.
[7] J.W. Nicholson, M.A. McKenzie, The properties of polymerizable luting cements, J. Oral Rehabil. 26 (1999) 767–774.
[8] H.F. Gruber, Photoinitiators for free radical polymerization, Prog. Polym. Sci. 17 (1992) 953–1044.
[9] D. Sustersic, P. Cevc, N. Funuk, M.M. Pintar, Determination of curing time in visible-light-cured composite resins of different thickness by electron paramagnetic resonance, J. Mater. Sci. Mater. Med. 8 (1997) 507–510.
[10] N.S. Koupis, L.C. Martens, R.M.H. Verbeeck, Relative curing degree of polyacid-modified and conventional resin composites determined by surface Knoop hardness, Dent. Mater. 22 (2006) 1045–1050.

[11] A.M. Young, S.A. Raffeka, J.A. Howlett, FTIR investigation of monomer polymerisation and polyacid neutralisation kinetics and mechanisms in various aesthetic dental restorative materials, Biomaterials 25 (2004) 823–833.
[12] N.S. Koupis, C.W. Vercruysse, L.A. Marks, L.C. Martens, R.M.H. Verbeeck, Curing depth of (polyacid-modified) composite resins determined by scraping and a penetrometer, Dent. Mater. 20 (2004) 908–914.
[13] H.V. Chen, K. Manhart, K.-H. Kunzelmann, R. Hickel, Polymerization contraction stress in light-cured packable composite resins, Dent. Mater. 19 (2003) 597–602.
[14] K.A. Schulze, A.A. Zaman, K. Soderholm, Effect of filler fraction on strength, viscosity and porosity of experimental compomer materials, J. Dent. 31 (2003) 373–382.
[15] J.W. Nicholson, Kinetic studies of water uptake and loss in glass-ionomer cements, J. Mater. Sci. Mater. Med. 19 (2008) 1713–1717.
[16] I. Sideridou, V. Tserki, G. Papanastasiou, Study of water sorption, solubility and modulus of elasticity of light-cured dimethacrylate-based dental resins, Biomaterials 24 (2003) 655–665.
[17] J.W. Nicholson, E. Gjorgievska, B. Bajraktarova, M.A. McKenzie, Changes in properties of polyacid-modified composite resins ('compomers') following storage in acidic solutions, J. Oral Rehabil. 30 (2003) 601–607.
[18] J.W. Nicholson, M. Alsarheed, Changes on storage of polyacid-modified composite resins, J. Oral Rehabil. 28 (1998) 616–620.
[19] R.L. Bowen, J.E. Rapson, G. Dickson, Hardening shrinkage and hygroscopic expansion of composite resins, J. Dent. Res. 61 (1982) 654–658.
[20] B. Torstenson, M. Brannstrom, Contraction gap under composite resin restorations: effect of hygroscopic expansion and thermal stress, Oper. Dent. 13 (1988) 24–31.
[21] G. Eliades, A. Kakaboura, G. Palaghias, Acid base reaction and fluoride release profiles in visible light-cured polyacid modified composite resin restorative materials (compomers), Dent. Mater. 14 (1998) 57–63.
[22] G.O. Adusei, S. Deb, J.W. Nicholson, The role of the ionomer glass component in polyacid-modified composite resin dental restorative materials, J. Mater. Sci. Mater. Med. 15 (2004) 751–754.
[23] A.J. Shaw, T. Carrick, J.F. McCabe, Fluoride release from glass-ionomer and compomer materials: 6 month data, J. Dent. 26 (1996) 355–356.
[24] X. Xu, J.O. Burgess, Compressive strength, fluoride release and recharge of fluoride-releasing materials, Biomaterials 24 (2003) 2451–2461.
[25] A. Piwowarczyk, P. Ottl, H.C. Lauer, A. Buchler, Laboratory strength of glass ionomer cement, compomers, and resin composites, J. Prosthodont. 11 (2002) 86–91.
[26] I.H. el-Kalla, F. Garcia-Gody, Mechanical properties of compomer restorative materials, Oper. Dent. 24 (1999) 2–8.
[27] A.U. Yap, S.M. Chung, W.S. Chow, K.T. Tsai, C.T. Lim, Short-term fluoride release from various aesthetic restorative materials, Oper. Dent. 29 (2004) 29–34.
[28] J.E. Dahl, J. Li, I.E. Ruyter, Long-term water uptake of compomers and its effect on mechanical properties, J. Dent. Res. 77 (1998) 657.
[29] A.J. Preston, L.H. Mair, E.A. Agalamanyi, S.M. Higham, Fluoride release from aesthetic dental materials, J. Oral Rehabil. 26 (1999) 123–129.
[30] N. Abu-bakr, L. Han, A. Okamoto, M. Iwaku, Changes in the mechanical properties and surface texture of compomer immersed in various media, J. Prosthet. Dent. 84 (2000) 444–452.
[31] M. Braden, K.W.M. Davy, Polymerization of methacrylate esters, Biomaterials 7 (1986) 474–475.

[32] G.O. Adusei, S. Deb, J.W. Nicholson, A preliminary study of experimental polyacid-modified composite resins ('compomers') containing vinyl phosphonic acid, Dent. Mater. 21 (2005) 491–497.
[33] D.C. Watts, B. Burtenshaw, J.S. Jugdev, pH and time-dependence of surface degradation in a compomer biomaterial, J. Dent. Res. 74 (1995) 912.
[34] S. Gladys, B. Van Meerbeck, M. Braem, P. Lambrechts, G. Vanherle, Comparative physico-mechanical characterization of new hybrid restorative materials with conventional glass-ionomer and resin composite restorative materials, J. Dent. Res. 76 (1997) 883–894.
[35] S.R. Grobler, R.J. Roussouw, K. Van Wyke, A comparison of fluoride release from various dental materials, J. Dent. 26 (1998) 256–265.
[36] D. Sales, D. Sae-Lee, S. Matsuya, I.D. Ana, Short-term fluoride and cations release from polyacid-modified composites in distilled water and an acidic lactate buffer, Biomaterials 21 (2003) 1687–1696.
[37] H. Forss, Release of fluoride and other elements from light-cured glass ionomers in neutral and acidic conditions, J. Dent. Res. 72 (1993) 1257–1262.
[38] R.M.H. Verbeeck, E.A. De Maeyer, L.A. Marks, R.J. De Moor, A.M. De Witte, L.M. Trimpeneers, Fluoride release process of (resin-modified) glass-ionomer cements versus (polyacid-modified) composite resins, Biomaterials 19 (1998) 509–519.
[39] A. Wiegand, W. Buchalla, T. Attin, Review on fluoride-releasing restorative materials – fluoride release and uptake characteristics, antibacterial activity and influence on caries formation, Dent. Mater. 23 (2007) 343–362.
[40] J.W. Nicholson, B. Czarnecka, Ion release from compomers under acidic and neutral conditions, J. Oral Rehabil. 31 (2004) 665–670.
[41] B.J. Millar, F. Abiden, J.W. Nicholson, *In vitro* caries inhibition by polyacid-modified composite resins ('compomers'), J. Dent. 26 (1998) 133–136.
[42] F. Trachtaberg, N.N. Maserejian, J.A. Soncini, C. Hayes, M. Tavares, Does fluoride in compomers prevent future caries in children? J. Dent. Res. 88 (2009) 276–279.
[43] J.W. Nicholson, B.J. Millar, B. Czarnecka, H. Limanowska-Shaw, The storage of polyacid-modified composite resins ('compomers') in lactic acid solution, Dent. Mater. 15 (1999) 413–416.
[44] V. Qvist, L. Laurberg, A. Poulsen, P.T. Teglers, Class II restorations in primary teeth: 7-year study on three resin-modified glass ionomer cements and a compomer, Eur. J. Oral Sci. 112 (2004) 188–196.
[45] M.A. Chinelatti, R.P. Ramos, D.T. Chimello, R.G. Palma-Dibb, Clinical performance of a resin-modified glass-ionomer and two polyacid-modified resin composites in cervical lesions restorations: 1-year follow-up, J. Oral Rehabil. 31 (2004) 1–7.
[46] M. Demirci, H. Erser, M. Topcubasi, M. Ucok, Clinical evaluation of a polyacid-modified resin composite in class V carious lesions: 3-year results, Dent. Mater. J. 24 (2005) 321–327.
[47] H.C. Gungor, N. Althay, R. Alpar, Clinical evaluation of a polyacid-modified resin composite-based fissure sealant: two-year results, Oper. Dent. 29 (2004) 254–260.
[48] P.H. Williams, M. Sherriff, A. Ireland, An investigation into the use of two polyacid-modified composite resins (compomers) and a resin-modified glass poly(alkenoate) cement used to retain orthodontic bands, Eur. J. Orthodont. 27 (2005) 245–251.
[49] D. Moodley, S.R. Grobler, Compomers: adhesion and setting reactions, S. Afr. Dent. J. 58 (2003) 24–28.
[50] F. Garcia-Gody, Resin-based composites and compomers in primary molars, Dent. Clin. North Am. 44 (2000) 541–570.

[51] J.C. Outiveros, S. Davies, J.M. Powers, A. Chow, J.C. McKee, Hardness of glitter compomer cured with LED and QTH lights, J. Dent. Res. 85 (Special issue A) (2006) Abstract 1928.
[52] I.E. Andersson-Wenket, U.H. Folkesson, J.W. van Duijken, Durability of a polyacid-modified composite resin (compomer) in primary molars. A multicenter study, Acta Odontol. Scand. 55 (1997) 255–260.
[53] R.J. Crisp, F.J.T. Burke, Evaluation of the handling of a new compomer and novel dispensing system in general practice, Quintessence Int. 31 (2000) 181–186.
[54] G. Ryge, Clinical criteria, Int. Dent. J. 30 (1980) 347–358.
[55] J. Knox, K.Y. Chye, P. Durning, An ex vivo evaluation of resin-modified glass polyalkenoates and polyacid-modified composite resins as orthodontic band cements, J. Orthodont. 31 (2004) 323–328.
[56] Y. Luo, E.C.M. Lo, D.T.S. Fang, R.J. Smales, S.H.Y. Wei, Clinical evaluation of polyacid-modified resin composite posterior restorations: one-year results, Am. J. Dent. 15 (2002) 402–406.
[57] C. Zantner, A.M. Kielbassa, P. Martins, K.H. Kunzelmann, Sliding wear of 19 commercially available composites and compomers, Dent. Mater. 20 (2004) 277–285.
[58] R.G. Lund, F.P. Shen, E. Piva, D. Detoni, F.R.R. Moura, P.E.C. Cardoso, F.F. Demarco, Clinical performance and wear resistance of two compomers in posterior occlusal restorations of permanent teeth: six-year follow-up, Oper. Dent. 32 (2007) 118–123.
[59] A.D. Lognercio, A. Reis, A.N. Barbosa, J.F. Roulet, Five-year double-blind randomized clinical evaluation of a resin-modified glass ionomer and a polyacid-modified resin in noncarious cervical lesions, J. Adhes. Dent. 5 (2003) 323–332.
[60] R.J. Smales, K.K.W. Ng, Longevity of a resin-modified glass ionomer cements and a polyacid-modified resin composite restoring non-carious cervical lesions in general dental practice, Aust. Dent. J. 49 (2004) 196–200.
[61] L.S. Türkün, E.U. Celik, Non carious class V lesions restored with a polyacid-modified composite and a nanocomposite: a two-year clinical trial, J. Adhes. Dent. 10 (2008) 399–405.
[62] M. Demirei, H.S. Sancakli, Ö. Uysal, Clinical evaluation of a polyacid-modifed resin composite (Dyract) in class V carious lesions: 5-year results, Clin. Oral Invest. 12 (2008) 157–163.
[63] M. Wucher, S.R. Grobler, P.J.C. Senekal, A 3-year clinical evaluation of a compomer, a composite and a compomer/composite (sandwich) in Class II restorations, Am. J. Dent. 15 (2002) 274–278.
[64] J.W.V. van Dijken, A 6-year clinical evaluation Class I poly-acid modified resin composite/resin composite laminate and resin composite restorations cured with a two-step curing technique, Dent. Mater. 19 (2003) 423–428.
[65] R.M. Puppin-Rontani, M.E. Baglioni-Gouvea, M.F. de Goes, F. Garcia-Godoy, Compomer as pit and fissure sealant; effectiveness and retention after 24 months, J. Dent. Child. 73 (2006) 31–36.
[66] M. Folwaczy, A. Mehl, K.H. Kunzelmann, R. Hickel, Clinical performance of a resin-modified glass-ionomer and a compomer in restoring non-carious cervical lesions. 5-year results, Am. J. Dent. 13 (2001) 153–156.
[67] A. Lindberg, J.W.V. van Dijken, M. Lindberg, Nine-year evaluation of a polyacid-modified resin composite/resin composite open sandwich technique in Class II cavities, J. Dent. 35 (2007) 124–129.

Dental adhesives

5

5.1 Introduction

Modern dentistry makes considerable use of adhesive materials and techniques in its treatments [1]. Although widely used in contemporary conservative dentistry, composite resins are not inherently adhesive to the tooth surface, but need to be used in association with specially designed adhesive substances. These adhesives are therefore critical for the success of these aesthetic materials in dentistry.

This chapter covers bonding agents in detail, and includes aspects of current understanding of surface treatments, and also of the clinical effects of bonding agents [2]. Using these materials requires an appreciation of their effects on both the hard and soft tissues. The chemicals employed in formulating bonding agents, such as 2-hydroxyethyl methacrylate (HEMA), can have adverse effects on the soft tissues of both the gingiva and the pulp, and these need to be understood and these effects mitigated as much as possible through careful handling of the adhesives during application.

The durability of these materials is also of critical importance. Repairs to the tooth using composite resins need to be able to survive for time periods of up to 15 years [3]. Materials used to fabricate the repair, including the bonding agent, need to be able to last for these sorts of time periods and to retain their function without being degraded or losing their adhesion. These are demanding requirements, and will be considered later in the present chapter.

Adhesive dentistry, specifically in association with the use of composite resins, has emerged as an important component of modern restorative dentistry. These are several reasons for this. First, as a result of the research into restorative materials of improved aesthetics, there are now polymeric and also ceramic materials that provide an excellent match for the natural tissue of the tooth. This is complemented by an increasing demand for aesthetic repairs by patients [3,4]. This is part of the trend within the developed world for cosmetic dental treatments, and for cosmetic dentistry to be seen as an acceptable part of the profession.

There are also sound clinical reasons for the shift towards aesthetic repairs. Patients are typically keeping their natural teeth well into old age, as a result of the substantial decline in the incidence of tooth decay in 'first world' populations since the 1970s [5]. Where people are able to retain their teeth for so long, when problems do emerge these people are increasingly reluctant to tolerate intrusive treatments, such as extraction or unsightly repair with silver amalgam. In general, too, these populations have experienced rising levels of affluence, so individuals are more prepared to fund costly and demanding dental procedures performed with more expensive materials.

These factors all favour materials such as composite resins, which exploit the growing technical knowledge of adhesion and the improved performance of bonding agents for their success. Current materials available for bonding are formulated with the aim of providing reliable adhesive bonds that are, in principle, capable of lasting for many

Materials for the Direct Restoration of Teeth. http://dx.doi.org/10.1016/B978-0-08-100491-3.00005-2

years in the demanding service environment of the mouth. Many types are available, and the topic is a complicated one.

In this chapter, we begin with an account of the basic principles of surface preparation, a vital aspect in obtaining a durable and reliable adhesive bond. We then consider the various types of bonding agent available, proposing a classification based on numbers of steps involved, rather than the widely used one based on numbering the 'generations' of products. However, we do explain the basis of the classification system based on generations and we also show how the two classification systems are related.

5.2 Adhesive bonding to the tooth

Most areas of technology in which adhesive techniques are used employ synthetic materials with reasonably well-defined surfaces. They also exclude water as far as possible, because water generally has deleterious effects on adhesive bonds [6]. Dental adhesion is completely different. It involves surfaces made of natural materials, and these tend to be of variable quality and composition. Adhesive bonds to these surfaces are also required to operate under very moist conditions, and the adhesive itself must resist both degradation and debonding when used in this way.

To understand some of these challenges, it is necessary to consider the anatomy of the tooth. In particular, the composition and structure of the two main tissues, enamel and dentine, need to be examined in order to understand how they influence adhesive bonds. Details of the composition of these tissues are shown in Table 5.1, from which it can be seen that the enamel comprises a much greater amount of mineral phase than the dentine. Consequently it is harder and stronger, and is also more brittle [4].

The two tissues, enamel and dentine, are connected by the dentino-enamel junction, which has distinctive characteristics of its own. It unites the thin and brittle enamel layer to the thicker, tougher underlying structure of dentine. Its mechanical properties make it ideal for the function of uniting two materials with such dissimilar properties, and one of its most important functions is to prevent cracks from passing through from the enamel to the dentine [7]. This feature protects the entire tooth from mechanical failure and is important in maintaining the tooth in service for long periods of time.

The mineral phase of the tooth is a type of hydroxyapatite [8]. True, chemically pure hydroxyapatite is a calcium phosphate mineral of composition $Ca_{10}(PO_4)_6(OH)_2$, which has a ratio of calcium to phosphate of 1.67. Naturally occurring hydroxyapatites

Table 5.1 Composition of tooth tissues

	Enamel	Dentine
Inorganic phase (mainly hydroxyapatite) (%)	94–96	70
Ca:P ratio	1.64	1.56
Organic phase (mainly collagen) (%)	4–5	20
Water (%)	1	10

of the type found in human teeth have similar crystal structures, but slightly different chemical compositions. They are typically deficient in calcium, with the extent of the deficiency varying between enamel hydroxyapatite and that found in dentine (see Table 10.1). Natural hydroxyapatites also typically have a small proportion of the phosphate groups replaced by carbonates [8,9]. These differences from the ideal composition make very little difference to the resulting mechanical properties, so that natural hydroxyapatite is still a hard and brittle mineral, a feature it retains in both dentine and enamel.

When a tooth is repaired, some sort of preparation is usually performed and this involves cutting with a rotary bur, the so-called dental drill. The cutting is carried out to contour the region of the teeth to accept the repair material and also to remove the tissue damaged by caries [1]. One result of cutting in this way is that the surface becomes covered with a coating known as the smear layer. This smear layer is only of the order of 1–2 μm thick, and it consists of natural hydroxyapatite embedded in a matrix of collagen that has become denatured by the cutting process [10]. The structure is thus essentially that of disorganized enamel or dentine. Despite its low level of organized, it is not a loose layer, but a firmly adherent layer of cutting debris that can be very tenacious.

One of the key research questions associated with the topic of bonding in dentistry is whether or not to leave the smear layer in place [10]. Its tenacity in remaining attached to the underlying tooth structure is advantageous, as is its high mineral content. However, its composition and structure are variable, and the bond strengths of bonding agents to it are affected by exactly how the tooth was cut to create the smear layer [11]. The structure of the smear layer can be fairly compacted or relatively open and porous and this affects the extent to which bonding agents in their liquid state are able to penetrate and form firm attachments. These differences explain the variability in measured bond strengths, and are also the reason that the durability of bonds formed by these bonding agents can differ so much.

During cutting of the tooth surface, in addition to forming the smear layer, cutting debris can be forced into dentinal tubules [10,11]. These are known as 'smear plugs' and they make the dentine less permeable than they would otherwise be. They also reduce the total surface through which bonding can occur. On the other hand, reducing the permeability may be helpful towards maintaining the adhesive bond, as the smear plugs may stop fluid being forced up the dentinal tubules and undermining the attachment.

Cut tooth surfaces may be treated to modify or remove the smear layer. This is done to provide a uniform surface to which reliable bonds can be formed. Such surface treatment may also attack the smear plugs, so removing them and re-opening the dentinal tubules. This permits the liquid bonding agent to penetrate the surface of the tooth more thoroughly. Again, this has advantages and disadvantages. It is advantageous in that it proves greater surface area for bonding, and thus may enhance the strength and durability of the adhesive bond. On the other hand, percolation of the liquid bonding agent down the tubules may lead to uncomfortable post-operative sensitivity for the patient.

5.2.1 Surface preparation

The first step in the history of adhesive dentistry was the introduction of acid-etching of enamel to promote bonding by Buonocore in 1955 [12]. The technique uses a solution of 37% phosphoric acid, and when applied to the enamel surfaces, this creates a surface with microscopic irregularities. Low viscosity resin formulations can flow into these irregularities. When hardened, such resins interlock with the irregular surface of the enamel, and this maintains the hardened resins in place. This type of bonding is known as micromechanical attachment, and it leads to shear bond strengths in the range 20–25 MPa. These values are high enough to keep the restoration in place despite the forces of biting and chewing, and restorations bonded in this way have very good rates of retention [13].

When this pioneering work was undertaken, the fact of the formation of the smear layer was not known. The results showed clearly that etching with acid was important in developing a surface to which strong and reliable bonds could be formed. The concentration of phosphoric acid was shown to be important. The final value, 37%, was chosen because it gave the best results. A concentration of 25% is too low to be effective, whereas 50% is so concentrated that it etches away too much tooth material. Such aggressive etching results in poor quality bonds, because there is insufficient roughened surface to create acceptable micromechanical bonds.

The success of acid-etching is due in part to the structure and composition of enamel [4]. As can be seen in Table 5.1, enamel contains almost no protein phase or water. Hence a fraction of the mineral phase can be removed without causing the enamel structure to collapse. This procedure produces a chalky appearance in the enamel, and once this develops, the etching process is considered to be complete and the enamel is ready to receive the liquid resin component. A scanning electron microscope (SEM) image of etched human dentine is shown in Fig. 5.1.

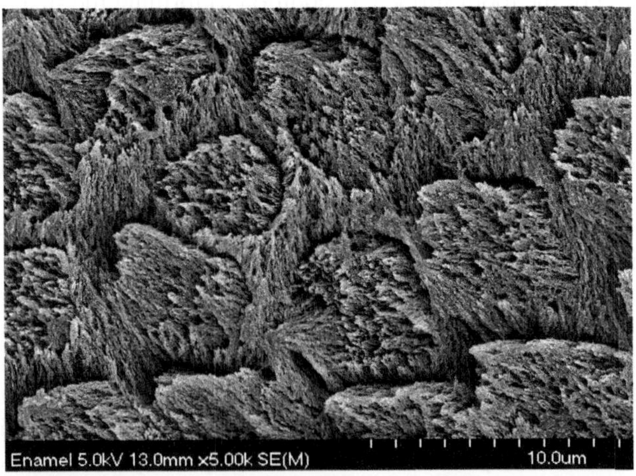

Fig. 5.1 Etched human enamel.
Image courtesy of Dr Jorge Perdigão, University of Minnesota. Used with permission.

For bonding to enamel to succeed, this liquid resin layer needs to penetrate well into the roughened etched tooth surface. This favours low viscosity systems, which implies in turn a composition without any filler. Unfilled resins can thus be used to provide the first layer of a bonded composite resin system. Unfortunately, such a layer experiences proportionately greater polymerization shrinkage than a filled composite system. To an extent, this problem is overcome by composite systems that have been formulated with at least some filler loading, but a low enough application viscosity to allow the liquid to flow into the roughened surface [3].

Bonding to dentine is more difficult than bonding to enamel, and it has been the subject of a considerable volume of research over the past 40 years or so. This is mainly due to the combination of its morphology and its composition. It contains more water than enamel (Table 10.1), and also more protein, which form the fibres of collagen that run through the structure. Dentine also contains numerous fluid-filled tubules running through the structure. Treating this tissue to obtain reliable surfaces for bonding is challenging, as is designing a material that is capable of wetting the surface but does not harden to form a substance that is susceptible to hydrolytic degradation.

A further consideration is that the surface is very hydrophilic, and the composite resins to be attached are hydrophobic. The aim is thus to create a union between two incompatible materials that is both strong and durable, an aim which is, by its nature, very challenging. The variety of procedures and materials that have been used and advocated by various authorities is a consequence of both the complexity and the difficulty of what is being attempted.

The acid-etch technique of Buonocore cannot be easily applied to dentine, because the process alters the surface of dentine unfavourably. It removes the mineral phase, and leaves behind a collagen-rich structure that is soft, and which tends to collapse when dried with air. The matted collagen fibre surface that is thereby formed forms weak bonds with organic substances, and this results in low values of bond strengths. These typically lie in the range 5–10 MPa [3].

Despite this, the acid-etch technique has been applied to dentine. Used in this way, the approach was originally known as 'total etch' [14], but now tends to be called 'etch-and-rinse' to reflect the clinical necessity of washing away the soluble products that are formed by the action of phosphoric acid on the dentine [15]. The concept of pre-treating dentine with phosphoric acid arose because of the difficulty, in practise, of etching only enamel when using a 37% phosphoric acid solution or gel [14]. The technique was quite fashionable a few years ago, and several authorities recommended it [16]. However, though still highly regarded by many practitioners [17], its use has been questioned, as experimental findings do not necessarily support its use. For example, in some studies bond durability using etch-and-rinse has been found to be inferior to that obtained with less aggressive pre-treatment techniques [18].

In practice, etch-and-rinse is a difficult technique because the etching step changes the nature of the dentine by selectively attacking the mineral phase. Once this is removed by washing, what is left behind is a structure that is relatively rich in collagen fibres. This is soft and has a tendency to collapse when dried. The mat of collagen fibres that results from such a collapse is able to form only weak adhesive bonds to the bonding agents used [4]. The extent to which this collapse of the collagen fibres takes place depends on the extent to which drying occurs, and the fact that it is a sensitive process explains the variation in shear bond strength values that have been recorded in the literature.

For some years, it was recommended that the newly prepared dentine surface should be air-dried prior to placement of the first layer of bonding agent. However, once its influence on reducing the bond strength was established, the recommendation changed, and the air-drying step was omitted. This led to what is known as 'wet-bonding' [14]. As far as practical bonding in the dental clinic was concerned, this simplified procedures and was beneficial for clinicians. However, it raised issues of what sort of liquid should be applied to the wet surface, and particularly which organic solvent was most appropriate. Favoured solvents are acetone and ethanol [19], both of which are reasonably hydrophilic, so can interact with a surface containing relatively large amounts of water. They are also sufficiently hydrophobic that the appropriate organic monomers can be dissolved in tem, ready to form the resin layer on the dentin surface where the tooth repair is being made.

A key part of creating a hydrophobic surface to which the composite resin monomers can bond is that the organic molecules of the liquid bonding agent should infiltrate the treated dentine surface. This has to take place immediately after the mineral phase is removed, or even possibly at the same time. The rapid application of liquid bonding agent is necessary in order to prevent the collagen fibres from collapsing, and to ensure that a structure consisting of resin-impregnated collagen fibres is formed. This is termed the hybrid layer [20]. It is of sufficiently hydrophobic character that the unset composite resin can bond to it readily, and it is also mechanically strong. It varies in depth, depending on how long the infiltration process is allowed to take place, with depths ranging from 2.1 to 4.1 μm [21].

Another important feature of the pre-treatment of the dentine surface is that the smear layer is removed and so also are the smear plugs. The latter is especially important as it opens to dentinal tubules, which means that liquid bonding agent can flow into the tubules (see Fig. 5.2). When polymerization occurs, this results in the formation of

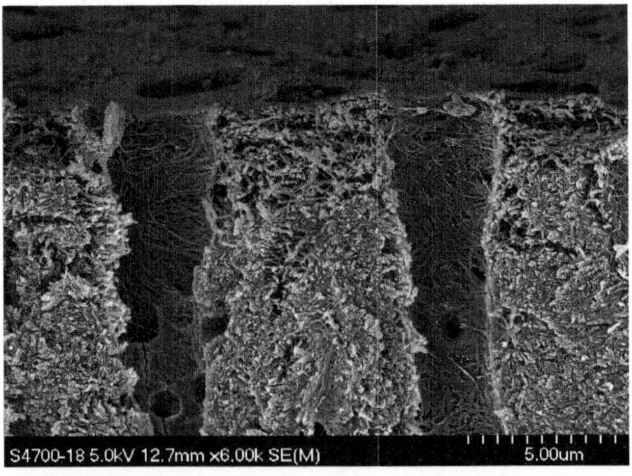

Fig. 5.2 Etched human dentine.
Image courtesy of Dr Jorge Perdigão, University of Minnesota. Used with permission.

hardened resin tags, and these provide an additional mechanism of attachment for the bonding agent. Studies suggest that this latter mechanism is less important than hybrid layer formation. The evidence for this is that even bonding agents that are too viscous in their liquid state to flow into the opened tubules and thereby form resin tags are able to bond strongly to dentine [22].

Pre-treatment of the newly cut dentine surface can also be carried out with weak organic acids, such as ethylene diamine tetra-acetic acid or citric acid. This is termed ‘conditioning’ and was the recommended approach for many years, with weak acids being advocated because of the need to protect the underlying pulp from damage by exposure to aggressive acid solutions. However, this is now less widely used than either the etch-and-rinse technique or by the deployment of self-etching primers (see Section 10.3). These claimed to give more reliable bonding under clinical conditions, and also stronger bonds when these are determined in vitro.

5.3 Dentine bonding agents

In the field of adhesive dentistry, we use the term ‘bonding agent’ for those materials that are used as adhesives, mainly for attaching composite resins to tooth surfaces. These are typically applied to the freshly cut tooth in the liquid state using a small brush, and either a dabbing or a painting action [22]. A wide variety of types of formulation have been available over the past 30–40 years, and still today, a bewildering array of brands and types are offered to the profession [23]. Information on their composition is not usually disclosed, though it is known that the monomer HEMA is widely used in these materials, typically blended with other monomers. Substances such as glutaraldehyde and various methacrylate monomers are used, with acetone, ethanol or water as solvents [22,23].

When dentine bonding began as a clinical technique, three layers were typically used in order to create an appropriately hydrophobic surface for the attachment of composite resins. These layers were as follows: (a) conditioning agent, (b) primer and (c) bonding agent. The conditioning agent had the role of removing the smear layer, either fully or partially. The primer then modified the surface to allow it to take the slightly less hydrophilic bonding agent. The overall effect was to produce a bond of high strength and good durability [22], and even today results obtained with such systems have not been surpassed by more modern systems. Their drawback, though, was that using a three-step system was time-consuming and difficult for the patient.

Modern formulations have been designed to simplify to their use in the clinic. They involve fewer layers, hence fewer application steps, which speeds up the treatment for the patient. However, this is generally regarded as being at the price of compromised bonding, either in terms of bond strength or durability. Typical materials involve a combined primer and adhesive within a single liquid mixture. Even with this degree of simplification, an acid-etch process is still needed as the initial step in creating an adhesive bond. As we have seen, this may involve either a separate etching step or the use of a self-etch primer.

Self-etching primers are blends that can both etch and prime the surface in one step. They contain at least one acidic monomer, in order to allow them to undertake the etching process. They also eliminate the need to rinse away the solubilized products to the etching step. Instead, these substances become incorporated into the primer layer. This has the advantage of reducing the technique sensitivity associated with the process of bonding [4]. However, there is some evidence that the resulting adhesive bonds are weaker than those with substances that do not incorporate any mineral components of the smear layer [24].

The acidity of self-etching primers allows them not only to penetrate the smear layer and incorporate its component, but also to interact with the underlying intact dentine. In doing so, it forms a hybrid layer of the type previously identified with three-layer bonding systems [20,21], and which is essential in promoting adhesion. This acidity varies between formulations, and can be classified as either strong or weak, depending on the acid involved in the blend and also its concentration [25].

Weak self-etch primers (sometimes described as 'mild') have pH values around 2, and as a result only partially attack the surface of the dentine and hence only solubilize a fraction of the available mineral phase. The hybrid layer formed with such primers is therefore relatively rich in mineral content, with bonding occurring by the interaction of carboxylic or phosphoric acid functional groups with the dentine surface.

On the other hand, strong self-etch primers have a pH of around 1, and hence contain strong acids based on phosphoric acid groups only. They interact more aggressively with the smear layer of the freshly cut tooth, removing more of it from the surface. Though these substances nonetheless include the components of the mineral phase, the resulting bonded surface closely resembles that created by the etch-and-rinse technique.

Bonding systems are typically applied as low viscosity liquids designed to infiltrate the surface layer to create the hybrid layer [15]. Having done so, they need to undergo some sort of setting process to harden to functional adhesives. Cure may be brought about either as a result of mixing two component adhesives, where polymerization is brought about by free radicals generated by reaction of a two-part initiator system, of by light-curing [26]. Dual-cure adhesive systems are also available and these combine both types of cure mechanism. Resulting solids typically have large coefficients of thermal expansion and also absorb significant quantities of water. Some modern brands are formulated with inorganic fillers, which have the dual function of reinforcing the set material and reducing the polymerization contraction [15]. However, filling loadings are limited by the need for the initial liquid formulation to have low application viscosity.

Because of the complexity of bonding agents, there are a variety of ways of classifying them. For some time, the concept of 'generations' was used [27], and this is still popular with manufacturers. This classification has arrived at the seventh generation, and the details of these are shown in Table 5.2. However, it is not derived from any fundamental properties, being essentially historically based, and for this reason some authorities consider it obsolete [15].

Table 5.2 Classification of dental bonding systems by generations [27]

Generation	Number of layers	Surface pre-treatment	Components	Shear bond strength (MPa)
1st	2	Enamel etch	2	2
2nd	2	Enamel etch	2	5
3rd	3	Dentine conditioning	2–3	12–15
4th	3	Total etch	3–5	25
5th	2	Total etch	2	25
6th	1	Self-etch adhesive	2	20
7th	1	Self-etch adhesive	1	25

At this stage, we propose an alternative classification of bonding systems, which reflects their essential mode of use, rather than their historical development. This classifies bonding systems as follows:

(a) 4-Step: Involving etch, rinse, prime and bond. These bonding systems are supplied as three bottles, one each from etchant, primer and bonding agent. These are the most complicated to use in the clinic, but result in highest bond strengths [13] and greatest durability.
(b) 3-Step: Here the steps are etch, rinse, then finally prime and bond in a single coating. Bonding systems of this type employ substances in two bottles, one consisting of etchant, and the other of the combined prime and bond formulation.
(c) 2-Step: For these systems, the two steps are etching and priming combined followed by bonding. It uses two bottles of components, the first containing a self-etching primer and the second the bonding agent. The self-etching primer modifies the smear layer on the surface of the dentine, and incorporates the products in the coating layer.
(d) 1-Step: This uses a single bottle containing a formulation that blends a self-etching primer and bond agent. Clinically, this is the easiest to use [28], and bond strengths are generally reported to be acceptable, despite the simplicity of the bonding operation [28,29].

From this detailed classification, two broad categories emerge, namely those which employ etch-and-rinse and those which are self-etching. Examples of each are shown in Table 5.3, which lists a representative range of current commercial products, with details of the number of steps that each involves and their mode of action. These basic types of bonding agent are now considered in detail in the following sections of the chapter.

5.3.1 Etch-and-rinse systems

As already mentioned, the etch-and-rinse technique should be employed in conjunction with the wet-bonding approach. This has been demonstrated by various in vitro studies [14,30,31], and is especially important when adhesives formulated with acetone are used [31,32]. However, this is difficult to achieve practically, as the enamel needs to be dried for bonding, and it is not straightforward to dry one without drying the other [15]. There is also uncertainty as to how wet the dentine needs to be in order

Table 5.3 Examples of commercially available bonding agents [15]

Brand	Type	Steps	Manufacturer
AdheSE	Self-etch	2	Ivoclar, Liechtenstein
AdheSE One F	Self-etch	1	Ivoclar, Liechtenstein
AdheSE	Multimode		Ivoclar, Liechtenstein
Adper Scotchbond 1XT	Etch-and-rinse	2	3M Oral Care, USA
Adper Single Bond Plus	Etch-and-rinse	2	3M Oral Care, USA
Adper Single Bond 2	Etch-and-rinse	2	3M Oral Care, USA
All-Bond 2	Etch-and-rinse	3	Bisco Inc, USA
All-Bond 3	Etch-and-rinse	3	Bisco Inc, USA
All-Bond SE	Self-etch	2	Bisco Inc, USA
ART Bond	Etch-and-rinse	3	Coltene/Whaledent, Switzerland
Clearfil New Bond	Etch-and-rinse	2	Kuraray, Japan
Clearfil SE Bond	Self-etch	2	Kuraray, Japan
Clearfil SE Protect	Self-etch	2	Kuraray, Japan
Clearfil S3 Bond Plus	Self-etch	2	Kuraray, Japan
Clearfil Universal Bond	Multimode		Kuraray, Japan
ExciTE	Etch-and-rinse	2	Ivoclar, Liechtenstein
G-Bond	Self-etch	1	GC, Japan
G-aenial Bond	Multimode		GC, Japan
Syntac	Etch-and-rinse	3	Ivoclar, Liechtenstein
One Coat Bond	Etch-and-rinse	2	Coltene/Whaledent, Switzerland
One Coat SE Bond	Self-etching	2	Coltene/Whaledent, Switzerland
One Coat 7.0	Self-etching	1	Coltene/Whaledent, Switzerland
One-step Plus	Etch-and-rinse	2	Bisco Inc, USA
Optibond All-In-One	Self-etch	1	Kerr, USA
Opitibond FL	Etch-and-rinse	3	Kerr, USA
Optibond Solo Plus	Etch-and-rinse	2	Kerr, USA
Optibond XTR	Self-etch	2	Kerr, USA
Prime & Bond NT	Etch-and-rinse	3	Dentsply, Germany
Scotchbond Universal	Multimode		3M Oral Care, USA
Unifil Bond	Multimode		GC, Japan
Xeno III	Self-etch	2	Dentsply, Germany
Xeno IV	Self-etch	1	Dentsply, Germany
XP Bond	Etch-and-rinse	2	Dentsply, Germany

to bond to it successfully [33,34] and there is some evidence that leaving the surface too wet leads to low bond strengths as the liquid adhesive becomes diluted by the excess moisture present [35].

Studies have shown that concerns about exactly how wet the surface needs to be can be overcome by rubbing the liquid etch-and-rinse adhesive into the dentine surface [36–39]. This causes the liquid adhesive to infiltrate the newly cut surface, regardless of its moisture content, or the nature of the solvent used in the adhesive. This results in good bond strengths [36–39] and highly durable adhesion in patients [40].

The infiltration step is critical for the development of sound adhesive bonds, as it is necessary to create the ideal hybrid layer with the demineralized dentine surface [36].

This hybrid layer modifies the surface characteristics, making it more hydrophobic and better able to form natural bonds to the polymer phase of composite resin restoratives. However, in practice it can be difficult to create a hybrid layer of adequate depth, even under favourable conditions, and this affects the resulting bond strengths that can be achieved [41–43]. As well as hybrid later formation, there may also be some development of resin tags at this stage, though as we have seen, these do not seem to be critical in developing strong and durable adhesive bonds [44,45].

Although the details of the compositions of bonding agents are not disclosed by the manufacturers, it is known that the primer/adhesive layer is made up of blends of relatively hydrophilic and more hydrophobic monomers. This prevents the wet coating from forming a completely integrated covering on the etched tooth surface [46]. Instead, the coating behaves as a semi-permeable film after setting, and this means that it allows dentinal fluid to pass through it, at least to an extent [47]. This leads to a degree of leakage, sometimes referred to as nano-leakage [15]. The clinical significance of this is not clear, though there is some evidence that it may facilitate the hydrolytic degradation of the bonding agent in situ [48]. Certain materials have been shown to exhibit very low nano-leakage, and these also give high bond strengths in vitro [49], so seem likely to provide the best clinical outcomes. Unfortunately, longer-term studies of the clinical performance of these materials are relatively uncommon, and there are many more in vitro studies of immediate bond strengths, with much debate centred on the relative importance of testing in shear and in micro-tensile modes.

There is also uncertainty on how important the solvent used in these systems is in practice. Some findings suggest that both acetone and ethanol give equivalent results [15], whereas others suggest that ethanol gives superior outcomes [50]. However, these solvents do have different characteristics, so that some differences in results are to be expected. Ideally the solvent should evaporate prior to polymerization of the adhesive, otherwise it will remain and act as plasticizer in the set material, altering the mechanical properties [15]. Acetone is more volatile and hence more easily evaporated. Against that, it is more sensitive to residual moisture in the dentine surface than ethanol [39]. This may reduce the extent to which acetone-based adhesives can interact with the hybrid layer [39] and has been suggested as the reason why ethanol-based adhesives have been found to give higher retention rates clinically than acetone-based ones [36,51].

In clinical practice, certain steps have been recommended to optimize the performance of etch-and-rinse adhesives [15]. In particular, extending the application time of the liquid primer/bonding mixture in order to allow maximum infiltration into the demineralized dentine is desirable [52,53]. It may also be helpful to apply more than one coat to achieve the best possible bonding, especially with acetone-based formulations [54,55].

5.3.2 Self-etch systems

Self-etch bonding systems provide a less sensitive approach to adhesion to dentine than etch-and-rinse systems. They have the additional advantages of using a simpler technique and therefore reduced application time [15]. As we have seen, self-etch bonding agents are available as one-step and two-step systems.

As formulated, liquid self-etch adhesives consist of aqueous solutions of functional monomers, cross-linkers and additives such as fillers and free radical initiators [56,57]. Water has to be present to allow the acid to ionize and thus be capable of carrying out its etching function [56]. The presence of water in the formulation means that self-etch adhesives less susceptible to variations in the moisture content of the substrate.

Self-etch adhesives vary in their acidity [58]. Some are very acidic, with a pH around 1 and interact quite strongly with the freshly cut tooth surface, penetrating several microns into the depth of either the dentine or the enamel. Some are considered only moderately strong, and these have a pH between 1 and 2. This allows them to penetrate to a depth of only about 1–2 μm [15]. Some are mild, with a pH of about 2, which permits penetration to a depth of about 1 μm only. Lastly, there are the ultra-mild adhesives, which have a pH of about 2.5. These penetrate the tooth surface to only a slight extent, typically in the nano-metre range [59].

The essential mechanism of action of self-etch adhesives is that they simultaneously etch and prime the freshly cut tooth surface, and in doing so, incorporate the components of the smear layer [58,60]. Because of the presence of the smear layer, and also because of smear plugs blocking the dentinal tubules, self-etch adhesives have been claimed to provoke less post-operative sensitivity in patients than the etch-and-rinse approach [61,62]. However, this has not been confirmed by scientific studies [63,64], but rather any reduction in patient discomfort has been attributed to operator technique [15].

The degree of interaction with the tooth surface varies with acidity of the self-etch formulation. Those systems with slightly higher pH, ie, mild or ultra-mild adhesives, interact with the dentine surface in two ways. Firstly, they develop a micromechanical interaction due to their infiltration into the dentine surface and, second, they form ionic bonds with the calcium ions present in the surface through reaction of the acid functional groups [65,66]. This reaction necessitates the displacement of the phosphate groups in the hydroxyapatite mineral phase by the acid functional group of the bonding agent [65]. This second step is effectively chemical adhesion, and is the same as that which seems to occur with glass-ionomer cements [67]. This reaction leads to good long-term stability of the adhesive bond, which has been demonstrated in both in vitro [68,69] and clinical studies [70–72]. Indeed, there is good evidence that mild self-etch systems give the best results, both in vitro and clinically, of all bonding agents, with one study demonstrating excellent clinical performance for one brand of material (Clearfil SE Bond, CSE, Kuraray, Japan) for up to 8 years with only minor leakage [62].

5.3.3 Universal bonding agents

Although there are two broad systems of bonding (etch-and-rinse and self-etch), generally with specific bespoke materials for use with them, there are also some bonding agents available that are described as 'universal', ie, they can be used in either etch-and-rinse or self-etch modes [15]. The most widely studied bonding agent of this type is Scotchbond Universal Adhesive (3M Oral Care) (Fig. 5.3), and there have been reports of its use in both etch-and-rinse and self-etch modes [73–75]. Testing the quality

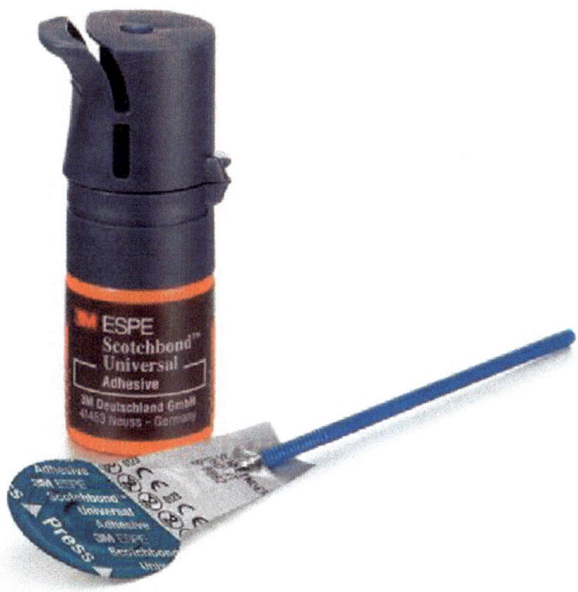

Fig. 5.3 Scotchbond™ Universal Adhesive (3M Oral Care).
Used with permission.

of the bond by measuring the micro-tensile strength showed that the mode of use did not alter the result [76,77]. Variations in the wetness of the dentine were also found to make no difference to the measured bond strengths, possibly because of the relatively high water content of the liquid formulation [78].

The good laboratory results obtained for Scotchbond Universal Adhesive have been confirmed in clinical use [71]. Like self-etch adhesives, universal bonding agents give their best results when rubbed into the freshly cut dentine surface [79]. They also perform better when coated with an extra layer of a hydrophobic resin prior to placing the composite resin. This improves both the immediate and the long-term bond strengths as well as reducing their nano-leakage [74,79].

5.4 Testing and evaluation of bonding agents

As can be seen from the earlier sections of this chapter, bonding agents are generally tested in the laboratory. These tests involve determination of the bond strength, either in shear or micro-tensile modes. They also involve leakage studies.

The issue of leakage is very important in evaluating bonding agents because a major function of these substances is to create a seal to the tooth surface. This is necessary to prevent the underlying dentine from being exposed to fluids from the mouth, since this could otherwise lead to bacterial infiltration leading to further decay and eventual damage to the pulp [4]. The leakage is generally referred to as micro-leakage, partly to indicate the size scale on which it occurs. It has conventionally been measured by dye-penetration experiments [80].

Even when there are no gaps, however, there can be leakage [81]. This can be demonstrated using aqueous solutions of silver nitrate, and the leakage is shown by passage of Ag^{+} ions between the bonding layer and the tooth surface. Silver ions are smaller than the dye molecules used conventionally, and the leakage detected is of a smaller size scale, hence termed nano-leakage [82].

The significance of regions of nano-leakage is not clear. Any voids at this scale are too small to admit bacteria, so there is no likelihood of infection and further tooth decay [83]. On the other hand, fluid can be admitted, and this may allow hydrolytic degradation of the hardened bonding agent to occur. If this happens, these nano-scale voids can grow so that eventually they are able to admit bacteria, with all their potential to create further substantial damage [4].

Laboratory results are not the only consideration when evaluating bonding agents. Their clinical effectiveness must be determined. Unfortunately, this is more demanding than carrying laboratory tests, and so fewer reports have been published on this important topic. Moreover, where such studies have been carried out, they are generally relatively short, typically no longer than 36 months and often shorter. While of some value, such studies are not able to answer the question of just how durable such bonding agents and their resulting adhesion are over the longer term. Adhesive bonds to the tooth surface are known to change with time, partly due to changes in the hybrid layer [84].

These changes occur as a result of several influences. The temperature fluctuations in the mouth put stresses on the hardened bonding agent, as do the presence of acids from certain foodstuffs. The moist environment can lead to hydrolytic degradation reactions, which, though by their nature slow, can lead to devastating changes over the longer term [84].

Clinical studies typically determine the retention, marginal integrity and marginal discoloration [85]. The latter is related to the extent to which micro-leakage occurs under clinical conditions. Post-operative sensitivity and the occurrence of secondary caries have also been considered in some studies, though they have not generally been found in association with modern bonding agents. Unfortunately, results of clinical studies do not show any correlation with results from laboratory studies, so that materials that show high bond strength and good marginal seal in vitro develop clear micro-leakage and distinct marginal gaps in vivo [86]. The reasons for this are not clear, but the results do show that the durability of bonding agents in patients is complex, and the various factors involved have not been properly identified in the current laboratory testing protocols.

There are also substantial differences between the findings of various clinical studies. For example, one comprehensive systematic review concluded that two-step etch-and-rinse systems were more effective than one-step self-etch ones [87], whereas other studies have suggested that the clinical performance of these two categories of bonding agent was similar [85]. These contradictions suggest that there is very little real difference in the overall performance of these two systems, and that any perceived differences are minor. Both seem appropriate approaches, and both are capable of giving acceptable clinical performance for reasonable lengths of time.

5.5 Biocompatibility of bonding agents

Bonding agents, by their nature, are used on relatively inert tissue, the dentine, and in close proximity to very delicate soft tissue, namely the pulp. For this reason, the question of their biocompatibility is complex, as well as being important [4].

One issue of concern is the extent to which monomers from the bonding agent can permeate through the dentine to reach the pulp. Related to this is the question of how much of these monomers can permeate, and whether the resulting concentration is sufficient to be damaging. The monomer HEMA is particularly important. It is present in many different brands of bonding agent, but has been shown to be capable of diffusing through the dentine into the pulp chamber when placed underneath a composite resin [88]. Diffusion has been shown to be more rapid in caries-affected teeth than in teeth with no caries, and once it occurs, it has a variety of adverse effects. These include cytotoxicity, the inhibition of cell proliferation and a decrease in mitochondrial activity [89]. The consequence of this latter effect is that the energy transduction processes within the cells are inhibited.

Despite these findings from in vitro biocompatibility studies, there do not appear to have been any reported incidents of adverse effects in patients [4]. This may be because only small amounts of monomer are released. In vivo, too, the fluid circulation within the living pulp may be capable of washing away any diffusing monomers, thus ensuring that damaging concentrations of monomer do not build up. Whatever the explanation, the reported in vivo biocompatibility of bonding agents is good and there appear to be no practical concerns with their use in patients.

5.6 Conclusions

This chapter has shown that the clinical performance of modern dental adhesives has reached the stage where they can be used reliably and predictably. Modern adhesive systems are better than their predecessors, showing good retention, low levels of leakage and sound clinical outcomes, regardless of whether they are designed for use as etch-and-rinse or self-etch systems. When placed properly, they are able to bond well to the cut tooth substrate and to retain that bond for considerable periods of time. Clinical outcomes, including biocompatibility, appear good though formal studies of durability are still needed to complement the shorter-term results obtained from laboratory studies.

Clinical summary

- The use of adhesives is essential for composite resins of all types, including polyacid-modified composite resins (compomers).
- Bonding to the tooth is technically difficult because it aims to unite the hydrophilic tooth surface with the hydrophobic organic resin system of the composite.
- Bonding to enamel is more straightforward than bonding to enamel. It can be done relatively simply with acid-etching, followed by rinsing, then attachment of the resin by means of the liquid resin flowing into the roughened surface, resulting in the so-called micromechanical attachment.

- Bonding to dentine is difficult, partly due to its moisture content and partly due to its stricture.
- There are two broad approaches to dentine bonding, namely etch-and-rinse and self-etching.
- Bonding agents come in a wide variety of presentations, with differing chemistry and varying numbers of coats required.
- In this chapter, a classification system based on number of steps rather than number of layers is proposed. This is to highlight the importance of the rinsing step in those systems that require this to be performed.
- Four-step bonding agents give the best results in terms of bond strength and durability. However, their use is time-consuming and not easily tolerated by some patients.

References

[1] G.J. Mount, W.R. Hume, Preservation and Restoration of Teeth, second ed., Knowledge Books and Software, Middlesbrough, 2005.
[2] G.J. Mount, Color Atlas of Glass Ionomer Cements, third ed., Martin Dunitz, London, 2002.
[3] J.-F. Roulet, G. Vanherle, Adhesive Technology for Restorative Dentistry, Quintessence Publishers, Chicago, 2004.
[4] J.W. Nicholson, Adhesive dentistry, in: L.F.M. da Aliva, A. Öchsner, R.D. Adams (Eds.), Handbook of Adhesion Technology, vol. 2, Springer-Verlag, Berlin and Heidelberg, 2011 (Chapter 56).
[5] T.M. Marthaler, Changes in dental caries 1953–2003, Caries Res. 38 (2004) 173–181.
[6] I.A. Ashcroft, J. Comyn, Effect of water and mechanical stress on durability, in: L.F.M. da Aliva, A. Öchsner, R.D. Adams (Eds.), Handbook of Adhesion Technology, vol. 2, Springer-Verlag, Berlin and Heidelberg, 2011 (Chapter 31).
[7] C.P. Lin, W.H. Douglas, Structure–property relations and crack resistance at the bovine dentin-enamel junction, J. Dent. Res. 73 (1994) 1072–1078.
[8] R.Z. Le Geros, Calcium Phosphates in Oral Biology and Medicine, Vol. 15 of Monographs in Oral Science, Karger, Basel, Switzerland, 1991.
[9] C. Robinson, J.A. Weatherell, A.S. Hallsworth, Variation in composition of dental enamel within thin ground tooth sections, Caries Res. 5 (1971) 44–57.
[10] M. Ogata, N. Harada, S. Yamaguchi, M. Nakajima, P.N. Periera, J. Tagami, Effect of different burs on bond strengths of self-etching primer bonding systems, Oper. Dent. 26 (2001) 375–382.
[11] H. Koibuchi, N. Yashuda, N. Nakabayashi, Bonding to dentin with a self-etching primer: the effect of smear layers, Dent. Mater. 17 (2001) 122–126.
[12] M.G. Buonocore, A simple method of increasing the adhesion of acrylic filling materials to enamel surfaces, J. Dent. Res. 34 (1955) 849–853.
[13] J. De Munk, K. Van Landuyt, M. Peumans, A. Pontevin, A. Lambrechts, M. Braem, B. Van Meerbeck, A critical review of the durability of adhesion to tooth tissue: methods and results, J. Dent. Res. 84 (2005) 118–132.
[14] J. Kanca, Resin bonding to wet substrate. I. Bonding to dentin, Quintessence Int. 23 (1992) 39–41.
[15] A. Sezinando, Looking for the ideal adhesive – a review, Rev. Port Estomatol. Med. Dent. Cir. Maxillofac. 55 (2014) 194–206.

[16] E.J. Swift Jr., Dentin/enamel adhesives: review of the literature, Pediatr. Dent. 24 (2002) 456–461.
[17] G. Alex, Is total etch dead? Evidence suggests otherwise, Compend. Contin. Educ. Dent. 33 (2012) 12–14.
[18] A. Sezinando, J. Perdigão, R. Regalheiro, Dentin bond strengths of four adhesion strategies after thermal fatigue and 6-month water storage, J. Esthet. Restor. Dent. 24 (2012) 345–356.
[19] F.R. Tay, A.J. Gwinnett, S.H.I. Wei, Relation between water content in acetone/alcohol-based primer and interfacial ultrastructure, J. Dent. 26 (1998) 147–156.
[20] N. Nakabayashi, K. Kojima, E. Masuhara, The promotion of adhesion by the infiltration of monomers into tooth substrates, J. Biomed. Mater. Res. 16 (1982) 265–273.
[21] N. Nakabayashi, Y. Saimi, Bonding to intact dentin, J. Dent. Res. 75 (1996) 1706–1715.
[22] J.W. Nicholson, Adhesive dental materials and their durability, Int. J. Adhes. Adhes. 20 (2000) 11–16.
[23] E.J. Swift Jr., Bonding systems for restorative materials – a comprehensive literature review, Pediatr. Dent. 20 (1998) 80–84.
[24] D. Pashley, R.M. Carvalho, Dentine permeability and dentine adhesive, J. Dent. 25 (1997) 355–373.
[25] B. Van Meerbeek, M. Vargas, S. Inoue, Y. Yoshida, M. Peumans, P. Lambrechts, G. Vanherle, Adhesives and cements to promote preservative dentistry, Oper. Dent. 26 (2001) 119–144.
[26] J.F. McCabe, A.W.G. Walls, Applied Dental Materials, ninth ed., Blackwell Munksgaard, Oxford, 2008.
[27] J.R. Dunn, iBond™: the seventh generation, one-bottle dental bonding agent, Compend. Contin. Educ. Dent. 24 (Suppl. 2) (2003) 14–18.
[28] A. Al-Ehaideb, H. Mohammed, Shear bond strength of 'one bottle' dentin adhesives, J. Prosthet. Dent. 84 (2000) 408–412.
[29] A.R. Yazici, Ç. Çelik, G. Özgünaltay, B. Dayangaç, Bond strength of different adhesive systems to dental hard tissues, Oper. Dent. 32 (2007) 166–172.
[30] J. Kanca, Effect resin primer solvents and surface wetness on resin composite bond strength to dentin, Am. J. Dent. 5 (1992) 213–215.
[31] A. Reis, R.H.M. Grande, G.M.S. Oliveira, G.C. Lopes, A.D. Loguercio, A 2-year evaluation of moisture on microtensile bond strength and nanoleakage, Dent. Mater. 23 (2007) 862–870.
[32] F.R. Tay, A.J. Gwinnett, K.M. Pang, S.H. Wei, Resin permeation into acid-conditioned, moist, and dry dentin: a paradigm using water-free adhesive primers, J. Dent. Res. 75 (1996) 1034–1044.
[33] A.J. Gwinnett, Dentin bond strengths after air-drying and re-wetting, Am. J. Dent. 7 (1994) 144–148.
[34] E.R. Van der Graaf, J.L. ten Bosch, Changes in dimension and weight of human dentine after different drying procedures and during subsequent rehydration, Arch. Oral Biol. 38 (1993) 97–99.
[35] M. Nakajima, N. Kanemura, P.N. Pereira, J. Tagami, D.H. Pashley, Comparative microtensile bond strength and SEM analysis of bonding to wet and dry dentin, Am. J. Dent. 13 (2000) 324–328.
[36] C. Zander-Grande, S.Q. Ferreira, T.R.F. da Costa, A.D. Loguetcio, A. Reiss, Application of etch-and-rinse adhesives on dry and rewet dentin under rubbing action: a 24-month clinical evaluation, J. Am. Dent. Assoc. 142 (2011) 828–835.

[37] A.D. Loguerio, F. Loeblein, T. Cherobin, F. Ogliari, E. Piva, A. Reiss, Effect of solvent removal on adhesive properties of simplified etch-and-rinse systems and on bond strengths to dry and wet dentin, J. Adhes. Dent. 11 (2009) 213–219.
[38] D.H. Pashley, K.A. Agee, M. Nakajima, F.R. Tay, R.M. Carvalho, R.A.S. Terada, F.J. Harmon, W.J. Lee, F.A. Rueggeberg, Solvent-induced dimensional changes in EDTA-demineralized dentin matrix, J. Biomed. Mater. Res. 56 (2001) 273–281.
[39] K. Dal-Bianco, A. Pellizzarro, A. Patzlaft, J.R. Bauer, A.D. Loguercio, Effects of moisture degree and rubbing action on the immediate resin-dentin bond strength, Dent. Mater. 22 (2006) 1150–1156.
[40] J. Perdgao, B. Van Meerbeek, M.M. Lopes, W.W. Ambrose, The effect of a re-wetting agent on dentin bonding, Dent. Mater. 15 (1999) 282–295.
[41] M. Hashimoto, H. Ohno, M. Kaga, H. Sano, K. Endo, H. Oguchi, Extent to which resin can infiltrate dentin bond in vitro, J. Dent. Res. 81 (2002) 74–78.
[42] Y. Wang, P. Spencer, Adhesive phase separation at the dentin interface under wet conditions, J. Biomed. Mater. Res. 62 (2002) 447–456.
[43] Y. Wang, P. Spencer, Hybridization efficiency of the adhesive/dentin interface with wet bonding, J. Dent. Res. 82 (2003) 141–145.
[44] J. Tagami, L. Tao, D.H. Pashley, Correlation among dentin depth, permeability, and bond strength of adhesive resins, Dent. Mater. 6 (1990) 45–50.
[45] F.R. Tay, A.J. Gwinnett, K.M. Pang, S.H. Wei, Micromorphologic relationship of the resin-dentin interface following a total-etch technique in vivo using a dentinal bonding system, Quintessence Int. 26 (1995) 63–70.
[46] F.R. Tay, R. Frankenberger, I. Krejci, S. Bouillaguet, D.H. Pashley, R.M. Carvalho, C.N.S. Lai, Single-bottle adhesives behave as permeable membranes after polymerization, I. In vivo evidence, J. Dent. 32 (2004) 611–621.
[47] F.R. Tay, D.H. Pashley, Water treeing: a potential mechanism for degradation of dentin adhesives, Am. J. Dent. 16 (2003) 6–12.
[48] M.R. Carrilho, R.M. Carvalho, M.F. de Goes, V. di Hipolito, S. Geraldeli, F.R. Tay, D.H. Pashley, L. Tjäderhane, Chlorhexidine preserves dentin bond in vitro, J. Dent. Res. 86 (2007) 90–94.
[49] A.D. Loguercio, I. Luque-Martinez, M. Munoz, A. Szesz, J. Cuadros-Sanchez, A. Reis, A comprehensive laboratory screening of three-step etch-and-rinse adhesives, Oper. Dent. 39 (2014) 652–662.
[50] K. Hosaka, Y. Nishitani, J. Tagami, M. Yoshiyama, W.W. Brackett, K.A. Agee, F.R. Tay, D.H. Pashley, Durability of resin-dentin bonds to water vs ethanol-saturated dentin, J. Dent. Res. 88 (2009) 146–151.
[51] A. Reis, A.D. Loguercio, A 36-month clinical evaluation of ethanol/water and acetone-based etch-and-rinse adhesives in non-carious cervical lesions, Oper. Dent. 34 (2009) 384–391.
[52] P. de Carvalho Cardoso, A.D. Loguercio, L.C.C. Viera, L.N. Baratieri, A. Reis, Effect of prolonged application times on resin-dentin bond strengths, J. Adhes. Dent. 7 (2005) 143–149.
[53] A. Reis, P. de Carvalho Cardoso, L.C.C. Viera, L.N. Baratieri, R.H.M. Grande, A.D. Loguercio, Effect of prolonged application times on the durability of resin-dentin bonds, Dent. Mater. 24 (2008) 639–644.
[54] J.A. Platt, J. Almeida, C. Gonzales, B. Rhodes, B.K. Moore, The effect of double adhesive application times on the shear bond to dentin of compomers using three one-bottle adhesive systems, Oper. Dent. 26 (2001) 313–317.

[55] A.D. Loguercio, A. Costenaro, A.P. Silveira, N.R. Ribeiro, T.R. Rossi, A. Reiss, A six-month clinical study of a self-etching and etch-and-rinse adhesive applied as recommended and after doubling the number of adhesive coats, J. Adhes. Dent. 8 (2006) 255–261.
[56] K.L. Van Landuyt, J. Snauwaert, J. De Munk, M. Peumans, Y. Yoshida, A. Poitevin, E. Coutinho, K. Suzuki, P. Lambrechts, B. van Meerbeek, Systematic review of the chemical composition of contemporary dental adhesives, Biomaterials 28 (2007) 757–785.
[57] S. Moszner, U. Salz, J. Zimmerman, Chemical aspects of self-etching enamel-dentin adhesives: a systematic review, Dent. Mater. 21 (2005) 895–910.
[58] F.R. Tay, D.H. Pashley, Aggressiveness of contemporary self-etching systems. I: Depth of penetration beyond dentin smear layers, Dent. Mater. 17 (2001) 296–308.
[59] K. Koshiro, S.K. Sidhu, S. Inoue, T. Ikeda, H. sano, New concept of resin-dentin interfacial adhesion: the nanointeraction zone, J. Biomed. Mater. Res. 77 (2006) 401–408.
[60] F.R. Tay, H. Sano, R. Carvalho, E.L. Pashley, D.H. Pashley, An ultrastructural study of the influence of acidity of self-etching primers and smear layer thickness on bonding to intact dentin, J. Adhes. Dent. 2 (2000) 83–98.
[61] N.J. Opdam, F.J. Roeters, A.J. Feilzer, E.H. Verdonschot, Marginal integrity and post-operative sensitivity in Class 2 resin composite restorations *in vivo*, J. Dent. 26 (1998) 555–562.
[62] M. Peumans, J. De Munck, K.L. Van Landuyt, A. Poitevin, P. Lambrechts, B. Van Meerbeek, Eight-year clinical evaluation of a 2-step self-etch adhesive with and without selective enamel etching, Dent. Mater. 26 (2010) 1176–1184.
[63] J. Perdigao, S. Geraldeli, J.S. Hodges, Total etch versus self-etch adhesive: effect on post-operative sensitivity, J. Am. Dent. Assoc. 134 (2003) 1621–1629.
[64] J. Perdigao, E.J. Swift, Critical appraisal: post-op sensitivity with direct composite restorations, J. Esthet. Restor. Dent. 25 (2013) 284–288.
[65] Y. Yoshida, B. van Meerbeek, Y. Nakayama, J. Snauwaert, L. Hellemans, P. Lambrechts, G. Vanherle, K. Wakasa, Evidence of chemical bonding at biomaterial-hard tissue interfaces, J. Dent. Res. 79 (2000) 709–714.
[66] M. Yoshioka, Y. Yoshida, S. Onoue, P. Lambrechts, G. Vanherle, Y. Nomura, M. Okazaki, H. Shintani, B. Van Meerbeek, Adhesion/decalcification mechanisms of acid interactions with human hard tissues, J. Biomed. Mater. Res. 59 (2002) 56–62.
[67] A. Lin, N.S. McIntyre, R.D. Davidson, Studies on the adhesion of glass-ionomer cements to dentin, J. Dent. Res. 71 (1992) 1836–1841.
[68] S.K. Mousa, A. Reis, A. Pelizzaro, K. Day-Bianco, A.D. Loguercio, V.E. Arana-Cahvez, R.H. Grande, Bond strength and morphology of enamel using self-etching adhesive systems with different acidities, J. Appl. Oral Sci. 17 (2009) 315–325.
[69] M. Sarr, A.W. Kane, M. Mine, J. Vreven, K.L. van Landuyt, M. Peumans, P. Lambrechts, B. van Meerbeek, J. De Munck, Microtensile bond strength and interfacial characterization of 11 contemporary adhesive systems bonded to bur-cut dentin, Oper. Dent. 35 (2010) 94–104.
[70] S. Kubo, K. Kawasaki, H. Yokota, Y. Hayashi, Five-year clinical evaluation of two adhesive systems in non-carious cervical lesions, J. Dent. 34 (2006) 97–105.
[71] J. Perdigao, C. Kose, A.P. Mena-Serrano, E.A. De Paula, L.Y. Tay, A. Reis, A.D. Loguercio, A new universal simplified adhesive: 18-month clinical evaluation, Oper. Dent. 39 (2014) 113–127.
[72] J. Perdigao, M. Dutra-Correa, C.H.C. Saraceni, M.T. Ciaramicoli, C.S. Queiroz, Randomized clinical trial of four adhesion strategies: 18-month results, Oper. Dent. 37 (2013) 3–111.

[73] J. Perdigao, A.D. Loguercio, Universal or multi-mode adhesives: why and how? J. Adhes. Dent. 16 (2014) 193–194.

[74] J. Perdigao, M. Munoz, A. Sezinando, I. Luque-Martinez, R. Staichak, A. Reis, A. Loguercio, Immediate adhesive properties to dentin and enamel of a universal adhesive associated with a hydrophobic resin coat, Oper. Dent. 39 (2014) 489–499.

[75] G. Marchesi, A. Frassetto, A. Mazzoni, A. Apolonio, M. Diolosa, M. Cadenaro, R. Di Lenarda, D.H. Pashley, F. Tay, L. Breschi, Adhesive performance of a multi-mode adhesive system: 1 year in vitro study, J. Dent. 42 (2014) 603–612.

[76] M. Hanabusa, A. Mine, T. Kuboki, Y. Momoi, A. Van Ende, B. Van Meerbeek, J. De Munck, Bonding effectiveness of a new multi-mode adhesive to enamel and dentine, J. Dent. 40 (2012) 475–484.

[77] M. Munoz, I. Luque, V. Hass, A. Reis, A.D. Loguercio, N.H. Bombarda, Immediate bonding properties of universal adhesives to dentine, J. Dent. 41 (2013) 404–411.

[78] J. Perdigao, A. Sezinando, P.C. Monteiro, Laboratory bonding ability of a multi-purpose dentin adhesive, Am. J. Dent. 25 (2012) 153–158.

[79] M. Munoz, A. Sezinando, I. Luque-Martinez, A. Szesz, A. Reis, A.D. Loguercio, N.H. Bombarda, J. Perdigão, Influence of a hydrophobic resin coating on the bonding efficacy of three universal adhesives, J. Dent. 42 (2014) 595–602.

[80] W.R.A. D'Hoore, S. Gonthier, M. Degrange, J. Dejou, Reliability of *in vitro* microleakage test: a literature review, J. Adhes. Dent. 3 (2001) 295–308.

[81] H. Sano, T. Takatsu, B. Ciucchi, J.A. Horner, W.G. Matthews, D.H. Pashley, Nanoleakage: leakage within the hybrid layer, Oper. Dent. 20 (1995) 18–35.

[82] C.E. Dörfer, H.J. Staehle, M.W. Wurst, H. Duschner, T. Pioch, The nanoleakage phenomenon: influence of different dentine bonding agents, thermocycling and etching time, Eur. J. Oral Sci. 108 (2000) 346–351.

[83] A.F. Reis, C.A.G. Arrais, P.D. Novaes, M. Giannini, Ultra-morphological analysis of the resin-dentin interface: nanoleakage patterns of simplified dental adhesives, Acta Microsc. 12 (2003) 575–576.

[84] L. Breschi, A. Mazzoni, A. Ruggeri, M. Cadenaro, R. Lenarda, E. De Stefano Dorigo, Dental adhesion review: aging and stability of bonded surfaces, Dent. Mater. 24 (2008) 90–101.

[85] J. Krithikadatta, Clinical effectiveness of contemporary dentin bonding agents, J. Conserv. Dent. 13 (2010) 173–183.

[86] S.D. Heintze, Systematic reviews. I. Correlation between laboratory tests on marginal quality and bond strength. II. The correlation between marginal quality and clinical outcome, J. Adhes. Dent. 9 (2007) 77–106.

[87] M. Peumans, P. Kanumilli, J. De Munck, K. Van Landuyt, P. Lambrechts, B. Van Meerbeek, Clinical effectiveness of contemporary adhesives: a systematic review of current clinical trials, Dent. Mater. 21 (2005) 864–881.

[88] A. Hamid, W.R. Hume, Diffusion of resin monomers through human carious dentin in vitro, J. Oral Rehabil. 24 (1997) 20–25.

[89] W.R. Hume, T.M. Gerzina, Bioavailability of components of resin-based materials which are applied to teeth, Crit. Rev. Oral Biol. Med. 7 (1996) 172–179.

Conventional glass-ionomer cements

6

6.1 Introduction

The glass-ionomer cement is an acid–base cement based on weak polymeric acids and powdered glasses that are basic in character [1]. Their setting takes place within water and results in a complex polysalt matrix, formed by chemical reaction of the acidic polymer solution with the basic glass. The structure also contains a substantial amount of unreacted glass that acts as reinforcing filler [2]. In terms of materials classification, this makes them composites, but convention in dentistry is to consider them distinct from composites, and to classify them as cements.

The term glass-ionomer was applied to them in the earliest publication [3], but is not strictly correct. An 'ionomer' is a polymer containing a minority of ionizable functional groups, for example the ethylene co-polymers known as 'surlyns' manufactured by the Du Pont company. These have been described in detail by MacKnight and Earnest [4]. In the case of the dental cements, the polymer contains a high density of ionizable functional, so that it is properly a polyelectrolyte cement, rather than an ionomer. This is recognized in the formally correct name of these materials, glass polyalkenoate cement, as defined in the appropriate international standard [5]. The term 'polyalkenoate' is derived from the type of acid used in these materials, which is a polyalkenoic acid, with the word polyalkenoate indicating that this acid forms a salt. The name 'glass-ionomer' (including the hyphen) for these cements is recognized as an acceptable trivial term [6], and is the one mainly within the dental profession. For this reason, it is the term used in the current chapter.

Glass-ionomers are one group of acid–base cements used clinically in dentistry. Others include the zinc phosphate, zinc polycarboxylate and zinc oxide eugenol cements [2]. Of these, glass-ionomer cements are much the most versatile, finding a variety of applications, including as direct restoratives, liners or bases, pit-and-fissure sealants and lutings cement for crowns and bridges [7].

Glass-ionomers were developed from the now obsolete dental silicate cement. This cement consisted of a basic glass of complex composition that was reacted with aqueous solutions of phosphoric acid [8]. These materials were originally developed at the beginning of the 20th century, and for almost 60 years were the only materials available for tooth repair that came close to matching the natural shade and translucency of the tooth, though compared with modern glass-ionomers, they were substantially opaque [9].

For many years, the dental silicate cement was thought to set by the formation of a silicate structure [9]. However, studies by Wilson et al. in the 1960s showed that it was, in fact, a phosphate cement [10–12]. Reaction of the glass with aqueous phosphoric acid was shown to yield a complex matrix that consisted of a mixture of calcium and aluminium phosphates. There was also some silica gel formed, though

Materials for the Direct Restoration of Teeth. http://dx.doi.org/10.1016/B978-0-08-100491-3.00006-4

this remained attached as a surface layer to the glass particles and was shown to be formed by extraction of cement-forming ions from the surface layers of the glass [13].

Several possible calcium and aluminium phosphates exist and they differ in their solubility in aqueous media and also in their resistance to acid attack. Among the factors determining which of these products are formed are powder:liquid ratio of the cement and concentration of the phosphoric acid solution. As a result, this material was easy to prepare in a soluble or acid-sensitive state. Incorrect metering of the powder to liquid components increased the solubility of the set cement, and leaving the bottle of phosphoric acid solution open to the air led to uptake of moisture from the atmosphere, with a corresponding reduction in acid concentration. This resulted in an increase in the proportion of more soluble metal salts in the set cement. These factors combined to make the dental silicate difficult to use in the clinic and gave the material a reputation for unreliability [8].

In 1968 Smith reported the invention of the zinc polycarboxylate cement [14]. This material was formed by reaction of deactivated zinc oxide powder with aqueous poly(acrylic acid). Since deactivated zinc oxide powder was the base used in conjunction with phosphoric acid solution in the zinc phosphate cement, the discovery suggested the possibility of combining dental silicate glass powder with aqueous poly(acrylic acid) as a route to forming novel cements. When the experiment was tried it was a failure [15]. The resulting cement set extremely slowly to form a weak, water-soluble material of no apparent promise whatsoever. This experiment was carried out as part of a study of alternative cement-forming liquids for use with dental silicate glasses, and results were so poor that they were not reported in the published account [16]. It was only many years later that Wilson confirmed that the experiment had been done, and how disappointing the results were [15].

In fact the invention of the glass-ionomer cement took considerably more work than simply mixing dental silicate glass powder with zinc polycarboxylate liquid. It began with the recognition of the mismatch between the strength of the acid involved and the basicity of the glass, which was followed by an extensive project aimed at preparing a workable glass of higher basicity, able to compensate for the reduced acidity of poly(acrylic acid) compared with phosphoric acid [15]. The search eventually yielded the first practical glass, the so-called G200, which formed the basis of the first commercial glass-ionomer cement. This material was launched in 1975 under the name ASPA (an acronym derived from alumino-silicate poly acrylic acid).

By modern standards, ASPA was a poor material [15]. Its setting was sluggish and its final appearance opaque. This latter property was a consequence of the relatively high fluoride content of G200, which was necessary to control the setting but which also caused to low translucency and overall poor appearance.

Since the days of the first commercial glass-ionomer cement there has been an enormous amount of research aimed at improving the properties to the extent that modern materials are superior in every aspect to the original ASPA material. An early critical discovery was the role of tartaric acid in moderating the setting reaction [17]. This allowed glasses of improved translucency and lower fluoride content to be developed.

Further improvements, mainly in terms of glass particle size and size distribution, have allowed glass-ionomers to be made with much greater strengths than the early materials, and also sharper setting properties, improved appearance and greater resistance to wear. These developments are described in the remaining sections of this chapter, together with accounts of the composition and setting of modern glass-ionomer materials, and discussion of their clinical applications and benefits. In addition, there was the major development of the resin-modified glass-ionomer cements, first reported in 1991 [18]. These are dealt with in detail in this chapter.

6.2 Composition of glass-ionomer cements

There are three essential ingredients to a glass-ionomer cement, namely polymeric acid, basic (ionleachable) glass and water [19]. Initially, these materials were formulated as an aqueous solution of acid that was mixed with the glass powder and allowed to harden. Since the launch of the earliest brand of glass-ionomer, alternative formulations have been produced, ranging from both the acid and the glass being present in the powder, with pure water being added to promote the setting reaction, to formulations in which a fraction of the acid is blended with the glass powder and the rest of the acid is present as a relatively dilute solution in water which is used as the liquid component.

Originally, too, the glass-ionomer was prepared for the so-called hand-mixing, using a spatula. Mixing of this type of material involved incorporating the powder into the liquid on either a waxed paper pad or a glass block, continuing until the powder was fully incorporated and a stiff homogeneous mixture had been achieved. Subsequently capsulated materials have been made available, where powder and liquid are supplied in the correct amounts in a bespoke capsule, separated by a membrane. The membrane is broken immediately prior to mixing, and the capsule is subjected to rapid vibratory mixing on a specially designed auto-mixer, after which the cement paste is immediately extruded from the capsule for placement.

It is often the case that a single brand is available as both a hand-mixed and capsulated version. However, this is slightly misleading, as the two types of cement have to be formulated differently. A cement formulation that sets in a satisfactory time when hand-mixed sets far too rapidly, possibly while still in the capsule, when subject to vibratory mixing. This is because the auto-mixing process is so efficient, and also because it effectively puts energy into the cement. Consequently, formulations for capsulation have to be deactivated relative to those for hand-mixing, and they rely on the accelerating effect of auto-mixing for their observed satisfactory working and setting times.

The components of the glass-ionomer cement have been the subject of considerable amounts of research over that years and a wide variety of materials are available that are capable of being used in glass-ionomer cements. These are considered in turn the following sections of the current chapter.

6.2.1 Polymeric acids

The polymers used in glass-ionomer cements are all polyelectrolytes [2]. This means that they are both polymeric in character and carry electrostatic charge. It is because of this charge that they are water soluble, although when they interact with di- and tri-valent ions, such as Ca^{2+} and Al^{3+} during the setting process, they become ionically crosslinked and lose the property of water-solubility.

The polyelectrolytes used in practical glass-ionomers are polyalkenoic acids, and two such substances are employed as the main polymer in these cements, namely the homopolymer poly(acrylic acid) and the 2:1 copolymer of acrylic acid and maleic acid. In addition, poly(vinyl phosphonic acid) has been studied as a potential cement former, but its practical use is restricted to a single brand, where it is used in a mixture with poly(acrylic acid) and effectively acts as a setting rate modifier.

There is confusion in the literature concerning the nature of the polymers used in glass-ionomers. This stems from the early research of Wilson et al., who studied a range of mono-, di- and tri-carboxylic acid monomers in polymers for cement formation, including itaconic and tricarballic acid [20] and this has led to the assumption that these must be used in practical cements. In fact proprietary materials are all based on the two polymers previously mentioned.

The features of the polymer influence the properties of the glass-ionomer cement formed from them. For cements prepared from the homopolymer of acrylic acid, compressive strength has been found to increase with increasing molecular weight (relative molar mass) [21]. Conversely, setting time is reduced. In order to obtain a cement with optimal properties, a balance needs to be struck between these two opposing trends. Early reports suggested that polymers of acrylic acid with average molar masses in the range 23,000–50,000 gave optimal results [22]. More recent studies have further determined the details of the optimized poly(acrylic acid) molar masses and suggest average values of 11,000 (number average) and 52,000 (mass average), giving a polydispersity of 4.7, are ideal [23].

Cements prepared from homopolymers of acrylic acid show increases in compressive strength with time for the first 4–6 weeks of the cement's life. By contrast, cements made from acrylic/maleic acid co-polymers show an increase in compressive strength up to a point, after which there is a decline before reaching an equilibrium value. This was initially attributed to hydrolytic instability of acrylic/maleic glass-ionomer cements [24]. However, there is no obvious reason why ion-carboxylate groups in the copolymer cements should be susceptible to hydrolysis when those in homopolymer cements are stable. Studies of copolymer cements stored in dry oil, rather than water, showed that they, too, achieve a maximum strength early in their life, and then decline somewhat [25]. This led to the alternative suggestion that the reduction in compressive strength is not due to chemical instability but to the higher crosslink density that develops within these cements. This causes them to become more brittle with time and for surface flaws to exercise a greater effect on reducing strength. Similar effects have been found to occur in experimental cements formulated from poly(vinyl phosphonic acid) which, due to the di-basic nature of the acid functional group, is also able to develop higher crosslink density than homopolymers of acrylic acid [26].

In practical clinical use, this difference between the homopolymer and copolymer cements does not seem significant. There is no evidence that cements made from acrylic/maleic acid copolymer are less satisfactory in clinical service, and brands containing this polymer, such as Ketac Molar, are proprietary glass-ionomer cements that are among the most respected brands within the profession.

6.2.2 Glasses

The essential feature of glasses for ionomer cements is that they are basic, ie, capable of reacting with an aqueous solution of an acid to form a salt. In principle, a wide variety of glass compositions can be prepared that fulfil this requirement and many different compositions have been reported in the research literature, including aluminoborates [27] and zinc silicates [28].

The only ones that have so far found practical application in glass-ionomers for dentistry are alumino-silicate glasses, with fluoride and phosphate additions. These are typically calcium based, with some extra sodium, though successful commercial materials exist in which calcium has been wholly or partly replaced by strontium.

The composition of the first successful glass, the so-called G200, is given in Table 6.1. It differs from modern glasses in that it is much higher in fluorite, CaF_2. As a consequence, its translucency is inferior, as is the translucency of the cements prepared from it.

Fluoride is a vital component of the glasses used in glass-ionomer cements. It was originally added to dental silicate glasses as a flux, ie, a substance that lowers the melting temperature, and was found to be leached from these cements when they had set. Because ionomer glasses were derived from dental silicate glasses, they too are formulated with fluoride present. Glasses containing fluoride were among the earliest reported when glass-ionomers were first described, and were either of the SiO_2–Al_2O_3–CaF_2 system or the more complex SiO_2–Al_2O_3–P_2O_5–CaO–CaF_2 system. The latter were especially important, as they combined basicity with translucency and thus gave cements that set at a clinically useful rate and yielded set materials with good appearance [29].

Preparing glasses for glass-ionomer cements was guided by the Random Network concept of Zacheriasen [30]. This concept models glasses as random assemblies of SiO_4 tetrahedra linked at their corners to form chains. The main rules of the Random Network concept are as follows:

(i) Each oxygen atom is linked to no more than two cations.
(ii) The co-ordination number of the network cation is small.
(iii) Oxygen polyhedra are connected only through the corners, not along the faces.
(iv) A three-dimensional network results from such polyhedra being shared by at least three corners.

Table 6.1 Composition of glass G200

Component	% by mass
SiO_2	30.1
Al_2O_3	19.9
AlF_3	2.6
CaF_2	34.5
NaF	3.7
$AlPO_4$	10.0

These rules need to be used in conjunction with Lowenstein's notion that while glasses consist of mainly of SiO_4 tetrahedra, inclusion of aluminium creates AlO_4 tetrahedra as the aluminium atoms are forced to adopt fourfold co-ordination [31]. In doing so, a species that is charge-deficient is formed, due to the fact that aluminium is formally Al^{3+} compared with the formal charge of silicon as Si^{4+}. Consequently additional cations such as Na^+, Ca^{2+} or Mg^{2+} are needed to compensate for the excess of negative charge on the glass network. The presence of these cations, plus the four-co-ordinate aluminium in the glass network confers basicity on the glass and makes it susceptible to acid attack. This explains the observation that the alumina:silica ratio controls the basicity of the glass.

The substitution of silicon by aluminium in oxygen tetrahedra can only occur up to a limit of a 1:1 ratio. Above this ratio, aluminium is no longer forced to take up fourfold co-ordination and its presence ceases to influence the basicity of the glass [2].

So far, all of the oxygen atoms considered have been bridging, ie, have been shared between tetrahedra. However, the introduction of components such as CaO creates an additional class of oxygen atoms, namely non-bridging oxygens. These occur as negatively charged ionic crosslinks between ions such as Ca^{2+}. Units of this type increase the susceptibility of the glass to reaction, since small species such as hydrated protons or water molecules can enter the glass structure at these points and solvate the ions involved [29].

There have been numerous studies of the structure of ionomer glasses, and their overall chemistry is reasonably well understood. In the case of the more complex glasses used in practical cements, the aluminium:silicon ratio had only a slight influence on the basicity of the glass [32]. One reason postulated to explain this is that, in addition to AlO_4 tetrahedra, there are also significant amounts of PO_4 tetrahedra. These have a reduced amount of formal negative charge, ie, are PO_4^{3-} compared with AlO_4^{3-}, and this balances the charge deficiency that arises from the inclusion of alumina. This reduces the number of Al–O–Si units available for acid attack [32].

Practical ionomer glasses are known to undergo at least partial phase separation as they cool [29]. This leads to regions of varying composition and typically to the occurrence of one phase that is more susceptible to acid attack than the others. Studies of ion release from phase-separated glasses show preferential attack on one phase, and removal of ions in a different ratio from that found in the overall glass composition [33,34]. An example is the glass G338, which has been widely studied and has the starting composition shown in Table 6.2. Acid washing studies were found to give the results shown in Table 6.3, where ratios in the acid washings are shown and compared with those in the complete glass [33]. By comparison, the oxide glass MP4, which is not phase-separated, gave ion release into acid solution that corresponded (within experimental error) that in the complete glass.

The inclusion of CaF_2 (fluorite) in the glass-forming mixture has interesting effects on the properties of the finished glass, and also on the mechanical properties of glass-ionomer cements prepared from that glass. The calcium ions from the fluorite disrupt the glass network by forming non-bridging oxygens and balancing the charge deficiency of the AlO_4 tetrahedra [35,36]. The fluorine, meanwhile, replaces the bridging oxygens with non-bridging fluoride ions. The net effect of these two behaviours

Table 6.2 **Composition of glass G338**

Component	% by mass
SiO_2	24.9
Al_2O_3	14.2
AlF_3	4.6
CaF_2	12.8
$NaAlF_6$	19.2
$AlPO_4$	24.2

Table 6.3 **Moles of ions released by glasses washed with 5% acetic acid for 5 min**

Ions released (moles) by 25 g glass in 100 cm³ of acid solution and mole ratio of ions	From glass MP4 (single-phase oxide glass)	From glass G338 (partially phase-separated fluoride glass)
Al	5.49×10^{-3}	4.11×10^{-3}
Ca	3.95×10^{-3}	1.85×10^{-3}
Si	3.75×10^{-3}	2.76×10^{-3}
Na	0.43×10^{-3}	3.04×10^{-3}
Al:Si ratio (ratio in glass)	1.39 (1.48)	1.49 (1.38)
Al:Ca ratio (ratio in glass)	1.46 (1.48)	2.22 (4.50)
Ca:Si ratio (ratio in glass)	1.05 (1.00)	0.67 (0.31)

is that the melting temperature of the glass is lowered and the susceptibility of the finished glass to acid attack is increased [35,37]. This gives the cements shorter working and setting times, but increased compressive strength and Young's modulus. This is an example of a general feature of glass-ionomer cements. Changes in composition and mixing conditions that increase the speed of setting (reduce working and setting times) generally improve compressive strength of the cement. Conversely, changes that slow down the speed of setting generally weaken the resulting cement.

Structural studies have been carried out using MAS-NMR spectroscopy and these have provided useful information on the co-ordination states of several of the elements in ionomer glasses. In particular, aluminium has been shown to occur in both four- and five-co-ordination in several glasses [38], which is attributed to reduction in the influence of silica on the co-ordination state of aluminium and an increase in the amount of species such as Al–F–Ca(*n*) in the glass [39].

Studies of the role of fluorine in ionomer glasses have shown that fluorine is bound exclusively to aluminium [40–43]. Previously the possibility of the occurrence of either CaF_2 clusters or SiF species had been postulated based in studies of related glasses [44,45], but there was no evidence for them in the specific glasses studied. However, although absent from these glasses, they may yet occur in practical cement-forming glasses if the fluoride content is high enough [46].

One important practical modification to ionomer glasses is the substitution of calcium with strontium. This is achieved by using the compounds SrO and SrF_2 in the place of CaO and CaF_2 in the glass-forming mixture [47]. Strontium has the effect of increasing radiopacity compared with calcium in these glasses without any adverse effect on the appearance of these cements. Fluoride release was enhanced from these cements, though the reason for this was unclear.

A number of other glasses have been studied as potential cement formers, but none apart from members of the fluoro-alumino-silicate system have found practical application in dental glass-ionomers. Some years ago, Combe et al. [27] studied aluminoborate glasses and found ways of heat-treating them to control their reactivity and improve the compressive strength of the set cements [48,49]. However, strengths remained too low for clinical application in dentistry and no further work on these glasses has been reported. There have also been reports of niobium silicate glasses as potential ionomer cement glasses [50]. They were fluoride-free and based on the SiO_2–Al_2O_3–Nb_2O_5–CaO system. Results have been satisfactory but resulting glasses do not seem to offer any advantage over the ones conventionally used in glass-ionomer cements.

Two other series of glasses have been made with orthopaedic (bone-contact) applications in mind, rather than dentistry. Consequently, they have been formed without aluminium present in the structure, a feature which is aimed at avoiding potentially harmful effects that may occur when aluminium is leached into bone [51]. One series was based in the replacement of aluminium by Fe^{3+} ions, a feature that was achieved by the incorporation of Fe_2O_3 into the glass-forming mixture [52]. Resulting glasses are black, as are the cements formed from them, a feature that could potentially be exploited in orthopaedics since the colour would leave no doubt where the cement ended and natural bone began. Properly formulated, these glasses were found to be capable of reacting with poly(acrylic acid) solutions to give cements of reasonable working and setting times, and acceptable strength [52].

The other aluminium-free series of glasses being studied are the zinc silicates. These are based on the system CaO–ZnO–SiO_2, which means that zinc effectively replaces aluminium compared with conventional ionomer glasses, despite the differences in charge on the respective metal ions. Compressive strengths of the first cements of this type proved low by comparison with dental glass-ionomers [53]. However, subsequent studies have shown that this property can be improved, albeit without reaching the level required for dentistry. The substitution of zinc for aluminium replaces a potentially harmful element (aluminium) with one possessing positive biological properties (zinc). The latter, for example, is capable of promoting increased bone mass in vivo, has an important role in immune system function, and is a useful antibacterial agent. It is thus promising as the basis of glass-ionomer cements for bone-contact applications, and research is continuing on this topic.

6.2.3 Chelating additives

The earliest practical glass for glass-ionomer cements, G200, was relatively high in fluoride. This led to the concept that, since aluminium-fluoro complexes form readily and are highly stable [54], the role of this excessive quantity of fluoride was to chelate

Table 6.4 Infrared absorption bands [57]

Salt	C–O asymmetric stretch (cm^{-1})	C–O symmetric stretch (cm^{-1})
Ca-PAA	1550	1410
Al-PAA	1559	1460
Ca-tartrate	1595	1385
Al-tartrate	1670	1410

the Al^{3+} ions and thereby prevent premature reaction with carboxylate groups on the polymer. Further consideration of this idea suggested that there may be alternative chelating agents that might have a similar effect. Several such compounds were studied as additives at either 5% or 10% by mass in cements [17]. Two proved highly successful, namely (+)-tartaric acid and citric acid and of these (+)-tartaric acid was the more effective.

The reasons for the exceptional properties of (+)-tartaric acid are not clear. In the past it was employed in the analysis of alumino-silicate rocks to prevent precipitation of aluminium salts, which it did by chelating Al^{3+} ions and keeping them in solution [55]. It may have the same effect in glass-ionomer cements, and act to prevent the premature formation of ionic crosslinks involving Al^{3+} [56]. There may be other effects, too. Tartaric acid is a stronger acid than poly(acrylic acid) as shown from its lower pK_a value and consequently, in a glass-ionomer cement, it is likely to attack the glass more readily and thereby remove a proportion of the cement-forming ions from the glass surface, retaining them so that they do not crosslink the polymer. Certainly this is consistent with the timing of the appearance of relevant bands in the infrared spectrum (Table 6.4).

The effect of this reaction on the setting of a glass-ionomer is to delay the onset of hardening. Later, when the poly(acrylic acid) is able to react with the glass, gelation occurs more readily. The overall result is a cement that has a delayed set, so is easier to mix, and which then sets sharply to give a hardened material that can be finished. The ability to promote these changes makes (+)-tartaric acid the ideal additive, though the effect varies somewhat between glasses, depending on their composition. Also, the effect owes something to stereochemistry, as meso-tartaric acid is not nearly so effective as the (+) isomer [15].

6.3 Setting of glass-ionomer cements

Glass-ionomers set rapidly by an acid–base (neutralization) reaction to form an insoluble salt. The first step involves attack by hydrated protons from the polyacid solution at susceptible sites on the surface of the glass particles. This liberates ions such as Na^+ and Ca^{2+} (or Sr^{2+}), to be followed quite quickly by Al^{3+}.

As part of this process, the polyacid molecule becomes progressively more charged and the resulting polyanion probably undergoes coil expansion to form a rigid rod. This is known to be what happens on neutralization of polyelectrolytes

Table 6.5 Viscosity of 45% poly(acrylic acid) progressively neutralized with sodium hydroxide

Neutralization (%)	pH	Viscosity (cP)
0	1.38	100
10	3.16	410
25	3.83	910
40	4.33	2210
55	4.71	4330
70	5.30	5330
85	5.84	13,100
100	7.83	51,550

such as poly(acrylic acid) in dilute solution [58]. Such effects are more complicated in highly concentrated solutions of the type used to prepare glass-ionomer cements, but they are consistent with the substantial increase in viscosity that develops as 45% poly(acrylic acid) solution is progressively neutralized with sodium hydroxide (Table 6.5).

As well as probable coil expansion of the polyacid molecules, there is rapid formation of ionic crosslinks based on Ca^{2+} (or Sr^{2+}) ions. The resulting ionically crosslinked polymer forms the basis of a rigid material. Also, at sufficiently high degrees of crosslinking the resulting polymer is no longer soluble in water. This stage was originally termed 'precipitation' by Wilson [59], but this is not strictly correct, because precipitation properly occurs when the insoluble product separates from the water. When a glass-ionomer cement sets there is no phase separation; all of the water becomes fully incorporated into the set cement.

The setting reaction has been studied by a variety of spectroscopic techniques, including infrared, fourier transform infrared (FTIR) and ^{13}C NMR spectroscopy. Setting appears to take place in two steps in what is, apparently, a diffusion-controlled reaction [60,61]. The initial step involves formation of ionic crosslinks following release of Ca^{2+} (or Sr^{2+}), and Al^{3+} ions [62,63]. The initial crosslinks are based on Ca^{2+} or Sr^{2+}, and form within the first minute or so of reaction following mixing. Subsequent crosslinking involves Al^{3+} ions but this cannot be identified unambiguously until about 10 min after mixing [64]. This step is relatively slow, and continues for about a day [65,66].

The second step is generally known as maturation, and is associated with a number of changes in the properties of the resulting glass-ionomer cement [19]. Translucency generally increases, as does strength, and also the proportion of water that is tightly bound within the structure increases. The precise mechanisms of these processes are not clear. A study many years ago showed that insoluble hard cements could be formed by reaction of ionomer glasses with acetic acid, despite the fact that the possible metal acetate salts that formed are all soluble in water [67]. Moreover, this type of cement became progressively stronger in compression up to 3 months, despite there being no discernible changes in the infrared spectra of the organic components. This led to the suggestion that there was some sort of inorganic setting reaction that complemented the setting of these cements. The initial suggestion was that this involved formation of metal silicates [68], but subsequent work on what became known as 'pseudo-cements' (ie, cements made from monomeric acids with ionomer glasses) showed that insoluble hard materials resulted only with phosphate glasses, and that phosphate-free silicate glasses did not undergo an equivalent setting reaction [69]. This suggested that the proposed inorganic network is phosphate-based, rather than silicate-based, a suggestion that is plausible, given that the former dental silicate cements were known to have this essential structure.

In practical terms, the setting of glass-ionomers has been studied either using Gillmore needles or using oscillating rheometry. Both distinguish between working and setting time [17]. These are considered to represent distinct phases of the overall setting process, and are respectively the time at which the cement is no longer able to be placed or moulded to the cavity, and the time at which the cement has hardened. Between these times, the cement has a rubbery consistency in which it is not properly hard but also will not flow and so cannot be adapted to the shape of a cavity.

Gillmore needles are recommended in the relevant ISO standard, ISO 9917 (dental water-based cements) [5], with different mass needles being used for working time and setting time. The approach with these devices is to place the needle, which has a flat circular end of 1 mm radius, onto the cement for 15 s, after which the specimen is examined for any trace of a mark. If a mark is visible, the relevant time (working or setting, depending on the mass of the needle) has not been reached.

The oscillating rheometer was originally described some years ago [70] and consists of a pair of metal plates, one of which is fixed rigidly in position, the other of which can be moved by a spring under tension, one end of which receives a reciprocating force from a small electric motor. Freshly mixed cement paste is placed between these plates and, as it hardens, so the spring-driven plate is able to move less and less in response to the force from the spring until it finally fails to move at all. At this point, the cement is considered to be fully set. What the device measures is actually a complex mixture of the spring constant (an instrument-dependent parameter), and the dynamic viscosity and the shear storage modulus of the setting cement [71]. However, despite this complexity, the result is useful because a trace can be printed out (Fig. 6.1) so that a permanent record of the setting profile is obtained. By arbitrarily taking the working time as the time from mixing until the amplitude reaches 95% of its initial value and setting time as the time to an amplitude of 5% of its initial value, results can be obtained that correspond to those obtained using Gillmore needles. The oscillating rheometer has been used in studies of additives for glass-ionomers [72] and in studies of novel glasses [36].

6.4 The role of water

As we have seen, water is the third essential component of the glass-ionomer cement, and it has several roles [73]. It is the solvent for the polymeric acid and as such allows the polymer to act as an acid by releasing protons, which in their hydrated form attack

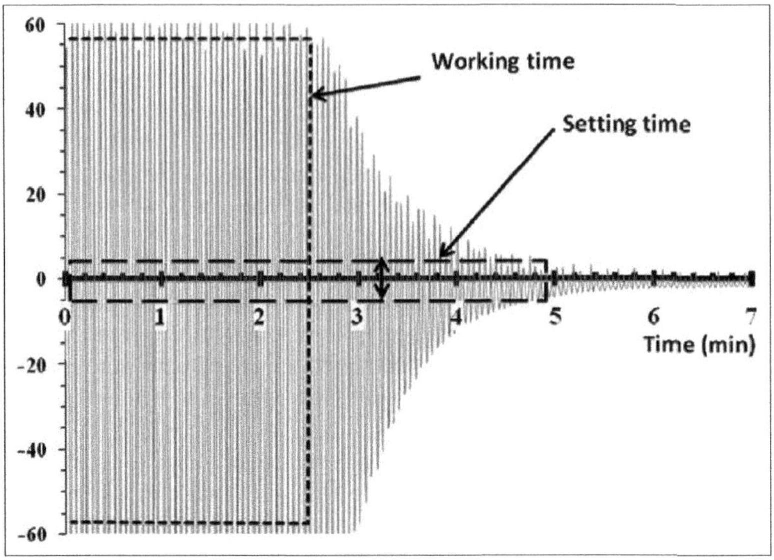

Fig. 6.1 Oscillating rheometer trace for setting glass-ionomer cement.

the basic glass powder to begin the setting process. It is also the medium in which the setting reaction takes place, and as setting proceeds, so it becomes incorporated into the cement structure without phase separation [73,74].

Binding of water is associated with increases in the translucency of the glass-ionomer cement. This change means that after some time, ranging from 1 week to 6 months, the restoration resembles the appearance of the natural enamel. Binding is likely to occur partly by the suggested mechanisms of co-ordination to metal ions [75] and hydration of the polyanion molecules [76–79]. In addition, there is the possibility of hydration of –Si–O–Si– units at the surface of the glass particles with formation of –Si–OH groups as the product. A few FTIR studies have examined the relevant region of the spectrum, and there is evidence of reduction in intensity of the band at 1060 cm^{-1} (from –Si–O–Si– groups) and development of a peak at 950 cm^{-1} [80,81] and one in the region 3435–3445 cm^{-1} [82,83], attributable to –Si–OH (silanol) groups.

The loosely bound water can be lost from the surface of freshly placed glass-ionomer cements by evaporation. This results in an unsightly chalky appearance as microscopic cracks form in the drying surface that compromise the aesthetics of the restoration. When such dehydrated restoration is subjected again to moisture, it is capable of regaining its original colour but only to an extent, never fully. Consequently it is very important to isolate the restoration by covering it with an appropriate varnish or petroleum jelly [84], especially if the restoration is visible while the patient is smiling. Isolation in this way allows the restoration to be carved to anatomical shape using hand instruments.

Varnishes are of two types, namely a simple solution of film-forming polymer in a solvent of a light-curable low viscosity monomer. There is some evidence that the latter give superior protection from drying out [85] as the absence of a solvent means that no porosities occur due to evaporation of the solvent.

The layer of varnish polymer may remain in place for some time, unlike petroleum jelly, with retention depending on several factors, including the vigour of the patient's toothbrushing technique [1]. Retention of such a layer probably inhibits release of fluoride to an extent, but as it does not last for long, it may not matter as much as allowing the glass-ionomer to develop its full physical and aesthetic properties [1].

6.5 Physical properties of glass-ionomers

The physical properties of glass-ionomer cements are influenced by several factors, including powder:liquid ratio, concentration of polyacid, particle size of the glass powder and age of the specimens. In addition, for hand-mixed cements, the experience of the operator has an influence, though the reasons for this are not completely clear [86]. Care is needed therefore in making generalizations about properties and part of the success of glass-ionomers may arise because they perform satisfactorily even when not properly mixed, or allowed to mature under optimum conditions.

The current ISO standard for glass-ionomers gives certain minimum values for physical properties, as shown Table 6.6. These vary depending on the clinical use for which the specific material is intended.

In addition to those properties specified in Table 6.6, there are other features of glass-ionomers that influence their clinical use, and these are now considered briefly.

The only type of strength that the ISO Standard deals with is compressive strength. Glass-ionomers also have reasonable flexural strengths [1]. As well as these values, their biaxial flexure [87] and their shear punch strengths [88] have been determined and, like compressive strength, these generally improve with higher powder:liquid ratios and concentration of polyacid. In all cases, failure is by brittle fracture, and this is a key feature of glass-ionomers; they are brittle materials and in this they differ from composite resins of all types. This is a limitation to their clinical use, and various techniques have been employed to reduce their brittleness and improve their toughness. These have included the addition of metal particles [89], mixing with nano-particles [90] and addition of resin to form the resin-modified glass-ionomer [18]. The latter material is the subject of Chapter 7, and is a widely used clinical material in its own right.

Table 6.6 ISO requirements for clinical grade glass-ionomer cements

Property	Luting cement	Restorative cement
Setting time (min)	2.5–8	2–6
Compressive strength (MPa)	70 (minimum)	130 (minimum)
Acid erosion (maximum) ($mm\,h^{-1}$)	–	0.05
Opacity, $C_{0.70}$	–	0.35–0.90
Acid-soluble As ($mg\,kg^{-1}$)	2	2
Acid-soluble Pb ($mg\,kg^{-1}$)	100	100

The inclusion of silver alloy metal powder led to materials of improved mechanical properties, including toughness. Unfortunately, these materials have substantially inferior aesthetics compared with unmodified conventional glass-ionomers. Nonetheless, metal-reinforced materials are still available and they occupy a niche role in specific clinical applications.

Another metal-containing glass-ionomer is based on a cermet, ie, a ceramic-metal hybrid [91]. In the case of the glass-ionomer cermet, fusing reactive ionomer glass with silver metal particles forms the hybrid material from which the cement is prepared. The resulting cement sets rapidly to form a hard material with improved toughness compared with conventional glass-ionomers. It is also strongly radiopaque, which is useful clinically. However, like the metal-reinforced glass-ionomers, its aesthetics are very poor (it is grey) and it cannot be used in anterior locations, because of its lack of a match in either colour or translucency with the appearance of the natural tooth.

6.6 Porosity

Glass-ionomer cements always contain a degree of porosity as a consequence of the need to mix the powder with the liquid at the preparation stage. Porosity varies with mixing technique. Hand-mixed cements contain a wide variety of pore sizes, whereas auto-mixed materials tend to show smaller pore sizes but the same overall pore volume. The problem of these pores is that they may promote crack propagation and hence act as sources of weakness in the cement. On the other hand, reducing the total porosity by mixing at reduced pressure, though improving strength of the resulting set cement, produced stiffer pastes that were difficult to place in a small cavity. Overall, therefore, this inherent porosity seems to be an inevitable feature of glass-ionomers, and one that must be tolerated.

The overall amount of porosity and size of the pores have been shown to have a significant effect on the strength of a glass-ionomer cement [92]. A porosity of approximately 3.5% of the total cement volume has been reported for a hand-mixed cement [93] and in an experimental study in which pores were deliberately introduced, a reduction of 50% in the strength of a luting grade glass-ionomer was reported for a 3% additional porosity [94].

Studies of porosity have generally been concerned with microscopic pores, ie, ones that can be viewed at reasonable magnifications using an optical or a scanning electron microscope. This limits the detection to pores larger than about 7 μm in diameter. More recent studies based on X-ray imaging have revealed the existence of nano-pores, ranging in size from 2 to 400 nm [95]. Their existence was confirmed using nitrogen adsorption to measure specific surface areas of cement specimens [95]. Studies suggest that these pores become smaller in mature specimens, a result that correlates with the measured increase in mechanical strength [92,96]. The gradual reduction in pore size, including the size of the nano-pores, on maturation is an interesting finding and appears to be the consequence of the mobility of important chemical species within the newly formed cement. Such mobility is a feature of these materials that is only just being investigated, and the recently observed changes in pore morphology are a new mechanism to explain the improvements in the strength of glass-ionomers on maturation.

6.7 Fluoride release

The ability of glass-ionomer cements to release fluoride is considered one of their important advantages [1]. Fluoride release can be sustained for very long periods of time, with up to 5 years having been demonstrated experimentally for specimens kept under running tap water [97]. The pattern of fluoride release from a glass-ionomer is of an initial rapid release ('early burst'), followed by a sustained, lower level release that occurs by a diffusion mechanism [98–100]. These processes have been quantified and shown to follow the pattern described by the equation [101]:

$$[F]_c = ([F]_1 \cdot t)/(t + t_{1/2}) + \beta \sqrt{t}$$

In this equation $[F]_c$ represents the cumulative fluoride release at time t seconds, $[F]_1$ represents the total amount of fluoride available, t is the time and $t_{1/2}$ is the time taken for fluoride release to drop by a half, the so-called half-life of the release process. The initial term in $[F]_c$ covers the 'early burst' phase, though this has been found to last for a surprisingly long time, up to 4 weeks having been indicated by the data. The second term, $\beta\sqrt{t}$, in this equation represents the long-term diffusion part of the release process.

Fluoride release from glass-ionomers changes in low pH environments, and increases compared with release in neutral conditions [102]. In addition, release at low pH is associated with an increase in pH of the external medium, a process that has been termed buffering. The ability to buffer acids such as lactic acid in active caries may be clinically beneficial and is a potential mechanism for the protection of the tooth from further tooth decay [103].

Release of fluoride under acidic conditions is associated with the occurrence of fluoride in complexed form. Under acidic conditions, aluminium ions are released in greater quantities than under neutral conditions, and it may be that the fluoride becomes complexed as species such as AlF_4^- [104]. There is also the possibility of the formation of the complex HF_2^- with protons from the acid; or, indeed, of forming undissociated HF [105]. None of the possible complexes of fluoride (nor undissociated HF) yields free fluoride ions, so they are not detectable with fluoride-ion selective electrodes. Instead, fluoride must be decomplexed and released as F^- ions by the addition of total ionic solubility acid buffer.

Studies of the interaction of hydroxyapatite with the acid washings from glass-ionomer cements show that fluoride is taken up readily by the mineral phase, despite the initial state of fluoride as a complex ion or covalent species [106]. There was no concomitant uptake of aluminium by the hydroxyapatite, suggesting that any complexes formed are dissociated by the mineral phase, allowing only fluoride to be taken up.

These results suggest that the elevated levels of fluoride release by glass-ionomers at low pH will deliver increased amounts of fluoride to the mineral phase of the tooth, despite the occurrence of complex species prior to incorporation into the mineral phase [106].

Fluoride release in vivo is generally considered to be beneficial clinically, though unambiguous evidence in its favour is lacking. It is known, however, that a continuous supply of low levels of fluoride to the saliva affects the hard dental tissues [107] and that sustained concentrations of fluoride at the parts per million level are sufficient to inhibit dentine demineralization to a measurable extent [108]. Fluoride release may also reduce or even eliminate hypersensitivity of the hard tissues, thus reducing the perception of cold foods and beverages. Such levels of fluoride release from glass-ionomers appear achievable [109], though actual measured levels have been found to be lower in artificial saliva than in pure water [110], which suggests that extrapolating likely clinical release performance from in vitro studies using pure water may not be valid.

Fluoride is not only released from glass-ionomer cements, it is also taken up, at least in the early stages of a cement's existence. The possibility was originally proposed by Walls [111] and early experiments confirmed the idea. Typical experiments involved preparing two groups of cement specimens and storing one in dilute fluoride solution and the other in deionized water. After a suitable time period, typically 24 h, both sets of specimens were placed in fresh volumes of deionized water, and their fluoride release measured. Samples previously exposed to fluoride released significantly greater amounts of fluoride under these circumstances [112–114]. A similar study was carried out using a fluoride-free glass-ionomer cement formation, and the samples exposed to fluoride were shown to become fluoride-releasing [115].

These experiments all measured fluoride uptake indirectly, and in fact, direct measurement of fluoride uptake has been undertaken only very rarely. One study in which fluoride uptake was measured directly determined reduction in fluoride content in fluoride solutions into which specimens of glass-ionomer cement had been placed. This enabled to uptake kinetics to be determined, and the process in this case was shown to be a pseudo-first order process [116], as are many technically important interactions of active solids with aqueous solutions of ions.

In another study where uptake was measured directly, two important findings emerged. These were (i) that the bulk of the fluoride taken up was not released again, at least, not in 24 h exposure to deionized water, and (ii) that maturation affected fluoride uptake, so that 1-month-old specimens of the brands Ketac Molar Quick and Fuji IX Fast did not take any measurable fluoride at all [117]. These results suggest that fluoride recharge is a more complicated phenomenon than may reports suggest [118].

6.8 Bioactivity of glass-ionomers

Glass-ionomer cements have a degree of natural bioactivity. They release certain key ions into surrounding aqueous media, not only fluoride, but also sodium, aluminium, phosphate and silicate [103]. Under mildly acidic conditions, they release all of these ions in larger quantities than in neutral conditions, and also release calcium (or strontium), ionic species which are insoluble in neutral solutions but which dissolve at low pH. This ion release is associated with increases in the pH of the surrounding storage medium, the so-called buffering. The relationship between extent of buffering and ions released is complicated because a cement specimen can repeatedly buffer volumes of storage medium to the same value of pH, yet have differing ionic content.

The ions released are generally beneficial biologically [119]. Phosphate is present in saliva and in balance with the mineral phase of the tooth. Silicate can also become incorporated into the mineral phase without adversely affecting the mineral structure. Calcium is an essential mineral element, and the main counterion in hydroxyapatite, and it may be that the associated release of calcium and phosphate ions in low pH conditions, together with fluoride release, promotes remineralization of the tooth in the immediate vicinity of the low pH region.

The ability to exchange ions with the surroundings also applies to the solid tooth. As will be described in more detail in Section 5.9, at the interface between the glass-ionomer cement and the tooth surface, an ion-exchange layer develops, due to diffusion of ions from each surface. The result is a distinctive structure that can be viewed under the scanning electron microscope, and which results from the mobility of key ions [120]. This ion-rich layer seems to be very resistant to acid attack, and secondary caries is very rarely observed around glass-ionomer restorations.

Glass-ionomers not only release ions, but are capable of taking them up. Studies have shown that cements exposed to natural saliva take up calcium and phosphate ions, and develop a surface of significantly increased hardness [121]. Also, when used as pit and fissure sealants, they interact with saliva to form a substance with increased content of calcium and phosphate that is considerably more resistant to cutting with a dental drill than the original material. Under these circumstances, the cement had become transformed into a material with enamel-like optical and mechanical properties [122]. This observation is the basis of the development of glass-ionomer type materials with even further enhanced bioactivity, the so-called glass carbomers, which are discussed in Chapter 8.

6.9 Adhesion

The ability of glass-ionomers to form a natural adhesive bond to the surface of the tooth is one of these material's most important clinical advantages. They were originally prepared from poly(acrylic acid), a substance chosen because of its use in the zinc polycarboxylate cement, a material known to adhere to the tooth surface [123]. The advantages of adhesion by these materials were apparent right from the start, when they were used for the repair of cervical erosion lesions and as pit and fissure sealants [124,125].

Tensile bond strengths to untreated enamel and dentine have been found to be good [126,127], with values on enamel varying from 2.6 to 9.6 MPa and on dentine from 1.1 to 4.1 MPa. The fact that results typically show higher bond strengths to enamel than to dentine suggests that the main interaction of the cement is with the hydroxyapatite mineral phase, rather than with the collagen component [19]. Bond strengths are known to develop quickly, about 80% of the eventual bond strength being achieved after 15 min [127]. It then continues to increase for several days [128].

There are several steps in mechanism of adhesion by these cements. First of all, when the fresh cement paste is placed on the surface of the tooth, wetting takes place. This means that the cement forms an intimate contact with the surface, driven by the fact that both the cement and the surface are hydrophilic. The adhesion that develops rapidly has been attributed to the formation of hydrogen bonds originating from the free carboxyl groups in the cement interacting with tightly bound water on the surface of the mineral phase of the tooth [129]. These hydrogen bonds seem to be gradually replaced by true ionic bonds formed from cations in the tooth interacting with polymeric anions in the cement [129]. This suggestion is consistent with results that show that an ion-exchange layer is slowly formed between the tooth and the cement [120,130]. The possibility of strong bonds involving carboxylate groups from the poly(acrylic acid) was also suggested by results using infrared spectroscopy to study the bonded surface [131].

The role of collagen in the tooth structure on the adhesion of glass-ionomers is unclear, though the finding that tensile bonds are stronger to enamel than to dentine suggests that the most important bonds are formed with the mineral phase of the tooth. Based on these results, and also those of infrared spectroscopy, it has been suggested that bonding involves the hydroxyapatite phase of the tooth only, and that collagen has no role at all [131]. However, as collagen is a protein that contains both amino and carboxylic acid groups, the possibility of an interaction with carboxylate groups is high, so that at least some of the adhesion seems likely to be due to this [132]. However, on balance, the evidence suggests that any bonds of this type are not particularly important in the overall adhesion of glass-ionomers to the tooth [128].

In the clinic, bonding is enhanced by surface conditioning, ie, treating the freshly cut tooth with a solution of 37% aqueous poly(acrylic acid) acid for 10–20 s followed by rinsing [128,133]. This technique is mild, and essentially acts to remove the smear layer and open the dentinal tubules. It also partially demineralizes the tooth surface, leading to an increase is surface area and exposure of micro-porosities in the surface, which allow micro-mechanical attachment and also hybrid-later formation [134]. These effects are not visible to the naked eye, but occur only on the microscopic level. However, conditioning is essential to promote sound bonding by glass-ionomers. Studies using both transmission electron microscopy (TEM) and X-ray photo-electron spectroscopy (XPS) have shown that the poly(acrylic acid) used for conditioning is not completely removed by rinsing [135,136], but instead remains present as a thin layer (up to 0.5 μm) on the tooth surface. This layer has been referred to as the gel phase [134].

Adhesion of glass-ionomer cements appears to be the result of two inter-related phenomena. These are:

(a) *Micromechanical interlocking*. This is caused by the formation of a shallow hybrid layer in which the hydroxyapatite-coated collagen fibrils at the tooth surface form a hybrid layer with the surface of the freshly placed glass-ionomer restoration. This suggests that glass-ionomers are effectively self-etching as a consequence of the presence of the polyacid component.

(b) *True chemical bonding*. This involves ionic bonds between the carboxylate functional groups on the polyacid molecules and calcium ions in the hydroxyapatite surface [137]. Such bonding has been observed experimentally on hydroxyapatite [137] and also on enamel and dentine [138] using XPS. However, some care is needed in interpreting these results. XPS is a high vacuum technique and consequently either the hydroxyapatite or the tooth surface was likely to have been more strongly desiccated in these experiments than they are under clinical conditions.

In the longer term, there is a substantial change in the interface between a glass-ionomer cement and a restored tooth. This appears to be the result of a diffusion process in which ions from the cement and ions from the tooth surface travel into the interfacial zone to create an ion-exchange layer (Fig. 6.2) [120]. This layer is clearly visible under the scanning electron microscope and is evidence of a chemical union between the tooth and the glass-ionomer cement. The image shown in Fig. 6.2 comes from a study in which the strontium-based glass-ionomer cement Fuji IX was placed in a tooth and allowed to mature. The interaction zone that resulted was not only a physically obvious structure, but analysis showed that it contained both strontium and calcium. These ions originated, respectively, in the cement and the tooth surface, and obviously travelled towards each other to create the interfacial zone. The resulting layer binds the cement and tooth together firmly.

Bond strengths of glass-ionomer cements to teeth have generally been measured on immature specimens in vitro [139]. The use of such specimens and the limited duration of the experiments mean that the diffusion layer has not had time to develop fully, and so resulting bond strengths are low, especially compared with those of composite resin systems. As we have seen, higher values are found for enamel than for dentine [19]. Slightly higher values have been reported for bonding to caries-affected dentine, ie, up to 8.3 MPa [140] compared with unaffected dentine, but values are still lower than for composite systems. Despite these results, there is evidence that bonds formed by glass-ionomer cements are durable in clinical use, and this may be a reflection of the strength of the interfacial ion-exchange zone that forms [140].

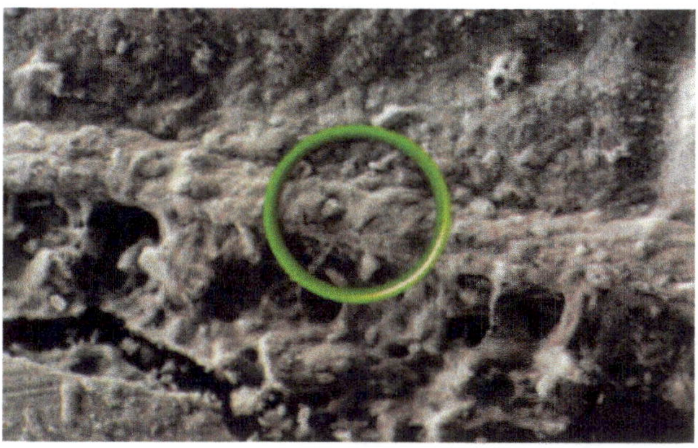

Fig. 6.2 Interfacial ion-exchange layer formed between tooth surface and glass-ionomer cement.

In vitro bonding studies typically show that failure of a glass-ionomer cement is cohesive, ie, occurs within the cement, rather than at the interface, which is adhesive failure [141]. This result is therefore not a measure of the true adhesive bond strength, but rather a measure of the tensile strength of the glass-ionomer material. This is low in immature specimens, and not representative of the final value that a fully matured cement is likely to have. The overall effect of these considerations is that determining the real strength of the adhesive bond formed by glass-ionomers to the tooth surface is difficult, and that values that have been quoted in the literature are almost certainly not the true strength of the adhesive bond formed.

Adhesion is significant because it not only aids the retention of glass-ionomer cements in the tooth, it also reduces the problem of marginal leakage and may eliminate it completely. Marginal leakage is a clinical problem because the gaps at the edges of restorations through which it occurs allow harmful micro-organisms to enter the space underneath the restoration. Their metabolism then gives rise to secondary caries below the restoration. Adhesion has been found to reduce this problem in in vitro studies [142–145].

6.10 Clinical applications of glass-ionomer cements

Glass-ionomers are used in a wide variety of clinical applications. They are generally considered to be inferior mechanically and aesthetically to composite resins, but they are nonetheless capable of being used as full restoratives and performing acceptably, especially in primary dentition.

Glass-ionomers have been classified into three types, depending on intended clinical use [19], and this remains a helpful system for describing uses and properties desired in the cement. The types are as follows:

Type I: Luting and bonding cements.

- Designed for cementation of crowns, bridges, inlays and orthodontic appliances.
- Relatively low powder:liquid ratio required (1.5:1 to 3.8:1), leading to set cements of moderate strength only.
- Fast setting with good early resistance to water.
- Radiopaque.

Type II: restorative cements.

There are two sub-divisions of Type II cements, depending on the importance of aesthetics.

For aesthetic (anterior) repairs, Type II (i):

- High powder:liquid ratio (at least 3:1, but up to 6.8:1).
- Excellent colour match and translucency.
- Protection needed from moisture for at least 24 h with varnish or petroleum jelly.
- Usually radiopaque.

For use where aesthetic considerations are not important (posterior repairs), Type II (ii):

- High powder:liquid ratio (3:1 to 4:1).
- Fast set and early resistance to water uptake.
- Radiopaque.

Type III: Lining or base cements
- Low powder:liquid ratio for liners (1.5:1) to allow good adaptation to the cavity walls.
- Higher powder:liquid ratio for bases (3:1 to 6.8:1), where base acts as a dentine substitute in the open sandwich technique in association with a composite resin.
- Radiopaque.

6.10.1 Pit and fissure sealants

Sealants are placed in pits and fissures of molars, either primary or permanent, in order to prevent the development of caries. By sealing a deep fissure in a newly erupted tooth, the space is filled and therefore cannot be occupied by plaque and pellicle [146]. This prevents caries in locations that are otherwise difficult to maintain in a clean and plaque-free condition.

Fissure sealing was first tried experimentally in the 1920s using amalgam as the sealant, but this procedure was never widely used in the profession [147]. Later, in the 1960s, unfilled resins based on cyanoacrylate chemistry were considered [148] but again without ever finding widespread use. It was not until the development of modern composite resins and glass-ionomers that fissure sealing became a widely used technique in clinical dentistry, as it continues to be, with particular emphasis on children's teeth. Glass-ionomer was first suggested for this purpose in 1977 [123], when it was shown that a properly formulated cement could successfully occlude fissures.

Since this time, there have been numerous studies to compare the clinical effectiveness of glass-ionomer cements with that of composite resin sealants. These have typically determined the relative retention rates, and they have usually found that glass-ionomer sealants show inferior performance [149]. However, when caries rate in teeth are compared it turns out that glass-ionomers are at least as effective as composite resins [150,151]. It has been suggested that this is due to retention of glass-ionomer cement deep within the fissure and also because of the fluoride release into the enamel prior to the loss of the bulk cement [1].

Glass-ionomers have other advantages over composites in this application, namely that they are hydrophilic and dimensionally stable. Their hydrophilic character enables them to absorb fluid that can be left at the bottom of the fissure without jeopardizing the adhesion to enamel. The dimensional stability is important because it allows the cement to retain its marginal adaption and seal, so that there is no risk of caries developing under the fissure sealing material. Fluoride release is also potentially advantageous.

More recent studies, using high-viscosity glass-ionomers, have reported significantly improved retention rates [123,152], so that they now compare favourably with those of composite sealants. There remains the fact that they are capable of conferring excellent protection against caries even following loss of most of the sealant and for this reason they continue to be used in this application.

6.10.2 Atraumatic restorative treatment technique

Glass-ionomers are the materials of choice for use in the atraumatic restorative treatment (ART) technique [153]. The technique was originally developed under the aegis of the World Health Organisation to provide dental care in low- and middle-income countries of the world. Typically in these countries, there is virtually no caries management and this can lead to serious physical and mental complications, especially in children. In these countries, toothache is generally dealt with by extraction of the offending tooth.

In addition to these features of lack of caries management and a ruthless policy of tooth extraction, low- and middle-income countries typically have unreliable or non-existent electrical power supplies. This means that electrically driven drills and burs cannot be used in routine clinical dentistry. The high price of such dental units is a further problem in low- and middle-income countries and contributes to their relative scarcity.

To address these issues, the ART technique has been developed and introduced to various countries throughout the world. It uses hand instruments to remove caries-affected dentine and enamel, and then employs high viscosity glass-ionomer cement to repair the tooth [154]. Glass-ionomer cement is used because of its adhesive properties, and the fact that the material can be applied to surfaces that have had only minimal preparation. The technique appears to be very successful, particularly in the repair of single-surface lesions. For example, in permanent teeth, after 2–3 years, success rates for Class I and Class V restorations have both been of the order of 90% [155]. ART has been widely used for children, who readily accept the treatment [156]. Overall, the technique has been responsible for the retention of many teeth that would otherwise have been extracted, and high viscosity glass-ionomers are important in achieving this overall success [157].

The ART technique can also be considered for dental practices in higher income countries, where it can be used for the treatment of children, especially those that are uncooperative. It can also be used for mentally handicapped patients and patients who have a phobia of the conventional dental drill.

Clinical summary

- Glass-ionomer cements are somewhat brittle and reasonably aesthetic materials for repairing teeth.
- They are acid–base materials and set by reaction between an aqueous solution of a polyalkenoic acid, such as poly(acrylic acid), with a special basic glass powder.
- The setting is a neutralization, which causes minimal shrinkage.
- Because of this setting reaction, glass-ionomers can be placed in full ('bulk fill') within a cavity.
- Glass-ionomers are adhesive to both enamel and dentine, so can be applied directly to the tooth surface after mild pre-treatment known as conditioning.
- Modern glass-ionomers have smaller particle size glasses and higher proportions of glass, and are sometimes called 'high-viscosity' glass-ionomers.
- Newly set glass-ionomers are susceptible to moisture loss, which causes surface crazing and the development of a 'chalky' appearance. This is overcome by applying a coating of varnish or petroleum jelly.
- Dental cure lamps have been used to assist cure of glass-ionomers, the effect being due to heating not the light which they emit.
- A wide range of repairs is possible with glass-ionomers, and they can be used as liners and bases, and as orthodontic adhesives.

- Glass-ionomers release fluoride, with a distinct pattern of high initial release ('early wash-out') and lower levels sustained release.
- Glass-ionomers are bioactive. They can buffer mouth acids (ie, shift their pH towards neutral) and also develop ion-exchange bonds with the tooth surface over time.
- Glass-ionomers are the material of choice for repairing teeth using the ART technique.

Clinical use of glass-ionomer cements

(i) Cavity preparation can be restricted to removal of caries and unsupported enamel only.
(ii) After cavity preparation, condition the cavity (remove the smear later) using a conditioning solution (typically 10% poly(acrylic acid) or 5% citric acid in water) using a cotton pellet saturated with conditioner placed in the cavity for 15–20 s, after which the surface is rinsed with water for 5 s, lightly dried but not dehydrated. This is achieved by swabbing with dry cotton pellets only.
(iii) In the case of deep caries, protect the pulpal floor with calcium hydroxide setting cement or zinc oxide-eugenol cement.
(iv) Mix the glass-ionomer cement according to the manufacturer's instructions. For hand-mixed cements, ensure that the correct powder:liquid ratio is used. For capsulated cements, ensure that mixing is carried out for the correct time.
(v) Completely fill the cavity in one portion, press the cement with an instrument or the finger until it has hardened, then remove excess using either hand instruments or a bur without water.
(vi) Cover the restoration with varnish, bonding agent or petroleum jelly, and where appropriate cure in accordance with manufacturer's instructions.
(vii) Check occlusion with articulation paper, and correct if necessary.
(viii) The patient should be asked not to eat and drink for 2 h after completion, and preferably to avoid biting on the tooth for 24 h.
(ix) If necessary, a final finishing of the restoration can be carried out after a minimum of 24 h following placement. This should use silicone rubber polishing discs and polishing pastes, and should be completed by further varnishing of the restoration.

References

[1] G.J. Mount, Color Atlas of Glass Ionomer Cement, second ed., Martin Dunitz, London, 2002.
[2] A.D. Wilson, J.W. Nicholson, Acid Base Cements, The University Press, Cambridge, 1993.
[3] A.D. Wilson, B.E. Kent, The glass-ionomer cement, a new translucent cement for dentistry, J. Appl. Chem. Biotechnol. 21 (1971) 313.
[4] W.J. MacKnight, T.R. Earnest Jr., The structure and properties of ionomers, J. Polym. Sci., Macromol. Rev. 16 (1981) 41–122.
[5] International Organization for Standardization, ISO 9917-1: Dental Water Based Cements, ISO, Geneva, Switzerland, 2003.
[6] J.W. McLean, J.W. Nicholson, A.D. Wilson, Guest Editorial: Proposed nomenclature for glass-ionomer dental cements and related materials, Quintessence Int. 25 (1994) 587–589.
[7] P.J. Knibbs, Glass-ionomer cement: ten years of clinical use, J. Oral Rehabil. 15 (1988) 103–115.
[8] A.D. Wilson, B.E. Kent, D. Clinton, R.P. Miller, The formation and microstructure of the dental silicate cement, J. Mater. Sci. 7 (1972) 220–238.

[9] A.D. Wilson, R.F. Batchelor, Dental silicate cements III. Environment and durability, J. Dent. Res. 47 (1968) 115–120.
[10] A.D. Wilson, R.F. Mesley, Dental silicate cements VI. Infrared studies, J. Dent. Res. 47 (1968) 644–652.
[11] A.D. Wilson, B.E. Kent, R.F. Mesley, R.P. Miller, D. Clinton, K.E. Fletcher, Formation of dental silicate cement, Nature 225 (1970) 272–273.
[12] B.E. Kent, A.D. Wilson, Dental silicate cements VIII. Acid–base aspect, J. Dent. Res. 48 (1969) 412–418.
[13] A.D. Wilson, B.E. Kent, Dental silicate cements, V. Electrical conductivity, J. Dent. Res. 47 (1968) 463–470.
[14] D.C. Smith, A new dental cement, Br. Dent. J. 125 (1968) 381–384.
[15] A.D. Wilson, A hard decade's work: steps in the invention of the glass-ionomer cement, J. Dent. Res. 75 (1996) 1723–1727.
[16] A.D. Wilson, Dental silicate cements VIII. Alternative liquid cement formers, J. Dent. Res. 47 (1968) 1133–1136.
[17] S. Crisp, A.D. Wilson, Reactions in glass ionomer cements. V. Effect of incorporating tartaric acid in the cement liquid, J. Dent. Res. 55 (1976) 1023–1031.
[18] S.B. Mitra, Adhesion to dentin and physical properties of a light-curable glass-ionomer liner/base, J. Dent. Res. 70 (1991) 72–74.
[19] A.D. Wilson, J.W. McLean, Glass-Ionomer Cement, Quintessence Publishing, Chicago, 1988.
[20] S. Crisp, B.E. Kent, B.G. Lewis, A.J. Ferner, A.D. Wilson, Glass ionomer cement formulations. II. The synthesis of novel polycarboxylic acids, J. Dent. Res. 59 (1980) 1055–1063.
[21] A.D. Wilson, S. Crisp, G. Abel, Characterization of glass-ionomer cements. 4. Effect of molecular weight on physical properties, J. Dent. 5 (1977) 117–120.
[22] A.D. Wilson, R.G. Hill, C.P. Warrens, B.G. Lewis, The influence of polymer molecular weight on some properties of glass-ionomer cements, J. Dent. Res. 68 (1989) 89–94.
[23] M.A. Fareed, A. Stamboulis, Nanoclay addition to conventional glass-ionomer cements: influence on properties, Eur. J. Dent. 8 (2014) 456–463.
[24] J.A. Williams, R.W. Billington, Increase in compressive strength of glass ionomer cements with respect to time periods of 1 day to 4 months, J. Oral Rehabil. 18 (1991) 475–479.
[25] J.W. Nicholson, F. Abiden, The effect of ageing in glass-ionomer cements prepared from acrylic/maleic acid copolymers, Biomaterials 18 (1997) 59–62.
[26] H.M. Anstice, J.W. Nicholson, Investigation of the post-hardening reaction in glass-ionomer cements based on poly(vinyl phosphonic acid), J. Mater. Sci. Mater. Med. 6 (1995) 420–423.
[27] A.D. Neve, V. Piddock, E.C. Combe, Development of novel dental cements. I. Formulation of aluminoborate glasses, Clin. Mater. 9 (1992) 7–12.
[28] M. Darling, R.G. Hill, Novel polyalkenoate [glass-ionomer] dental cements based on zinc silicate glasses, Biomaterials 15 (1994) 289–294.
[29] R.G. Hill, A.D. Wilson, Some structural aspects of glasses used in ionomer cements, Glass Technol. 29 (1988) 150–188.
[30] W.H. Zachariasen, The atomic arrangement in glass, J. Am. Chem. Soc. 54 (1932) 3841–3851.
[31] W. Lowenstein, The distribution of aluminium in the tetrahedral of silicates and aluminates, Am. Mineral. 39 (1954) 92–96.
[32] S.C. Griffin, R.G. Hill, Influence of glass composition on the properties of glass polyalkenoate cements. Part I: influence of aluminium to silicon ratio, Biomaterials 20 (1999) 1579–1586.

[33] E.A. Wasson, J.W. Nicholson, A study of the relationship between setting chemistry and properties of modified glass polyalkenoate cements, Br. Polym. J. 23 (1990) 179–183.
[34] E.A. Wasson, J.W. Nicholson, Studies in the setting of glass-ionomer cements, Clin. Mater. 7 (1991) 289–293.
[35] E. De Barra, R.G. Hill, Influence of glass composition on the properties of glass polyalkenoate cements. Part III: influence of fluorite content, Biomaterials 21 (2000) 563–569.
[36] S.C. Griffin, R.G. Hill, Influence of glass composition on the properties of glass polyalkenoate cements. Part IV: influence of fluorine content, Biomaterials 21 (2000) 693–698.
[37] A.D. Wilson, S. Crisp, H.J. Prosser, B.G. Lewis, S.A. Merson, Aluminosilicate glasses for polyelectrolyte cements, Ind. Eng. Chem. Prod. Res. Dev. 19 (1980) 263–270.
[38] J.F. Stebbins, S. Kroeker, S.K. Lee, T.J. Kiczenski, Quantification of five- and six-coordinated aluminium ions in aluminosilicate and fluoride-containing glasses by high-field, high-resolution Al-27 NMR, J. Non-Cryst. Solids 275 (2000) 1–6.
[39] A. Stamboulis, R.G. Hill, R.V. Law, Structural characterization of fluorine-containing glasses by F-19, Al-27, Si-29 and P-31 MAS-NMR spectroscopy, J. Non-Cryst. Solids 351 (2005) 3289–3295.
[40] A. Stamboulis, R.V. Law, R.G. Hill, Characterisation of commercial ionomer glasses using magic angle nuclear magnetic resonance (MAS-NMR), Biomaterials 25 (2004) 3907–3913.
[41] R.G. Hill, A. Stamboulis, R.V. Law, Characterisation of fluorine-containing glasses by F-19, Al-27, Si-29 and P-31 MAS-NMR spectroscopy, J. Dent. 34 (2006) 525–534.
[42] S. Matsuya, A. Stamboulis, R.G. Hill, R.V. Law, Structural characterization of ionomer glasses by multinuclear solid state MAS-NMR spectroscopy, J. Non-Cryst. Solids 353 (2007) 237–243.
[43] R. Hill, D. Wood, M. Thomas, Trimethylsilylation analysis of the silicate structure of fluoro-alumino-silicate glasses and the structural role of fluorine, J. Mater. Sci. 34 (1999) 1767–1774.
[44] C.M. Gorman, R.G. Hill, Heat-pressed ionomer glass-ceramics. Part II. Mechanical property evaluation, Dent. Mater. 20 (2004) 252–261.
[45] J.F. Stebbin, Q. Zeng, Cation ordering at fluorite sites in silicate glasses; a high-resolution F-19 NMR study, J. Non-Cryst. Solids 262 (2000) 1–5.
[46] A. Stamboulis, F. Wang, Ionomer glasses: design and characterisation, in: D.S. Katti, A. Kumar (Eds.), Advanced Biomaterials: Fundamentals, Processing and Applications, American Ceramic Society, Ohio, USA, 2009 (Chapter 12).
[47] S. Shahid, U. Hassan, R.W. Billington, R.G. Hill, P. Anderson, Glass ionomer cements: effect of strontium substitution on esthetics, radiopacity and fluoride release, Dent. Mater. 30 (2014) 308–313.
[48] A.D. Neve, V. Piddock, E.C. Combe, The effect of glass heat treatment on the properties of a novel polyalkenoate cement, Clin. Mater. 12 (1993) 113–115.
[49] A.D. Neve, V. Piddock, E.C. Combe, Development of novel dental cements. II. Cement properties, Clin. Mater. 9 (1992) 13–20.
[50] M.J. Bertolini, R.G. Palma-Gibb, M.A. Zaghete, R. Gimenes, Evaluation of glass ionomer cements properties obtained from niobium silicate glasses prepared by chemical process, J. Non-Cryst. Solids 351 (2005) 466–471.
[51] P.V. Hatton, K. Hurrell-Gillingham, I.M. Brook, Biocompatibility of glass-ionomer bone cements, J. Dent. 34 (2006) 598–601.
[52] K. Hurrell-Gillingham, I.M. Reaney, I. Brook, P.V. Hatton, In vitro biocompatibility of a novel Fe_2O_3 based glass ionomer cement, J. Dent. 34 (2006) 533–538.

[53] D. Boyd, A. Wren, O.M. Clarkin, M.R. Towler, Zinc-based glass polyalkenoate cements with improved setting times and mechanical properties, Acta Biomater. 4 (2008) 425–431.
[54] J.W. Akitt, N.N. Greenwood, G.D. Lester, Nuclear magnetic resonance and Raman studies of aluminium complexes formed in aqueous solutions of aluminium salts containing phosphoric acids and fluoride ions, J. Chem. Soc. A (1971) 2450–2457.
[55] P.J. Potts, Handbook of Silicate Rock Analysis, Blackie and Son, Glasgow and London, 1987.
[56] H.J. Prosser, C.P. Richards, A.D. Wilson, NMR spectroscopy of dental materials. II. The role of tartaric acid in glass-ionomer cements, J. Biomed. Mater. Res. 16 (1982) 431–445.
[57] J.W. Nicholson, P.J. Brookman, O.M. Lacy, A.D. Wilson, The influence of (+)-tartaric acid on the setting of glass-ionomer dental cements, J. Dent. Res. 67 (1988) 1451–1454.
[58] P.J. Kay, F.E. Treloar, The intrinsic viscosity of poly(acrylic acid) at different ionic strengths: random coil and rigid rod behaviour, Die Makromol. Chem. 175 (1974) 3207–3223.
[59] S. Crisp, A.D. Wilson, Reactions in glass ionomer cements. III. The precipitation reaction, J. Dent. Res. 53 (1974) 1420–1424.
[60] S. Crisp, M.A. Pringuer, D. Wardleworth, A.D. Wilson, Reactions in glass-ionomer cements: II. An infrared spectroscopic study, J. Dent. Res. 53 (1974) 1414–1419.
[61] L.H. Prentice, M.J. Tyas, M.F. Burrow, Ion leaching of a glass-ionomer glass: an empirical model and effects on setting characteristics and strength, J. Mater. Sci. Mater. Med. 18 (2007) 127–131.
[62] W.D. Cook, Degradative analysis of glass-ionomer polyelectrolyte cements, J. Biomed. Mater. Res. 17 (1983) 1015–1017.
[63] R.A. Pires, T.G. Nunes, I. Abrahams, G.E. Hawkes, The role of aluminium and silicon in the setting chemistry of glass ionomer cements, J. Mater. Sci. Mater. Med. 19 (2008) 1687–1692.
[64] R. Pires, T.G. Nunes, I. Abrahams, G.E. Hawkes, C.M. Morais, C. Fernandez, Stray-field imaging and multinuclear magnetic resonance spectroscopy studies on the setting of a commercial glass-ionomer cement, J. Mater. Sci. Mater. Med. 15 (2004) 201–208.
[65] N. Zainuddin, N. Karpukhina, R.G. Hill, R.V. Law, A long-term study on the setting reaction of glass ionomer cements by ^{27}Al MAS-NMR spectroscopy, Dent. Mater. 25 (2009) 290–295.
[66] S. Matsuya, T. Maeda, M. Ohta, IR and NMR analysis of hardening and maturation of glass-ionomer cement, J. Dent. Res. 75 (1996) 1920–1927.
[67] E.A. Wasson, J.W. Nicholson, New aspects of the setting of glass-ionomer cements, J. Dent. Res. 72 (1993) 481–483.
[68] J.W. Nicholson, H. Tawfik, B. Czarnecka, Cements made from lactic acid and ion-leachable glasses, J. Mater. Sci. Mater. Med. 13 (2002) 417–419.
[69] S. Shahid, R.W. Billington, G.J. Pearson, The role of glass composition in the glass acetic acid and glass lactic acid cements, J. Mater. Sci. Mater. Med. 19 (2008) 541–545.
[70] S.C. Bovis, E. Harrington, H.J. Wilson, Setting characteristics of composite filling materials, Br. Dent. J. 131 (1971) 352–356.
[71] W.D. Cook, P. Brocklehurst, The oscillating rheometer – what does it measure? J. Dent. Res. 59 (1980) 795–799.
[72] J.W. Nicholson, Studies in the setting of polyelectrolyte materials, Part 3: effect sodium salts on the setting and properties of glass polyalkenoate and zinc polycarboxylate dental cements, J. Mater. Sci. Mater. Med. 6 (1995) 404–408.

[73] J.W. Nicholson, Chemistry of glass-ionomer cements: a review, Biomaterials 6 (1998) 485–494.
[74] T.I. Barry, D.J. Clinton, A.D. Wilson, The structure of a glass-ionomer cement and its relationship to the setting process, J. Dent. Res. 58 (1979) 1072–1079.
[75] G.W. Neilson, J.E. Enderby, in: The Coordination of Metal Aquaions, vol. 34, Academic Press, Orlando, 1989, pp. 195–218.
[76] A. Ikegami, Hydration and ion binding of polyelectrolytes, J. Polym. Sci. A 2 (1964) 907–921.
[77] M. Satoh, J. Komiyama, A new model of counterion condensation in polyelectrolyte solutions, I. Applications to potentiometric titration of weak acids, Polym. J. 19 (1987) 1201–1208.
[78] A.D. Wilson, S. Crisp, J.M. Paddon, Hydration of a glass-ionomer (ASPA) cement, Br. Polym. J. 13 (1981) 66–70.
[79] J.W. Nicholson, B. Czarnecka, Kinetic studies of water uptake and loss in glass-ionomer cements, J. Mater. Sci. Mater. Med. 19 (2008) 1723–1727.
[80] L.T. Zhuravlev, The surface chemistry of amorphous silica. Zhuravlev model, Colloids Surf A Physicochem. Eng Asp. 173 (2000) 1–38.
[81] D. Tadjiev, R.J. Hand, Surface hydration and nano-indentation of silicate glasses, J. Non-Cryst. Solids 356 (2010) 102–108.
[82] J.W. Nicholson, B. Czarnecka, Kinetic studies of the effect of varnish on water loss by glass-ionomer cements, Dent. Mater. 23 (2007) 1549–1552.
[83] M.A. Fareed, A. Stamboulis, Nanoclay addition to a conventional glass ionomer cements: influence on physical properties, Eur. J. Dent. 8 (2014) 456–463.
[84] B. Czarnecka, J.W. Nicholson, Kinetic studies of the effect of varnish on water loss by glass-ionomer cements, Dent. Mater. 23 (2007) 1549–1552.
[85] M.S.A. Earl, G.J. Mount, W.R. Hume, Effect of varnishes and other surface treatments on water movement across the glass-ionomer cement surface II, Aust. Dent. J. 34 (1989) 326–329.
[86] E.A. Wasson, J.W. Nicholson, Effect of operator skill in determining the physical properties of glass-ionomer cements, Clin. Mater. 15 (1994) 169–173.
[87] W.J. Higgs, P. Lucksanasombool, R.J.E.D. Higgs, M.V. Swain, Evaluating acrylic and glass-ionomer cement strength using the biaxial flexure test, Biomaterials 22 (2001) 1583–1590.
[88] G.J. Mount, O.F. Makinson, M.C.R.B. Peters, The strength of auto-cured and light-cured materials. The shear punch test, Aust. Dent. J. 41 (1996) 118–123.
[89] N.K. Sarkar, Metal-matrix interface in reinforced glass ionomers, Dent. Mater. 14 (1999) 421–425.
[90] E.S. Gjorgievska, G. van Tendaloo, J.W. Nicholson, N.J. Coleman, I.J. Slipper, S.E. Booth, The incorporation of nano-particles into conventional glass ionomer dental restorative cements, Microsc. Microanal. 21 (2015) 1–15.
[91] J.W. McLean, Cermet cements, J. Am. Dent. Assoc. 120 (1990) 43–47.
[92] D. Xie, W.A. Brantley, B.M. Culbertson, G. Wang, Mechanical properties and microstructures of glass-ionomer cements, Dent. Mater. 17 (2001) 456–470.
[93] B.W. Burtenshaw, V. Piddock, Porosity in water-based dental luting cement, J. Mater. Sci. Mater. Med. 4 (1993) 415–417.
[94] R. Nomoto, M. Komoriyama, J.F. McCabe, S. Hirano, Effect of mixing method on the porosity of encapsulated glass ionomer cement, Dent. Mater. 20 (2004) 972–978.
[95] A.R. Benetti, J. Jacobsen, B. Lehnoff, N.C.R. Momsen, D.V. Okhrimenko, M.T.F. Telling, N. Kardjilov, M. Strobl, T. Seydel, I. Manke, H.N. Bordallo, How mobile are protons in the structure of dental glass ionomer cements? Sci. Rep. 5 (2015). Article 8972.

[96] R.G. Hill, The fracture properties of glass polyalkenoate cements as a function of cement age, J. Mater. Sci. 28 (1993) 3851–3858.
[97] L. Forsten, Short- and long-term fluoride release from glass ionomers, Scand. J. Dent. Res. 99 (1991) 241–245.
[98] A.D. Wilson, D.M. Groffman, A.T. Kuhn, The release of fluoride and other chemical species from a glass-ionomer cement, Biomaterials 6 (1985) 431–433.
[99] W.M. Tay, M. Braden, Fluoride ion diffusion from polyalkenoate (glass-ionomer) cements, Biomaterials 9 (1988) 454–459.
[100] A.M. De Witte, E.A. De Maeyer, R.M.H. Verbeeck, L.C. Martens, Fluoride release profiles of mature restorative glass ionomer cements after fluoride application, Biomaterials 21 (2000) 475–482.
[101] R.G.J. De Moor, R.M.H. Verbeeck, E.A.P. De Maeyer, Fluoride release profiles of restorative glass ionomer formulations, Dent. Mater. 12 (1996) 88–95.
[102] S.M. Mousavinasab, I. Meyers, Fluoride release and uptake by glass-ionomer cements, compomers and giomers, Res. J. Biol. Sci. 4 (2009) 609–616.
[103] J.W. Nicholson, B. Czarnecka, H. Limanowska-Shaw, The long term interaction of dental cements with lactic acid solutions, J. Mater. Sci. Mater. Med. 10 (1999) 449–452.
[104] G.E. Jackson, The existence of AlF_4^- in aqueous solution and its relevance to phosphorylase reaction, Inorg. Chim. Acta 151 (1988) 273–276.
[105] G. Nagy, L. Nagy, in: L.M.L. Nollet (Ed.), Handbook of Water Analysis, second ed., CRC Press, Boca Raton, FL, 2007, pp. 157–200 (Chapter 6).
[106] S.M. Lewis, B. Czarnecka, N.J. Coleman, J.W. Nicholson, Interaction of aluminium fluoride complexes derived from glass-ionomer cements with hydroxyapatite, Ceram. Silikaty 57 (2013) 196–200.
[107] J.D. Featherstone, Prevention and reversal of dental caries: role of low level fluoride, Community Dent. Oral Epidemiol. 27 (1999) 31–40.
[108] J. Hicks, F. Garcia-Gody, C. Flaitz, Biological factors in dental caries: role of remineralization and fluoride in the dynamic process of demineralization and remineralization (part 3), J. Clin. Pediatr. Dent. 28 (2004) 203–214.
[109] H. Hsu, G. Huang, H. Chang, Y. Hang, M. Guo, A continuous flow system for assessing fluoride release/uptake of fluoride-containing restorative materials, Dent. Mater. 20 (2004) 740–749.
[110] B.F. El Mallak, N.K. Sarker, Fluoride release from glass ionomer cements in deionised water and artificial saliva, Dent. Mater. 6 (1990) 118–122.
[111] A.W.G. Walls, Glass polyalkenoate (glass-ionomer) cements: a review, J. Dent. 14 (1986) 231–246.
[112] S.L. Creanor, L.M.C. Carruthers, W.P. Saunders, R. Strang, R.H. Foye, Fluoride uptake and release characteristics of glass ionomer cements, Caries Res. 28 (1994) 322–328.
[113] P. Weidlich, L.A. Miranda, M. Maltz, S.M.W. Samuel, Fluoride release and uptake from glass ionomer cements and composite resin, Braz. Dent. J. 11 (2000) 89–92.
[114] W. Gao, R.J. Smales, Fluoride release/uptake of conventional and resin-modified glass-ionomers and compomers, J. Dent. 29 (2001) 301–306.
[115] R.W. Billington, P.C. Hadley, M.R. Towler, G.J. Pearson, J.A. Williams, Effects of adding sodium and fluoride ions to glass ionomer on its interactions with sodium fluoride solution, Biomaterials 21 (2000) 377–383.
[116] K. Pawluk, S.E. Booth, N.J. Coleman, J.W. Nicholson, The kinetics of fluoride uptake by immature glass-ionomer dental cements, Dent. Forum 36 (2008) 11–14.
[117] B. Czarnecka, J.W. Nicholson, Maturation affects fluoride uptake by glass-ionomer dental cements, Dent. Mater. 28 (2012) e1–e5.

[118] F. Arbabzadek-Zavareh, T. Gibbs, I.A. Meyers, M. Bouzari, S. Mortazavi, L.J. Walsh, Recharge pattern of contemporary glass ionomer restoratives, Dent. Res. J. (Isfahan) 9 (2012) 139–145.

[119] J.W. Nicholson, J.H. Braybrook, E.A. Wasson, The biocompatibility of glass-ionomer cements: a review, J. Biomater. Sci. Polym. Ed. 2 (1991) 277–285.

[120] N.G. Ngo, G.J. Mount, M.C.R.B. Peters, A study of glass-ionomer cement and its interface with enamel and dentin using a low-temperature, high-resolution scanning electron microscopic technique, Quintessence Int. 28 (1997) 63–69.

[121] K. Okada, S. Tosaki, K. Hirota, W.R. Hume, Surface hardness change of restorative filling materials stored in saliva, Dent. Mat. 17 (2001) 34–39.

[122] R.N.B. Van Duinen, C.L. Davidson, A. de Gee, A.J. Feilzer, In situ transformation of glass-ionomer into an enamel-like material, Am. J. Dent. 17 (2004) 223–227.

[123] J.W. McLean, A.D. Wilson, Fissure sealing and filling with an adhesive glass-ionomer cement, Br. Dent. J. 136 (1974) 269–276.

[124] J.W. McLean, A.D. Wilson, The clinical development of the glass-ionomer cement. II. Some clinical applications, Aust. Dent. J. 22 (1977) 120–127.

[125] J.W. McLean, A.D. Wilson, The clinical development of the glass-ionomer cement. III. The erosion lesion, Aust. Dent. J. 22 (1977) 190–195.

[126] P.R. Perondi, P.H.C. Oliveira, A. Cassoni, A.F. Reis, J.A. Rodrigues, Ultimate tensile strength and microhardness of glass ionomer materials, Braz. Dent. Sci. 17 (2014) 16–22.

[127] J.W. McLean, A.D. Wilson, The clinical development of the glass-ionomer cement. I. Formulations and properties, Aust. Dent. J. 22 (1977) 31–36.

[128] D.R. Powis, T. Folleras, S.A. Merson, A.D. Wilson, Improved adhesion of a glass ionomer cement to dentin and enamel, J. Dent. Res. 61 (1982) 1416–1422.

[129] A.D. Wilson, Alumino-silicate polyacrylic acid cement, Br. Polym. J. 6 (1974) 165–179.

[130] N. Hien-Chi, G. Mount, J. McIntyre, J. Tuisuva, R.J. Von Doussa, Chemical exchange between glass-ionomer restorations and residual carious dentine in permanent molars: an in vivo study, J. Dent. 34 (2006) 608–613.

[131] D.R. Beech, Improvement in the adhesion of polyacrylate cements to human dentine, Br. Dent. J. 135 (1973) 442–445.

[132] M. Brannstrom, Pretreatment before the placement of restorations, in: Dentin and Pulp in Restorative Dentistry, Dental Therapeutics, Nacka, Sweden, 1981.

[133] T.E. Long, E.S. Duke, B.K. Norling, Polyacrylic acid cleaning of dentin and glass ionomer bond strengths, J. Dent. Res. 65 (Special issue) (1986) 345. Abstract 1583.

[134] B. Van Meerbeek, Y. Yoshida, S. Inoue, J. De Munck, K. van Landuyt, P. Lambrechts, Glass-ionomer adhesion: the mechanisms at the interface, J. Dent. 34 (2006) 615–617.

[135] B. Van Meerbeek, Y. Yoshida, S. Inoue, R. Fukada, M. Okazaki, P. Lambrechts, G. Vanherle, Interfacial characterization of resin-modified glass-ionomers to dentin, J. Dent. Res. 80 (2001) 739. Abstract 1701.

[136] B. Van Meerbeek, Y. Yoshida, J. De Munck, S. Inoue, M. Vargas, P. Lambrechts, G. Vanherle, in: J. Tagami (Ed.), Self-etching Primer: Current Status and Its Evolution, Proceedings of the International Symposium '01 in Tokyo, Dental Materials Department, Kuraray Medical Inc., Tokyo, 2003, pp. 41–55.

[137] R. Fukada, Y. Yoshida, Y. Nakayama, M. Okazaki, S. Inoue, H. Sano, H. Shintani, J. Snauwaert, B. Van Meerbeek, Bonding efficacy of polyalkenoic acids to hydroxyapatite, enamel and dentin, Biomaterials 24 (2003) 1861–1867.

[138] Y. Yoshida, B. Van Meerbeek, Y. Nakayama, J. Snauwaert, L. Hellmans, P. Lambrechts, G. Vanherle, K. Wakasa, Evidence of chemical bonding at biomaterial-hard tissue interfaces, J. Dent. Res. 79 (2000) 709–714.

[139] R.G. Palma-Dibb, C.G. de Castro, R.P. Ramos, D.T. Chimello, M.A. Chinelatti, Bond strength of glass-ionomer cements to caries-affected dentin, J. Adhes. Dent. 5 (2003) 52–62.
[140] G.J. Mount, Longevity in glass-ionomer restorations: review of a successful technique, Quintessence Int. 28 (1997) 643–650.
[141] P.O. Glantz, Adhesion to teeth, Int. Dent. J. 27 (1977) 324–332.
[142] A. Maldonado, M.L. Swartz, R.W. Phillips, An in vitro study of certain properties of a glass-ionomer cement, J. Am. Dent. Assoc. 96 (1978) 785–791.
[143] J.H. Hembree, J.T. Andrews, Microleakage of several class V anterior restorative materials, J. Am. Dent. Assoc. 97 (1978) 179–183.
[144] E.A.M. Kidd, Cavity sealing ability of composite resin and glass ionomer restorations: an assessment in vitro, Br. Dent. J. 144 (1978) 139–142.
[145] D.R. Powis, Unpublished report, 1986, cited in Wilson and McLean [131].
[146] J.A. Weintraub, The effectiveness of pit and fissure sealants, J. Public Health Dent. 49 (1989) 317–330.
[147] J. Avinash, C.M. Marya, S. Dhingra, P. Gupta, S. Kataria, Meenu, H.P. Bhatia, Pit and fissure sealants: an unused caries prevention tool, J. Oral Health Comm. Dent. 4 (2010) 1–6.
[148] E.I. Cueto, M.G. Buonocore, Sealing of pits and fissures with an adhesive resin: its use in caries prevention, J. Am. Dent. Assoc. 75 (1967) 121–128.
[149] S. Kervanto-Seppala, E. Lavonius, I. Pietila, J. Pitkaniemi, J.H. Meuman, E. Kerosuo, Comparing the caries-preventive effect of two fissure sealing modalities in public health care: a single application of glass ionomer and a routine resin-based sealant programme. A randomized split-mouth clinical trial, Int. J. Paediatr. Dent. 18 (2008) 56–61.
[150] V. Yengopal, S. Mickenautsch, A.C. Bezerra, S.C. Leal, Caries-preventive effect of glass ionomer and resin-based fissure sealants on permanent teeth: a meta-analysis, J. Oral Sci. 51 (2009) 373–382.
[151] F. Barja-Fidalgo, S. Maroun, B.H. de Oliveira, Effectiveness of a glass ionomer used as a pit and fissure sealant in recently erupted permanent first molars, J. Dent. Child. (Chicago) 76 (2009) 34–40.
[152] M.C. Morales-Chavez, Z.C. Nualart-Grollmus, Retention of a resin-based sealant and a glass ionomer used as a fissure sealant in children with special needs, J. Clin. Exp. Dent. 6 (2014) e551–e555.
[153] J.E. Frencken, S.C. Leal, M.F. Navarro, Twenty-five-year atraumatic restorative treatment (ART) approach: a comprehensive overview, Clin. Oral Invest. 16 (2012) 1337–1346.
[154] J.E. Frencken, The ART approach using glass-ionomers in relation to global oral health care, Dent. Mater. 26 (2010) 1–6.
[155] R.J. Smales, H.K. Yip, The atraumatic restorative treatment (ART) approach for the management of dental caries, Quintessence Int. 33 (2002) 427–432.
[156] R.J. Smales, H.K. Yip, The atraumatic restorative treatment (ART) approach for primary teeth: review of the literature, Pediatr. Dent. 22 (2000) 294–298.
[157] J.E. Frencken, C.J. Holmgren, Atraumatic Restorative Treatment (ART) Approach for Dental Caries, STI Books, Nijmegen, 1999.

Resin-modified glass-ionomer cements

7

7.1 Introduction

Resin-modified glass-ionomers are materials that fall within the glass-ionomer family in that they contain basic glass, water and an acidic polymer and are capable of setting by an acid–base reaction [1]. They also contain a resin component (ie, a monomer) and the ingredients necessary to cause these to undergo polymerization. Various terms have been used to describe them, including 'light-cured glass-ionomers', 'dual-cured glass-ionomers', and quite unacceptably, 'resin-reinforced glass-ionomers', but the preferred term is the one applied to this type of material in the earliest patent on them [2], namely 'resin-modified glass-ionomers'.

As for conventional glass-ionomers, there are problems with the 'glass-ionomer' part of the term. For this reason, the strictly correct nomenclature for these materials is resin-modified glass polyalkenoate [1]. However, the trivial name of 'resin-modified glass-ionomer' is correct, and is widely used and accepted. It is the term that we shall use throughout this chapter, and which is preferred in the profession.

The reason that the designation 'resin-modified' is preferred to 'light-cured' (or 'light-curable') is that these latter terms incorrectly imply that the characteristic acid–base reaction is initiated by irradiation with light. It should be noted, however, that unfortunately this term has been widely used for these materials, including in the first two scientific papers describing the properties of the first commercially successful formulation [3,4]. The option 'dual-cure' is rendered inappropriate because of the possibility of 'tri-cure' formulations, where the monomer is polymerized both by photo-initiators and two-component free radical initiators, both of which complement the acid–base cure process. Consequently, it is possible in principle to have a 'dual-cure' material in which there is no acid–base reaction, and the system is not a glass-ionomer at all.

Finally, the term 'resin-reinforced' is completely unacceptable because the resulting materials are not in any meaningful sense reinforced. They are not, in general, stronger than conventional (resin-free) glass-ionomers. The word 'reinforced' simply cannot be appropriated in this way, and its meaning changed so radically.

As a result of these considerations, the term 'resin-modified' has become the most widely used in the literature on these materials, and is widely used for commercial materials. This does not mean that there are not occasional uses of the alternatives; but there is no justification for these terms, and their use really should discontinue completely.

For any of the materials to be considered to be glass-ionomers, it is essential that the acid–base reaction contributes to the setting process of the cement [1]. This means that for a formulation to be considered a resin-modified glass-ionomer, it should contain

Materials for the Direct Restoration of Teeth. http://dx.doi.org/10.1016/B978-0-08-100491-3.00007-6

sufficient numbers of acid-functional groups on the polymer to react significantly with the basic glass filler, and for that setting to occur in a reasonable time. In the past, materials were available that were marketed as 'light-cured glass-ionomers' that did not undergo such acid–base reaction, and which probably contained no acid-functional polymer. This latter feature is not known for certain, though, given that the full details of proprietary formulations are not generally reported in the open literature. However, it seems likely as the materials in question would not cure away from light, suggesting that there was no reaction to supplement the light-initiated polymerization reaction.

An essential feature of genuine resin-modified glass-ionomers is that they undergo some sort of acid–base reaction and therefore will set in the dark. Such setting must be caused only be the acid–base reaction, not by a two-part polymerization process analogous to those which occur in two-paste composite resins. Where an acid–base reaction occurs, it is slower than the light-initiated reaction and results in a cement with inferior mechanical properties. Dark-curing on its own is not sufficient to confirm that a material is a resin-modified glass-ionomer, but failure to set in the dark is proof that the material is not any sort of glass-ionomer cement [1].

Having established the essential features of resin-modified glass-ionomers, in the rest of the chapter we consider their composition, properties and clinical applications in modern clinical practice.

7.2 Composition of resin-modified glass-ionomers

The essential feature of resin-modified glass-ionomers is that they include polymerizable components with an acid–base system [2–4]. They therefore comprise a complex blend of components, as follows:

(i) An ion-leachable (basic) glass powder.
(ii) A polymeric acid, either poly(acrylic acid) or acrylic/maleic acid copolymer.
(iii) A monomer, typically 2-hydroxyethyl methacrylate, HEMA (Fig. 7.1), which is water soluble and capable of undergoing rapid free radical addition polymerization to create part of the matrix of the set cement–polymeric matrix.
(iv) Possibly a polymerizable side chain grafted onto the polymeric acid molecules that are capable of undergoing addition polymerization with the HEMA and thereby becoming incorporated into the set matrix.
(v) Water.

Resin-modified glass-ionomers can thus be seen to contain more components than conventional glass-ionomers. They set by a number of competing reactions between these components, and these reactions are influenced by each other in complex ways.

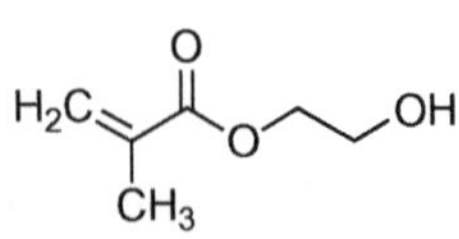

Fig. 7.1 The monomer 2-hydroxyethyl methacrylate, HEMA.

They result in a set material with a complicated interlocking structure [5]. Their individual components are considered in detail in this section of the chapter and the interactions that result in setting are considered in Section 7.3.

7.2.1 Glasses for resin-modified glass-ionomers

The glasses employed in resin-modified glass-ionomer cements are essentially the same as those used in conventional glass-ionomers. Their key requirement is that they are basic in character. They are therefore capable of reacting with the acidic polymer component to form ionically crosslinked polymeric salts that are structurally rigid and insoluble in aqueous media. The details of the composition and structure of these glasses are discussed in Chapter 6, and the methods used to optimize their reactivity are explained. For resin-modified glass-ionomers, glasses of the alumino-silicate type, either calcium- or strontium-based, with added phosphate, are also suitable, and these are the glasses used in these cements. If modifications in reactivity are needed for optimal clinical performance, reactivity may be altered slightly by the manufacturers, but any resulting differences from glasses used in conventional glass-ionomers are minor. Essentially the glass component does not differ in any significant way in conventional or resin-modified glass-ionomers.

7.2.2 The acidic polymer component

As in conventional glass-ionomers, the acidic component in resin-modified glass-ionomers is either poly(acrylic acid) or acrylic/maleic acid copolymer. In many brands, this polymer is simply blended with the monomer HEMA in aqueous solution. However, in certain brands, the polymeric acid is modified with side chains that allow it to participate in the addition polymerization process and thereby form a copolymer network with the HEMA.

Although the main acidic polymers used in resin-modified glass-ionomers are the same as in conventional glass-ionomers, they behave differently due to the presence of the HEMA component [6]. In particular, HEMA seems to affect the spatial arrangement of the polymers in solution, which in turn affects their acidity. These effects lead to a slower acid–base reaction than in conventional glass-ionomers.

The effect of HEMA on the conformation of poly(acrylic acid) or acrylic/maleic acid copolymer has not been studied in detail, but its effect in glass-ionomers has been compared with that of methanol, whose influence on the extent of coiling of poly(acrylic acid) molecules in solution has been studied [7]. Methanol is a less effective solvent than water for poly(acrylic acid), so that where it partly replaces water in a solvent system, it causes the poly(acrylic acid) molecules to coil more tightly in solution than they do in pure water [7]. This, in turn, means the system is closer to undergoing phase separation than it is in pure water.

The experiments on the effect of methanol on poly(acrylic acid) in solution were carried out at low concentrations, in the so-called 'semi-dilute' region [7]. However, the effects observed almost certainly happen at the higher concentrations used in practical poly(acrylic acid) solutions for preparing glass-ionomer cements. When included in

Table 7.1 Effect of organic compounds on the working and setting times of a water-activated conventional glass-ionomer cement [6]

Liquid component	Working time (min)	Setting time (min)
Water	3.6 (0.1)	9.1 (0.6)
Water/methanol: 50/50	12.8 (1.3)	28.0 (2.4)
Water/HEMA: 50/50	6.6 (0.4)	19.1 (0.1)

Standard deviations in parentheses.

a glass-ionomer cement formulation, methanol was found to reduce the rate of the acid–base reaction, an effect that is consistent with the polyacid molecules adopting a more tightly coiled conformation [6]. The tighter the coiling, the harder it is to ionize the polyacid, which means that its acidity will be reduced. This reduced acidity causes the setting to occur more slowly (see Table 7.1).

HEMA has been shown to have similar effects to methanol on the rate of setting of the conventional glass-ionomer cement, so can be assumed to cause the same effect on the coiled structure of the polyacid molecules [6]. In addition, as can be seen in Table 7.1, the compressive strengths of the resulting cements are reduced. This reduction is significant compared with cements containing only water as solvent ($p < 0.01$). However, as the difference between HEMA and methanol is also significant (also to $p < 0.01$), results show that HEMA has less effect than methanol. Compressive strengths in the presence of the organic additives did not differ significantly, though both gave significantly weaker cements ($p < 0.01$) than the original conventional glass-ionomer cement [6].

As noted earlier, some brands of resin-modified glass-ionomer contain chemically modified polyacid molecules [3,4]. These are prepared by reacting a minority of carboxylic acid-functional groups with either amine- or alcohol-terminated molecules that also contain a double bond (vinyl group) [8]. The resulting side chains are sufficiently long and flexible that the vinyl groups can react with HEMA during the addition polymerization phase of the setting process. In other words, they effectively copolymerize with the HEMA.

There do not appear to be any technical advantages with these graft copolymers, and very satisfactory materials are available that do not contain them. From considerations of fundamental chemistry, they seem likely to be less soluble in pure water than the parent polyacids, though their behaviour in the water/HEMA mixtures that they find themselves in as part of resin-modified glass-ionomer formulations is unclear.

The earliest patent on resin-modified glass-ionomer cements also included bisGMA [2], with HEMA acting partly as a co-solvent for this substance, which would not otherwise dissolve in water. Such organic-rich blends have not been developed commercially, and no resin-modified glass-ionomer cement in current clinical use contains bisGMA or similar polymers. However, this approach is being reconsidered experimentally [9], and it may be that in the future resin-modified glass-ionomers consisting of more elaborate blends of components become available to the dental profession.

7.2.3 Polymerization initiators

Two sorts of initiator systems are used in resin-modified glass-ionomer cements, depending on whether or not they are designed to be photo-cured. The full details of the initiator systems used in commercial cements are confidential, but an indication of the type of chemistry used is available from the patent literature.

For light-cured materials, the initiator system can be based on camphorquinone, so that cements can be cured with a conventional dental cure lamp emitting at a maximum wavelength around 470 nm. Unlike formulations of composite resin, these materials cannot deploy amines as activators, because they would react with the carboxylic acid groups on the polymer, forming salts. Instead, a substance such as sodium *p*-toluene sulfinide is used as the activator. In addition, a photo-accelerator such as ethyl 4-*N,N′*-dimethylamino benzoate is included [10].

Resin-modified glass-ionomers may also be formulated with a two-part free radical initiator system that generates active centres simply on mixing. Appropriate substances for this are redox systems consisting of an oxidizing agent and a reducing agent [11]. Reaction of these components together in water leads to formation of free radicals. Possible oxidizing agents are potassium or ammonium persulfate, and reducing agents may be compounds such as ascorbic acid or urea [11]. These may either by included separately, one in the glass powder and one in the polymer solution; or they may be present together in the dry glass powder, and only react together when the glass is added to the aqueous polymer solution [11]. These could be considered to be self-cured resin-modified glass-ionomers.

Such a system may be included alongside a photo-initiator system to create a so-called 'tri-cure' system. Because these materials undergo a polymerization that is independent of a light source, it has been suggested that there are no problems with depth of cure, as both polymerization and acid–base reactions can occur throughout the material [12]. Alternatively, this type of redox system can be the sole free radical initiator in a resin-modified glass-ionomer. A material of this type does not need a cure lamp to bring about free radical polymerization, and such cements are available for clinical use as luting cements [13].

7.3 Setting of resin-modified glass-ionomers

The process of setting in resin-modified glass-ionomers is complicated because of the variety of reactions involved [6]. In principle it consists of two distinct parts, namely an acid–base reaction as in conventional glass-ionomers, and a free radial polymerization reaction. However, the two reactions influence each other in various ways. The acid–base reaction is slowed down in these materials for two reasons. One is that, as we have seen, the presence of HEMA causes the molecules to adopt a more coiled configuration and this reduces the ease with which they donate protons and behave as acids. The other reason is that the reduced polarity of the HEMA/water mixture compared with pure water inhibits the activation step of the acid–base reaction. This step involves electronically charged species, namely hydrogen ions from the acid and metal ions (Ca^{2+} or Sr^{2+}, Al^{3+}) from the glass, and these dissolve more readily in polar solvents (eg, pure water) than in non-polar ones (such as HEMA/water mixtures).

Once either reaction has been able to proceed to any extent, the reaction mixture has an increased viscosity and this has the effect of reducing the mobility of the reacting species. This type of inhibition is especially significant in photo-initiated resin-modified glass-ionomers, since the longer the delay between mixing and irradiation with light, the further the acid–base reaction will have proceeded. This will present a barrier to diffusion of the monomer molecules and the free radical centres, and hence will reduce the rate and extent of the polymerization reaction.

Experimental studies have shown that the acid–base reaction and the free radical polymerization both compete with each other and inhibit each other during the early stages of setting [14]. Spectroscopic studies have confirmed that the acid–base reaction is slower in resin-modified glass-ionomers than in conventional ones, presumably due to the lower polarity of the solvent mixture compared to that of pure water [15]. Studies have also shown that the reaction is significantly inhibited by the occurrence of the polymerization reaction, due to the reduced diffusion rates of the necessary reacting species through the polymer network [15]. Spectroscopic studies have also shown that the acid–base reaction is more affected in light-cured resin-modified glass-ionomers than in dark cured ones [16]. However, as different commercial brands were used in this work, the significance of the observation is not clear.

When HEMA undergoes free radical polymerization, there is a substantial exotherm. In resin-modified glass-ionomers, this has been shown to lead to temperature rises of around 20°C in light-cured specimens [17], a rise that undoubtedly affects the rate of the acid–base reaction [14]. The acceleration that would result from such a temperature rise might go some way to offsetting the inhibition caused by the difficulties of reactants diffusing through the polymerized HEMA, though to what extent is not known.

Polymerization of HEMA is affected by the presence of the other components of resin-modified glass-ionomers. It has been shown that HEMA itself will undergo addition polymerization more rapidly in the presence of poly(acrylic acid) than on its own [18]. However, in resin-modified glass-ionomers, pure unreacted poly(acrylic acid) may not be present for very long, and the effect of metal polyacrylate salts on the rate of polymerization of HEMA has not been studied.

Formation of at least part of the polysalt matrix from the acid–base components has been shown to reduce the efficiency of the polymerization process [19]. In a study in which the application of the dental cure lamp was delayed for 20 min following mixing of the cement, the degree of conversion was found to be substantially reduced and the overall rate of polymerization to be lower than in systems that were irradiated immediately after mixing [19]. It is worth noting that conversion of HEMA to polymer is never particularly efficient in these systems, and that the maximum reported conversion in this study was only about 60%, and this was for a specific material, namely Fuji II LC (Fig. 7.2).

Delaying the light-initiation step in this way has been shown to affect a number of physical properties of resin-modified glass-ionomers. These include diametral tensile and compressive strength [20,21], both of which are reduced, and wear rates, which are increased [22]. Chemical properties, namely fluoride release [23], water uptake

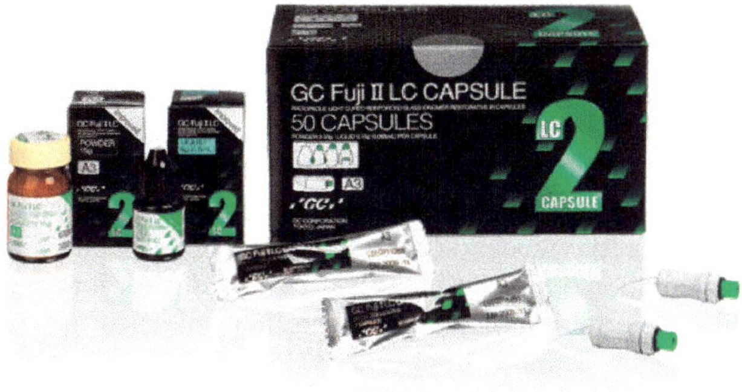

Fig. 7.2 Commercial resin-modified glass-ionomer cement (Fuji II LC).
GC Japan, image used with permission.

[21] and erosion [24], have also been found to be affected by such a delay, confirming the importance of light-curing these materials as soon as possible following mixing and placement. Fluoride release is enhanced by allowing the acid–base reaction to proceed as far as possible without being hindered by formation of poly(HEMA), whereas water uptake and erosion are both minimized by allowing HEMA polymerization to occur as early as possible. From these results, it can be seen that the overall properties represent a compromise between those which are improved by delaying the exposure to light, hence polymerization, and those which are made worse by such a delay. On balance, it seems desirable to light-cure resin-modified glass-ionomers as soon as possible after mixing, since this will allow the material to form that has been optimized by the manufacturers for a range of properties, both physical and chemical.

The setting reaction of resin-modified glass-ionomers is characterized by one further feature, ie, the tendency for the cement mixture to undergo phase separation as the reaction proceeds. There are two reasons for this. First, that poly(HEMA) is insoluble in water, unlike monomeric HEMA. Consequently, mere polymerization of the monomer is sufficient to drive the phase separation. Second, as the neutralization reaction proceeds, and poly(acrylic acid) is converted to calcium (or strontium) and aluminium polyacrylate, so the relatively hydrophobic organic substance, HEMA becomes less soluble in the aqueous solvent [6]. This tendency to phase-separate must be less pronounced with grated polymeric acids, because part of the organic phase and the polar component are on the same molecule. Nonetheless, the tendency is undoubtedly there in other types of resin-modified glass-ionomers. It has been suggested that this likely to result in the existence of different domains containing different phases within the set material. However, such domains have not been observed experimentally, and no physical properties of resin-modified glass-ionomers have been attributed to them.

7.4 Mechanical properties

Given the complexity of the relationship between the two setting reactions in these materials, it is difficult to make definitive statements about the mechanical properties of resin-modified glass-ionomer cements. Even a single formulation can give rise to a variety of values of a mechanical property, such as compressive strength, depending on its age, the speed with which it was light-cured following mixing and how it has been stored.

A particular problem, which is explored in detail in Section 7.5.1, is that the storage environment itself is able to influence the properties of these materials, since they are susceptible to moisture uptake. In extreme cases, storage in water has been found to cause the mechanical failure mode to change from brittle to tough [25].

The relevant International Standard for resin-modified glass-ionomer cements uses flexural strength as the criterion of acceptable mechanical performance [26], and further specifies a minimum flexural strength of 20 MPa for these materials. No distinction is made between values required for liner/base materials and full restoratives, or indeed for materials intended for any other application, such as luting, but most brands of resin-modified glass-ionomer cement comfortable exceed this minimum value [27].

Like conventional glass-ionomers, resin-modified glass-ionomers may improve in strength as they age, which indicates that they, too, undergo slow maturation reactions [25,28]. In a study of compressive strength on early commercial resin-modified glass-ionomer cements, the values shown in Table 7.2 were obtained for specimens stored in air at ambient humidity [25]. Storage in an aqueous solution of sodium chloride or in water masked this effect, for reasons explained in Section 7.5.1.

The compressive strength of conventional glass-ionomer cements is known to vary with the powder:liquid ratio, with high relative amounts of powder leading to stronger cements [29]. Similar effects have been demonstrated for resin-modified glass-ionomer cements, as shown in Table 7.3. The experiments reported in this table were carried out with specimens stored in distilled water for 24 h prior to testing.

Table 7.2 Variation in compressive strength of resin-modified glass-ionomers with age when stored in air at ambient humidity [25]

Storage time (days)	RX Ionomer	Vitrebond
1	73 (5)	80 (10)
7	83 (8)	73 (5)
90	126 (30)	100 (14)

Standard deviations in parentheses.

Table 7.3 Variation of compressive strength of resin-modified glass-ionomers with powder:liquid ratio when stored in distilled water for 24 h [27]

Powder:liquid ratio	Vitremer	Fuji II LC
1:1	218.46 (7.72)	183.88 (18.34)
1:2	130.70 (8.63)	129.76 (9.33)
1:3	98.79 (4.88)	95.54 (7.51)

Standard deviations in parentheses.

A further mechanical property that has been reported for these materials is fracture toughness [30,31]. In an early study, four brands of resin-modified glass-ionomer cement were employed and compared with a composite resin and two metal-reinforced conventional glass-ionomers [30]. Specimens were stored for 2 weeks at 100% relative humidity prior to testing. The resin-modified glass-ionomers all had higher fracture toughness values than the metal-reinforced glass-ionomers, with values ranging from 0.88 to 1.37 MPs $m^{1/2}$ and two brands (Fuji II LC and Photac-Fil) proved to be significantly tougher than the composite resin studied.

Fracture toughness of resin-modified glass-ionomers has been found to vary only slightly with the powder:liquid ratio [31]. By contrast, the particle size of the glass did influence the fracture toughness, with finer particles leading to reduced fracture toughness.

Resin-modified glass-ionomers generally have higher fracture toughness than conventional glass-ionomers [31]. This is clearly due to the contribution of the polyHEMA phase, since this is known to be a tough substance, and therefore imparts a degree of toughness to resin-modified glass-ionomers which they would otherwise lack. This feature may be important in obtaining good clinical outcomes when the materials are sued in regions of high stress within the mouth.

Overall, the mechanical properties of resin-modified glass-ionomers make them suitable for their varied clinical applications, and they now have been employed clinically for well over 20 years, generally with good results. Their mechanical properties are influenced by similar compositional factors to those influencing the behaviour of conventional glass-ionomers. The broad conclusion from many years of study is that the occurrence of the two competing reactions does not necessarily improve the strength of resin-modified glass-ionomer compared with conventional materials [21,32], though the presence of the polyHEMA phase has a beneficial effect on toughness.

7.5 Interaction with water

In this section, three aspects of the interaction of resin-modified glass-ionomers with water are dealt with, namely water uptake, fluoride release and other ion release and its associated buffering effect. Like conventional glass-ionomer cements, resin-modified glass-ionomers are deployed in an essentially wet environment and their behaviour in terms of each of these features differs more or less from that of conventional glass-ionomers, due to the presence of the polyHEMA phase. These are considered in turn.

7.5.1 Water uptake

From soon after they were made available to the dental profession, resin-modified glass-ionomers have been reported to take up water when stored in aqueous media, either pure water [33–36] or in physiological saline [25]. Typical results are shown in Table 7.4.

Results in Table 7.4 show that specimens both gained mass and swelled when stored in pure water, whereas they lost mass and shrank somewhat when stored in air

Table 7.4 Changes (%) in resin-modified glass-ionomers stored in air at ambient humidity or deionized water for 90 days [33]

	XR Ionomer	Vitrebond
Mass gain		
Air	−2.8 (0.4)	−4.4 (0.4)
Water	2.9 (0.3)	2.3 (0.4)
Volume gain		
Air	−5.9 (0.9)	−7.6 (0.9)
Water	3.8 (1.0)	2.3 (0.8)

Standard deviations in parentheses.
NB: Negative values mean there was a mass or volume loss.

at ambient humidity. Although not shown in Table 7.4, published results shown that specimens underwent smaller changes in these properties that were distinct after only 1 day of storage in the respective environments [33]. These results have been confirmed in several other studies [34–37]. Specimens stored under these conditions have also been tested for compressive strength [25] and shown to become weaker on storage in water, and to change from being brittle to tough materials.

In physiological saline, uptake effects and weakening were less marked [25]. In all cases, specimens took up less water from the physiological saline solution than they did from pure water, and their dimensions changed less. They were stronger in compression than specimens stored in pure water, though they were also weaker than those specimens stored in air at ambient humidity. They also changed from brittle materials to tough ones.

The reason for this behaviour is that the polyHEMA component of the set resin-modified glass-ionomer cement is a hydrogel, ie, a material capable of taking up large amounts of water to form a soft gel. Pure polyHEMA is able to take up about 80% of its mass of water [38], though data suggest that it does begin to approach this figure when it is part of a resin-modified glass-ionomer. Hydrogels typically have low mechanical strengths when swollen with water, with strength varying inversely with the amount of water taken up [39].

Swelling of hydrogels is an osmotic effect, driven by the chemical potentials of water in the gel phase and in the surrounding storage medium. It continues until these chemical potentials are the same, at which point the hydrogel reaches its equilibrium water uptake [39]. Because the chemical potential of water in the pure state is greater than it is in a solution such as physiological saline, swelling is greater in pure water than in the latter solution.

The lower swelling when stored in solution is useful because it means that resin-modified glass-ionomers will swell less in saliva than in the pure water typically employed for in vitro experiments. Indeed, the relevance of many of the in vitro studies is unclear, because swelling is so great, and no comparable dimensional changes have been reported for resin-modified glass-ionomers when used in patients. It may well be that swelling is negligible when these materials are exposed to natural saliva, and that under clinical conditions the hydrogel character of the polyHEMA phase does not impart unacceptable properties to these materials.

7.6 Fluoride release and recharge

The ability of resin-modified glass-ionomers to release fluoride was reported in one of the earliest accounts of these materials [4], and it is considered one of their key clinical advantages [40]. The fluoride release behaviour is found to be similar between resin-modified and conventional glass-ionomers in that release is greatest in the first day, and declines from the second day, finally stabilizing to a steady release by about 7 days [41–44]. This pattern is that described previously for conventional glass-ionomers in Chapter 6, and involves early wash-out of readily available soluble fluoride, followed by steady low levels of fluoride released more slowly by a diffusion process as fluoride ions move gradually through the cement and out through pores and cracks [45]. The early wash-out phase is considered to involve fluoride present in the matrix of the cement as a result of the acid–base reaction during the setting process [40].

There is some evidence that resin-modified glass-ionomers may release more fluoride than conventional glass-ionomers [46]. However, this may simply be a result of the details of the glass formulations involved, rather than a fundamental feature of these materials.

Because identical phases of release are involved, fluoride release follows the same kinetics from resin-modified glass-ionomers as it does from conventional cements [47]. Consequently it, too, can be described by the equation [48]:

$$[\mathrm{F}]_c = [\mathrm{F}]_1 \frac{t}{\left(t_{1/2} + t\right)} + \alpha t^{1/2}$$

Like studies of conventional glass-ionomers, studies of fluoride release from resin-modified glass-ionomers have used a range of methodologies and materials, and consequently results obtained show considerable variation. There is not even agreement on the units of release to be used, nor whether they should be quoted relative to the total mass of the specimens involved, or their surface area.

Nonetheless, some clear patterns do emerge from these studies. Not only are the two processes of early wash-out and steady diffusion observed in all published studies, other features have been identified. Resin-modified glass-ionomers release more fluoride in acid media than neutral ones [49–53], and also release greater amounts in pure water than into solutions including artificial saliva [53–55]. In these features, resin-modified glass-ionomers also resemble conventional glass-ionomers.

Resin-modified glass-ionomers are also able to take up fluoride from external solutions [53–55], including fluoridated toothpaste [56]. Experiments have typically been carried out indirectly, ie, by determining fluoride release from specimens following exposure to a fluoride-containing solution. This means there is no data available on what proportion of fluoride taken up is subsequently released, nor whether the ability to resin-modified glass-ionomers to take up fluoride declines with maturation.

The current consensus is that this fluoride recharge is a useful feature of resin-modified glass-ionomers. There is certainly evidence that this release has beneficial effects on the surrounding tooth tissue, and it is one of the reasons that certain authors advocate these materials for restorative dentistry [29,57].

7.7 Release of other ions and buffering

In aqueous solution, resin-modified glass-ionomers have been found to release not only fluoride but also other ions [58,59]. Under neutral conditions, ions released were sodium, aluminium, phosphorus (as some sort of phosphate) and silicon (as silicate). Under acidic conditions, in addition to these ions, either calcium or strontium was released as well [58,59]. Acidic conditions also caused much higher concentrations of all ions to be released [59]. This behaviour is similar to that of conventional glass-ionomers, though levels of phosphorus were much lower for resin-modified glass-ionomers for reasons that are not clear [59].

The ion release in acidic conditions was found to be associated with a buffering effect, ie, an increase in pH towards neutral, with pH changes of the order of 1 unto being recorded after 1 week [59]. There may be clinical benefit in this phenomenon, since the difference in pH between active caries (pH 4.9) and arrested caries (pH 5.7) is only 0.8 of a pH unit [60]. This means that the measured changes in pH by resin-modified glass-ionomers (pH 2.7–3.7) would be sufficient to arrest nearby caries in vivo and, were such buffering to occur in the mouth of a caries-prone patient, it could have an effect of reducing the extent of caries in the tooth surface adjacent to a restoration.

7.8 Biocompatibility of resin-modified glass-ionomers

The biocompatibility of resin-modified glass-ionomers has been assessed partly in terms of their cytotoxicity towards the pulp and partly in terms of their effects on dental personnel exposed to these materials in a regular basis [61].

As we have seen, inorganic ions (Sr^{2+}, Al^{3+}, F^-) are released from set resin-modified glass-ionomers, but at levels too low to have any cytotoxic effect [62]. However, several studies have shown that HEMA is released by resin-modified glass-ionomers [62–64] and this is the substance that compromises the biocompatibility of these materials [65]. HEMA released by fully set resin-modified glass-ionomers can penetrate the dentine and adversely affect the pulp [66–69]. It can also be distributed systemically from its location in the mouth, and can have the potential to cause damage [61]. Dental personnel may risk a variety of adverse effects from manual contact with the skin, ranging in severity from mild to severe dermatitis [70,71]. They are also at risk from inhalation of the volatile HEMA vapour.

A variety of in vitro studies have shown the problems caused by HEMA release from these materials. HEMA release occurs mainly in the first 24 h after setting, with degree of light-curing affecting the total amount released [63,64,72]. This makes it imperative to follow manufacturer's instructions closely, in order to minimize the amount of HEMA released.

The diffusion of HEMA through extracted human molars has been studied in detail [73,74], though for HEMA released from a dentine bonding agent rather than a resin-modified glass-ionomer. However, the ability of HEMA to diffuse through dentine logically must be independent of which sort of material it was released by. These studies showed that dentine in all conditions was permeable to HEMA, and that in teeth with either mild or moderate caries, diffusion took place significantly quicker [73]. Thickness of dentine influenced the result with thicker layers (ie, 3.4–3.6 mm) showing much lower rates of diffusion than very thin layers (eg, 1.4–1.6 mm or 0.4–0.6 mm) [74]. Overall, these results showed that dentine is a poor barrier to the passage of HEMA, and that thin layers of dentine will allow the ready movement of HEMA into the pulp.

Cell culture studies have shown that HEMA is unquestionably cytotoxic towards cells [75,76]. In one study using the resin-modified glass-ionomer Vitremer, severe cytotoxic effects were shown to occur on exposure to mouse 3T3 fibroblast cells [77]. Surprisingly, the authors attributed this finding to release of the monomer TEGDMA, but in view of the relative amounts of monomers released, and their generally known biological effects, it seems more likely that HEMA was responsible.

Studies in which resin-modified glass-ionomers were placed in the teeth of monkeys confirmed that there were issues of biocompatibility with these materials [77,78]. In a number of cases, pulps showed distinct inflammatory responses. However, these were of limited duration and the effects disappeared within a week or two, and there appeared to be no long-term damage [77,78]. These results are consistent with the known pattern of HEMA release from resin-modified glass-ionomers.

HEMA is a known contact allergen [70,71], but despite this there do not seem to have been any reports of dermatitis among dental personnel, either dentists or their assistants [61]. Latex gloves are inadequate to protect the skin because they are permeable to HEMA [79]. The volatility HEMA may also cause problems with these materials, and inhalation of the vapour should be avoided [61]. There are anecdotal reports of dental personnel developing allergies to resin-modified glass-ionomers, but again there seem to be no detailed reports or case studies in the literature about this.

Despite this, and in view of the known biological hazard of HEMA and the knowledge that it is far from fully polymerized in these materials, certain safety procedures are essential. The following have been recommended [61]:

- **(a)** Ensure a well-ventilated workspace.
- **(b)** Avoid inhalation of HEMA vapour.
- **(c)** Only touch unset materials with instruments, and avoid touching with the hands, even when wearing gloves.
- **(d)** Avoid contact of resin-modified glass-ionomer (cured or uncured) with the oral mucosa of the patient.
- **(e)** Use resin-modified glass-ionomers in the tooth with a liner.
- **(f)** Build up restorations in increments of ~1 mm and fully cure each layer before applying the next.
- **(g)** Light-cure all unused remnants of resin-modified glass-ionomer before disposal in order to minimize exposure to HEMA vapour.

Overall, these precautions have been shown to be necessary in studies of the biocompatibility of resin-modified glass-ionomers. Used in this way, they are able to perform satisfactorily and to cause only minimal, short-term damage to the pulp, if any. However, it is clear that these materials are much less biocompatible for their intended clinical use than conventional glass-ionomers, and that it is the monomer HEMA that is responsible for this difference [61].

7.9 Adhesion of resin-modified glass-ionomers

Resin-modified glass-ionomers show good inherent adhesion to freshly cut tooth surfaces [80]. This property was reported early on, when Mitra observed shear bond strengths of the first commercial material, Vitremer liner/base to bovine dentine of 12 ± 3 MPa after 24 h in distilled water [3]. Like conventional glass-ionomers, resin-modified glass-ionomers can be used with only minimal surface preparation, for example, conditioning with dilute aqueous poly(acrylic acid) followed by rinsing [81], though other workers prefer etching with phosphoric acid as the surface treatment. As well as shear bond strength, micro-tensile bond strengths have also been determined for these materials [82,83].

Good bonding by resin-modified glass-ionomers is partly a function of the fact that they contain a polymeric acid such as poly(acrylic acid), which as we have seen is capable of interacting strongly with the mineral phase of the tooth [84]. In addition, they contain HEMA, a substance that is also currently used as a component of dentine bonding agents [85]. The effect of this combination is not known for certain, but is likely to result in high bond strengths and durable bonding to the tooth surface. Unlike conventional glass-ionomers, there is evidence that resin-modified glass-ionomers bond more strongly to the dentine than to the enamel [86,87], and this may be a function of their HEMA content.

The bonding of resin-modified glass-ionomer cements is associated with the formation of a gel phase at the interface between the material and the tooth surface [82,88]. This phase seems to originate from the acid–base part of the formulation, as it consists substantially of calcium polyacrylate, a substance that forms as the cement sets. However, the gel phase is more substantial in these materials than in conventional glass-ionomers, so that its occurrence owes something to the overall composition of resin-modified glass-ionomers [89].

Since the earliest report on the adhesion of resin-modified glass-ionomers, a variety of studies have been reported. Comparisons have been made with conventional glass-ionomers, but findings have been inconclusive. This is partly because both materials often fail cohesively, so that results of bond testing turn out to be strongly influenced by the strength (either shear or tensile) of the specific materials employed. There is some evidence that these materials do show definite differences in bond strength [89], as illustrated by the results shown in Table 7.5, where the resin-modified glass-ionomer Fuji II LC exhibited significantly higher

Table 7.5 Micro-tensile bond strengths of conventional and resin-modified glass-ionomer to human teeth [89]

Substrate	Conventional glass-ionomer (Fuji IX)	Resin-modified glass-ionomer (Fuji II LC)
Enamel	5.19 (1.38) MPa	11.08 (2.45) MPa
Dentine	4.82 (1.68) MPa	11.37 (2.64) MPa

Standard deviations in parentheses.

micro-tensile bond strength than the conventional glass-ionomer Fiji IX. Against that, it showed no significant difference when bonded to enamel or dentine.

Attempts have been made to improve the bond strengths of resin-modified glass-ionomers to dentine by using them in association with dentine bonding agents [90,91]. However, using shear bond testing, such bonding agents have been found to make no significant difference to the measured bond strength [91], a result that a more recent study confirms [90].

Microleakage of resin-modified glass-ionomers has been reported as being better than that of conventional glass-ionomer [92]. This is consistent with findings about the quality of the interface and its resistance to permeability [93], and probably results from improved wetting of the tooth surface caused by the presence of HEMA. However, differences were slight [92], and the study used samples that were only 24 h old. Given that conventional glass-ionomers are known to develop dense ion-exchange interfaces with the tooth surface as they age, it may be that over the longer term, any differences between the microleakage of the two types of glass-ionomer become negligible.

7.10 Clinical applications of resin-modified glass-ionomers

Resin-modified glass-ionomers have more or less the same clinical applications as conventional glass-ionomers, with the possible exception of their use in the ART technique [94]. Thus, they have been widely used in Class I, Class II, Class III and Class V restorations as the full restorative material. They have also been used as liners and bases and, despite the issues with biocompatibility, have found particular application in children's dentistry [94].

For Class I restorations, resin-modified glass-ionomers have been used in both primary [95] and permanent teeth [96]. Good results have been obtained for small, minimally invasive preparations, though for larger repairs, physical properties of resin-modified glass-ionomers are considered inferior to those of composite resins, so that the latter materials are preferred for this type of repair [96].

Resin-modified glass-ionomer cements have been used for both Class II and Class III restorations in primary teeth [97,98]. Their lower brittleness compared with conventional glass-ionomers make them appropriate for these applications, though composite resin again appears preferred for these types of cavity in permanent teeth [94]. Various clinical studies have shown resin-modified glass-ionomers to perform well in these restorations [99,100], and in addition they have been shown to have useful caries inhibition properties as a result of their fluoride release [101].

Resin-modified glass-ionomer cements have been used in Class V cavities, again with much of this use being in primary dentition [94]. For this type of repair, there do not appear to be any advantages of resin-modified over conventional glass-ionomers cements. Both types of material have proved effective in this application [57,102].

Other clinical uses of resin-modified include as pit and fissure sealants [103–105], as orthodontic adhesives and as luting cements [106]. Materials for the latter two applications need to be self-curing, ie, not to need light activation. Rather, the free radical polymerization part of the setting process needs to be activated by bringing the two parts of the initiator together on mixing, as described in Section 7.2. Resin-modified materials of this type perform satisfactorily, even though they do not offer any particular advantages over well-established conventional materials, such as zinc phosphate luting cements or resin-based adhesives.

7.11 Recent developments

A relatively new development of resin-modified glass-ionomers is to have them presented as a paste-liquid system [107]. Such a presentation makes the material easier to mix at the chair-side than the conventional powder-liquid system, though there are difficulties in producing stable systems of this type. This material contains a modified polyacid, which is a methacrylated copolymer [107], and it also contains what have been described as 'nano-fillers' [108]. However, the exact state of division of these fillers has not been reported in the scientific literature, and there is evidence that such fillers are in fact of larger size than the nanometre scale, and consist of clusters of nanoparticles [109] or even nanocrystallites within more conventionally sized particles.

Properties of this material have been reported. It has been found to bond to enamel and dentine, and to do so reliably and with good durability [107]. Results from X-ray photoelectron spectroscopy (XPS) and fourier transform infrared spectroscopy (FTIR) show that this bonding is the same as for conventional glass-ionomers, and involves the formation of chemical bonds to calcium in the mineral phase of the tooth. There is also evidence of micromechanical adhesion in this material [107].

Fluoride release and recharge have been reported as well [108]. Release follows the same kinetics as for other types of resin-modified glass-ionomer, namely an early burst followed by a steady release based on diffusion which has a square root of time dependency. The new type of resin-modified glass-ionomer showed similar recharge behaviour to other types of resin-modified glass-ionomer, and was able to take up and release reasonable amounts of fluoride after ageing for 3 months. Surprising, coating the material with its proprietary primer did not alter the fluoride release rate significantly.

Overall, the results show that the material presented as a paste-liquid system has satisfactory in vitro properties. Further work is necessary to determine how it performs clinically over reasonable periods of time.

Clinical summary

- Resin-modified glass-ionomer cements are aesthetic materials for repairing teeth.
- To be a true resin-modified glass-ionomer, the material must be capable of undergoing an acid–base setting reaction. Such a reaction will occur without light-initiation, though does not provide a satisfactory material in its own right, as it is mechanically weak and able to leach considerable amounts of the monomer HEMA.

- The setting is a mixture of addition polymerization and neutralization, and there is some shrinkage due to the polymerization process.
- Self-cure versions are available, where polymerization is initiated by a two-part initiator system that comes together when the material is mixed. This type of resin-modified glass-ionomer can be placed in full ('bulk fill') within a cavity.
- Resin-modified glass-ionomers are adhesive to both enamel and dentine.
- Set resin-modified glass-ionomers are able to take up moisture to an extent, which may lead to slight swelling.
- A wide range of repairs is possible with resin-modified glass-ionomers, and they can also be used as liners and bases, and as orthodontic adhesives.
- Resin-modified glass-ionomers release fluoride, showing a similar pattern of release to conventional glass-ionomers.
- Resin-modified glass-ionomers are much less biocompatible than conventional glass-ionomers. This is due to the HEMA that they contain. This monomer may cause sensitization to dental personnel, and can be leached from set cements and pass through thin layers of dentine to damage the pulp of the patient. They should be used with care.

Clinical use of resin-modified glass-ionomer cements

(a) Light-cured RMGICs

(i) Cavity preparation can be restricted to removal of caries and unsupported enamel only (the same as for conventional glass-ionomer).

(ii) After cavity preparation, condition the cavity (remove the smear later) using a conditioning solution (typically 10% poly(acrylic acid) or 5% citric acid in water) using a cotton pellet saturated with conditioner placed in the cavity for 15–20 s, after which the surface is rinsed with water for 5 s, lightly dried but not dehydrated. This is achieved by swabbing with dry cotton pellets only.

(iii) In the case of deep caries, protect the pulpal floor with calcium hydroxide setting cement. Note: zinc oxide-eugenol cement must not be used because it inhibits the polymerization reaction.

(iv) Mix the glass-ionomer cement according to the manufacturer's instructions. For hand-mixed cements, ensure that the correct powder:liquid ratio is used. For capsulated cements, ensure that mixing is carried out for the correct time.

(v) Apply first layer of cement to a maximum depth of 2 mm and light cure for 40 s.

(vi) Apply next layers, curing each one for 40 s.

(vii) Complete the restoration with either diamond bur or finishing bur with a high-speed handpiece, then polish.

(viii) The patient can rinse, eat and drink immediately.

(b) Self-cure RMGICs

(i) Cavity preparation can be restricted to removal of caries and unsupported enamel only (the same as for conventional glass-ionomer).

(ii) After cavity preparation, condition the cavity (remove the smear later) using a conditioning solution (typically 10% poly(acrylic acid) or 5% citric acid in water) using a cotton pellet saturated with conditioner placed in the cavity for 15–20 s, after which the surface is rinsed with water for 5 s, lightly dried but not dehydrated. This is achieved by swabbing with dry cotton pellets only.

(iii) In the case of deep caries, protect the pulpal floor with calcium hydroxide setting cement. Note: zinc oxide-eugenol cement must not be used because it inhibits the polymerization reaction.

(iv) Mix the glass-ionomer cement according to the manufacturer's instructions. For hand-mixed cements, ensure that the correct powder:liquid ratio is used. For capsulated cements, ensure that mixing is carried out for the correct time.
(v) Fill to cavity using a single portion of mixed resin-modified glass-ionomers.
(vi) Complete the restoration with either diamond bur or finishing bur with a high-speed handpiece, then polish.
(vii) The patient can rinse, eat and drink immediately.

References

[1] J.W. McLean, J.W. Nicholson, A.D. Wilson, Proposed nomenclature for glass-ionomer dental cements and related materials, Quintessence Int. 25 (1994) 587–589.
[2] J.M. Antonucci, J.E. McKinney, J.W. Stansbury, Resin-modified glass-ionomer cement, US Patent Application 160856, 1988.
[3] S.B. Mitra, Adhesion to dentin and physical properties of a light-cured glass-ionomer liner/base, J. Dent. Res. 70 (1991) 72–74.
[4] S.B. Mitra, In vitro fluoride release from a light-cured glass-ionomer liner/base, J. Dent. Res. 70 (1991) 75–78.
[5] J.W. Nicholson, H.M. Anstice, The physical chemistry of light-curable glass-ionomers, J. Mater. Sci. Mater. Med. 5 (1994) 119–122.
[6] H.M. Anstice, J.W. Nicholson, Studies in the setting of polyelectrolyte materials, Part 2: the effect of organic compounds on a glass polyalkenoate cement, J. Mater. Sci. Mater. Med. 5 (1994) 299–302.
[7] N.T.M. Klooster, F. Vandertouw, M. Mandel, Solvent effects in poly-electrolyte solutions. 1. Potentiometric and viscometric titration of poly(acrylic acid) in methanol and counterion specificity, Macromolecules 17 (1984) 2070–2078.
[8] B.M. Culbertson, Glass-ionomer dental restoratives, Prog. Polym. Sci. 26 (2001) 577–604.
[9] J. Gaviria, C.G. Garcia, E. Velez, J. Quijano, The mechanism of formation of glass-ionomer cement: a theoretical study, Model. Numer. Simul. Mater. Sci. 3 (2013) 149–154.
[10] X. Quan, X. Chen, Dental resin-modified glass-ionomer cement composition, Eur. Patent 2764859 A2, 2014.
[11] S.B. Mitra, S. Mitra, Universal water-based medical and dental cement, US Patent 5154762, 1992.
[12] Y.K. Kim, K.-H. Kim, T.-Y. Kwon, Setting reaction of dental resin-modified glass ionomer restoratives as a function of curing depth and post-irradiation time, J. Spectroscopy 2015 (2015), Article ID 462687.
[13] C.H. Pameijer, Crown retention with three resin-modified glass ionomer luting agents, J. Am. Dent. Assoc. 143 (2012) 1218–1222.
[14] D.W. Berzin, S. Abey, M.C. Costache, C.A. Wilkie, H.W. Roberts, Resin-modified glass-ionomer setting reaction competition, J. Dent. Res. 89 (2010) 82–86.
[15] A.M. Young, S.A. Rafeeka, J.A. Howlett, FTIR investigation of monomer polymerisation and polyacid neutralisation kinetics and mechanisms in various aesthetic dental restorative materials, Biomaterials 25 (2004) 823–833.
[16] G. Eliades, G. Palaghias, In vitro characterization of visible light-cured glass ionomer liners, Dent. Mater. 6 (1993) 198–203.

[17] W. Kanchanavasita, G.J. Pearson, H.M. Anstice, Temperature rise in ion-leachable cements during setting reaction, Biomaterials 16 (1995) 1261–1265.
[18] E. Andrzejewska, M. Andrzejewski, M. Socha, S. Zych-Tomkowiak, Effect of polyacid aqueous solutions on photocuring of polymerizable components of resin-modified glass ionomer cements, Dent. Mater. 19 (2003) 501–509.
[19] A. Kakaboura, G. Eliades, G. Palaghias, An FTIR study on the setting mechanism of resin-modified glass ionomer restoratives, Dent. Mater. 12 (1996) 173–178.
[20] J. Li, M. von Beetzen, F. Sundstrom, Strength and setting behaviour of resin-modified glass ionomer cements, Acta Odontol. Scand. 53 (1995) 311–317.
[21] A.M. Hegarty, G.J. Pearson, Erosion and compressive strength of hybrid glass ionomer cements when light activated or chemically set, Biomaterials 14 (1993) 349–352.
[22] A.J. de Gee, G. Lehoup, A. Werner, J. Vreven, C.L. Davidson, Structural integrity of resin-modified glass ionomers as affected by the delay or omission of light activation, J. Dent. Res. 77 (1998) 1658–1663.
[23] P. Jevnikar, O. Jarh, A. Sepe, M.M. Pintar, N. Dunduk, Micro magnetic resonance imaging of water uptake by glass ionomer cements, Dent. Mater. 13 (1997) 20–23.
[24] A. Yoda, T. Nakaido, M. Ikeda, H. Sonada, R.M. Foxton, J. Tagami, Effect of curing method and storage condition on fluoride ion release from a fluoride-releasing resin cement, Dent. Mater. 25 (2006) 261–266.
[25] H.M. Anstice, J.W. Nicholson, Studies on the structure of light-cured glass-ionomer cements, J. Mater. Sci. Mater. Med. 3 (1992) 447–451.
[26] International Organization for Standardization, ISO 9917-2: Dentistry – Water-Based Cements, Part 2: Resin-Modified Cements, ISO, Geneva, Switzerland, 2010.
[27] J.F. McCabe, A.W.G. Walls, Applied Dental Materials, ninth ed., Blackwell Munksgaard, Oxford, 2008.
[28] M. Aratani, A.C. Periera, L. Correr-Sobrinho, M.A.C. Sinhorett, S. Consani, Compressive strength of resin-modified glass ionomer restorative materials: effect of the p/l ratio and storage time, J. Appl. Oral Sci. 13 (2005) 356–359.
[29] G.J. Mount, Color Atlas of Glass Ionomer Cement, second ed., Martin Dunitz, London, 2002.
[30] R.E. Kovarik, M.V. Muncy, Fracture toughness of resin-modified glass ionomers, Am. J. Dent. 8 (1995) 145–148.
[31] A. Mitsuhashi, K. Hanaoka, T. Teranaka, Fracture toughness of resin-modified glass ionomer restorative materials: effect of powder/liquid ratio and powder particle size reduction on fracture toughness, Dent. Mater. 19 (2003) 747–757.
[32] R.E. Kerby, J. Knobloch, A. Thakur, Strength properties of visible-light-cured resin-modified glass-ionomer cements, Oper. Dent. 22 (1997) 79–83.
[33] J.W. Nicholson, H.M. Anstice, J.W. McLean, A preliminary report on the effect of storage in water on the properties of commercial light-cured glass-ionomer cements, Br. Dent. J. 173 (1992) 98–101.
[34] A. Yap, C.M. Lee, Water sorption and solubility of resin-modified polyalkenoate, J. Oral Rehabil. 24 (1997) 310–314.
[35] W. Kanchanavasita, G.J. Pearson, H.M. Anstice, Water sorption characteristics of resin-modified glass-ionomer cements, Biomaterials 18 (1997) 343–349.
[36] A. Akashi, Y. Matsuya, M. Unemori, A. Akamine, The relationship between water absorption characteristics and the mechanical strength of resin-modified glass-ionomer cements in long-term water storage, Biomaterials 20 (1999) 1573–1578.
[37] N.C. Beriai, D. Nalbant, Water absorption and HEMA release of resin-modified glass-ionomers, Eur. J. Dent. 3 (2009) 267–272.

[38] D.G. Pedley, P.J. Skelly, B. Tighe, Hydrogels in biomedical applications, Br. Polym. J. 12 (1980) 99–110.
[39] J. Kalal, Water sensitive chemically cross-linked gels, in: C.A. Finch (Ed.), The Chemistry and Technology of Water-Soluble Polymers, Plenum Press, New York and London, 1983.
[40] A. Weigand, W. Buchalla, T. Attin, Review on fluoride-releasing restorative materials – fluoride release and uptake characteristics, antibacterial activity and influence on caries formation, Dent. Mater. 23 (2007) 343–362.
[41] A.M. Diaz-Arnold, D.C. Holmes, D.W. Wistrom, E.J. Swift Jr., Short-term fluoride release/uptake of glass ionomer restoratives, Dent. Mater. 11 (1995) 96–101.
[42] D.C. Can-Karabulut, I. Batmaz, H. Solak, M. Tastekin, Linear regression modeling to compare fluoride release profiles of various restorative materials, Dent. Mater. 23 (2007) 1057–1065.
[43] W.D. Chan, L. Yang, W. Lan, A.S. Rizkalla, Fluoride release from dental cements and composites: a mechanistic study, Dent. Mater. 22 (2006) 366–373.
[44] M.F. Costa Cabral, R.L. de Menezes Martinho, M.V. Guedes-Neto, M.A.B. Rebelo, D.G. Pontes, F. Cohen-Carneiro, Do conventional glass ionomer cements release more fluoride than resin-modified glass ionomer cements? Restor. Dent. Endod. 40 (2015) 209–215.
[45] S.M. Mousavinasab, I. Meyers, Fluoride release by glass ionomer cements, compomer and giomer, Dent. Res. J. (Isfahan) 6 (2009) 75–81.
[46] M.A. Paschoal, C.V. Gurgel, D. Rios, A.C. Magalhaes, M.A. Buzalaf, M.A. Machado, Fluoride release profile of a nanofilled resin-modified glass ionomer, Braz. Dent. J. 22 (2011) 275–279.
[47] R.M.H. Verbeeck, E.A.P. De Maeyer, L.A.M. Marks, R.J.G. De Moor, A.M.J.C. De Witte, L.M. Trimpeers, Fluoride release process of (resin-modified) glass-ionomer cements versus (polyacid-modified) composite resins, Biomaterials 19 (1998) 509–519.
[48] C.L. Dhont, E.A.P. De Maeyer, R.M.H. Verbeeck, Fluoride release from glass-ionomer activated with fluoride solution, J. Dent. Res. 80 (2001) 1402–1406.
[49] R.N. Bahadure, R.K. Pandy, R. Kumar, K. Gopal, R.K. Singh, An estimation of fluoride release from various dental restorative materials at different pH: *in vitro* study, J. Indian Soc. Pedod. Prev. Dent. 30 (2012) 122–126.
[50] J.L. Moreau, H.H. Xu, Fluoride releasing restorative materials: effects of pH on mechanical properties and ion release, Dent. Mater. 26 (2010) e227–e235.
[51] A.S. Carvalho, J.A. Cury, Fluoride release from dental materials in difficult solutions, Oper. Dent. 24 (1999) 14–19.
[52] M.G. Gandolfi, S. Chersoni, G.L. Acquaviva, G. Piana, C. Prati, R. Mongiorgi, Fluoride release and absorption at different pH from glass-ionomer cements, Dent. Mater. 22 (2006) 441–449.
[53] B. Levallois, Y. Fovet, L. Lapeyre, J.Y. Gal, *In vitro* fluoride release from restorative materials in water versus artificial saliva medium (SAGF), Dent. Mater. 14 (1998) 441–447.
[54] M.F. Hayacibara, G.M. Ambrosano, J.A. Cury, Simultaneous release of fluoride and aluminium from dental materials in various materials, Oper. Dent. 29 (2004) 16–22.
[55] X. Xu, J.O. Burgess, Compressive strength, fluoride release and recharge of fluoride-releasing materials, Biomaterials 24 (2003) 2451–2461.
[56] M. Rothwell, H.M. Anstice, G.J. Pearson, The uptake and release of fluoride by ion-leaching cements after exposure to toothpaste, J. Dent. 26 (1998) 591–597.

[57] T.P. Croll, Y. Bar-Zion, A. Segura, K.J. Donly, Clinical performance of resin-modified glass ionomer cement restorations in primary teeth: a retrospective evaluation, J. Am. Dent. Assoc. 132 (2001) 1110–1116.
[58] H. Forss, Release of fluoride and other elements from light-cured glass ionomers in neutral and acidic conditions, J. Dent. Res. 72 (1993) 1257–1262.
[59] B. Czarnecka, J.W. Nicholson, Ion release by resin-modified glass-ionomer cements into water and lactic acid solutions, J. Dent. 34 (2006) 539–543.
[60] S. Hojo, M. Komatsu, N. Takahashi, T. Yamada, Acid profiles and pH of carious dentine in active and arrested lesions, J. Dent. Res. 73 (1994) 1853–1857.
[61] J.W. Nicholson, B. Czarnecka, The biocompatibility of resin-modified glass-ionomer cements for dentistry, Dent. Mater. 24 (2008) 1702–1708.
[62] L. Stanislawski, X. Daniau, A. Lautie, M. Goldberg, Factors responsible for pulp cytotoxicity induced by resin-modified glass ionomer cements, J. Biomed. Mater. Res. (Appl. Biomater.) 48 (1999) 277–288.
[63] G. Palmer, H.M. Anstice, G.J. Pearson, The effect of curing regime on the release of hydroxethyl methacylate (HEMA) from resin-modified glass-ionomer cements, J. Dent. 27 (1999) 303–311.
[64] K. Kawai, T. Takaoka, Fluoride, hydrogen ion and HEMA release from light-cured GIC restorations, Am. J. Dent. 15 (2002) 149–152.
[65] W. Guertsen, Biocompatibility of resin-modified filling materials, Crit. Rev. Oral Biol. Med. 11 (2000) 333–335.
[66] W.R. Hume, T.M. Gerzina, Bioavailability of components of resin-based materials which are applied to teeth, Crit. Rev. Oral Biol. Med. 7 (1996) 172–179.
[67] V. Qvist, K. Stoltze, J. Qvist, Cytotoxicity of a bisGMA dental composite before and after leaching in organic solvent, J. Biomed. Mater. Res. 25 (1989) 443–457.
[68] A.B. Fuks, P. Cleaton-Jones, Pulp response to a composite resin inserted in deep cavities with and without a surface seal, J. Prosthet. Dent. 63 (1990) 129–134.
[69] M. Fujitani, S. Inokoshi, H. Hosada, Effect of acid etching on the dental pulp in adhesive composite restorations, Int. Dent. J. 42 (1992) 3–11.
[70] H. Schweikl, C. Spagnuolo, G. Schmalz, Genetic and cellular toxicology of dental resin monomers, J. Dent. Res. 85 (2006) 870–877.
[71] L. Kanerva, R. Jolanki, T. Leino, T. Estlander, Occupational allergic contact dermatitis from 2-hydroxethyl methacrylate and ethylene glycol dimethacrylate in a modified acrylic structural adhesive, Contact Dermat. 33 (1995) 84–89.
[72] A.M.F. Aranha, E.M.A. Giro, P.P.C. Souza, J. Hebling, C.A. Costa, Effect of curing regime on the cytotoxicity of resin-modified glass-ionomer lining cements applied to an odontoblast cell line, Dent. Mater. 22 (2006) 864–869.
[73] A. Hamid, W.R. Hume, Diffusion of resin monomers through human carious dentin *in vitro*, Endod. Dent. Traumatol. 13 (1997) 1–5.
[74] A. Hamid, W.R. Hume, The effect of dentine thickness on diffusion of resin monomers *in vitro*, J. Oral Rehabil. 24 (1997) 20–25.
[75] P.P. Souza, A.M. Aranha, J. Hebling, E.M. Giro, C.A. Costa, In vitro cytotoxicity and in vivo biocompatibility of contemporary resin-modified glass-ionomer cements, Dent. Mater. 22 (2006) 838–844.
[76] E. Yoshii, Cytotoxic effects of acrylates and methacrylates: relationships of monomer structures and cytotoxicity, J. Biomed. Mater. Res. 37 (1998) 517–524.
[77] K.C. Kan, L.B. Messer, H.H. Messer, Variability in cytotoxicity and fluoride release of resin-modified glass-ionomer cements, J. Dent. Res. 76 (1997) 1502–1507.

[78] B. Tarim, A.A. Hafez, C.F. Cox, Pulpal response to a resin-modified glass-ionomer material on non-exposed and exposed monkey pulps, Quintessence Int. 29 (1998) 535–542.
[79] H. Andreasson, A. Boman, S. Johnsson, S. Karlsson, L. Barregard, On permeability of methyl methacrylate, 2-hydroxyethyl methacrylate and triethylenegycol dimethacrylate through protective gloves in dentistry, Eur. J. Oral Sci. 111 (2003) 529–535.
[80] S.K. Sidhu, T.F. Watson, Resin-modified glass ionomer materials: a status report, Am. J. Dent. 8 (1995) 59–67.
[81] V. Sattabanasuk, V. Vachiramon, F. Qian, S.R. Armstrong, Resin-dentin bonding strength as related to different surface preparation methods, J. Dent. 35 (2007) 467–475.
[82] S. Inoue, B. Van Meerbeek, Y. Abe, Y. Yoshida, P. Lambrechts, G. Vanherle, H. Sano, Effect of remaining dentin thickness and the use of conditioner on micro-tensile bond strength of a glass-ionomer adhesive, Dent. Mater. 17 (2001) 445–455.
[83] P. Wangpermtam, M.G. Botelho, J.E. Dyson, Effect of contamination and decontamination on adhesion of a resin-modified glass-ionomer cement to bovine dentin, J. Adhes. Dent. 13 (2011) 445–453.
[84] D.N. Misra, Adsorption of polyacrylic acids and their sodium salts on hydroxyapatite: effect of relative molar mass, J. Colloid Interface Sci. 181 (1996) 289–296.
[85] A. Cetinguc, S. Olmez, N. Vural, HEMA diffusion from dentine bonding agents in young and old primary molars in vitro, Dent. Mater. 23 (2007) 302–307.
[86] P.N.R. Pereira, T. Yamada, R. Tei, J. Tagami, Bond strength and interface micromorphology of an improved resin-modified glass ionomer cement, Am. J. Dent. 10 (1997) 128–132.
[87] V.V. Gordan, D. Bover, K. Söderholm, Enamel and dentine shear bond strength of two resin modified glass ionomers and two resin based adhesives, J. Dent. 26 (1998) 497–503.
[88] E. Coutinho, Y. Yoshida, S. Inoue, R. Fukuda, J. Snauwaert, R. Nakayama, J. De Munck, P. Lambrechts, K. Suzuki, B. Van Meerbeek, Gel phase formation at resin-modified glass ionomer/tooth interfaces, J. Dent. Res. 86 (2007) 656–661.
[89] A.M. El Wakeel, D.W. Elkassas, M.M. Yousry, Bonding of contemporary glass ionomer cements to different tooth substrates; microshear bond strength and scanning electron microscope study, Eur. J. Dent. 9 (2015) 176–182.
[90] L. Wang, V.T. Sakai, E.S. Kawai, M.A. Buzalaf, M.T. Atta, Effect of adhesive systems associated with resin-modified glass ionomer cements, J. Oral Rehabil. 33 (2006) 110–116.
[91] P.N.R. Periera, T. Yamada, S. Inokoshi, M.F. Burrow, H. Sano, J. Tagami, Adhesion of resin-modified glass ionomer cements using resin bonding systems, J. Dent. 26 (1998) 479–486.
[92] A. Diwanji, V. Dhar, R. Arora, A. Madhusudan, A.S. Rathore, Comparative evaluation of microleakage of three restorative glass ionomer cements: an in vitro study, J. Nat. Sci. Biol. Med. 5 (2014) 373–377.
[93] S.K. Sidhu, T.F. Watson, Interfacial characteristics of resin-modified glass ionomer materials: a study on fluid permeability using confocal fluorescence microscopy, J. Dent. Res. 77 (1998) 1749–1759.
[94] J.H. Berg, Glass ionomer cements, Pediatr. Dent. 24 (2002) 430–438.
[95] M.E. Curzon, M.A. Pollard, M.S. Duggal, Restoration of primary molars, Br. Dent. J. 180 (1996) 246.
[96] T.P. Croll, M.L. Helpin, Class II Vitremer restoration of primary molars, ASDC J. Dent. Child. 64 (1997) 131–134.

[97] S. Hübel, I. Mejàre, Conventional versus resin-modified glass-ionomer cement for Class II restorations in primary molars. A 3-year clinical study, Int. J. Paediatr. Dent. 13 (2003) 2–8.
[98] J. Rutar, L. MacAllan, M.J. Tyas, Three-year clinical performance of glass ionomer cement in primary molars, Int. J. Paediatr. Dent. 12 (2002) 146–147.
[99] K.J. Donly, T.W. Wild, M.E. Jensen, Posterior composite Class II restorations: *in vitro* comparison of preparation designs and restoration techniques, Dent. Mater. 6 (1990) 88–93.
[100] V. Vilkinis, P. Horsted-Bindslev, V. Baelum, Two-year evaluation of Class II resin-modified glass ionomer cement/composite resin open sandwich and composite restorations, Clin. Oral Invest. 4 (2000) 133–139.
[101] K.J. Donly, C. Ingram, An in vitro caries inhibition of photopolymerized glass ionomer liners, ASDC J. Dent. Child. 64 (1997) 128–130.
[102] V. Qvist, L. Laurberg, A. Poulsen, P.T. Teglers, Longevity and cariostatic effects of everyday conventional glass-ionomer and amalgam restorations in primary teeth: 3-year results, J. Dent. Res. 76 (1997) 1387–1396.
[103] S. Karvanto-Seppala, E. Lavonius, E. Kerosuo, I. Pietila, Clinical evaluation of a glass-ionomer/resin-based hybrid materials used as pit-and-fissure sealants, Quintessence Int. 32 (2001) 463–468.
[104] R.J. Smales, K.C. Wong, Two-year clinical performance of a resin-modified glass ionomer sealant, Am. J. Dent. 12 (1999) 62–64.
[105] M. Raadal, A.B. Urkilen, O.L. Nilsen, Fissure sealing with a light-cured resin-modified glass-ionomer cement (Vitrebond) compared with a resin sealant, Int. J. Paediatr. Dent. 6 (1996) 235–239.
[106] C.H. Pameijer, Crown retention with three resin-modified glass ionomer luting cements, J. Am. Dent. Assoc. 143 (2012) 1218–1222.
[107] S.B. Mitra, C.-Y. Ling, H.T. Bui, D. Tantbiroin, R.P. Rusin, Long-term adhesion and mechanism of bonding of a paste-liquid resin-modified glass-ionomer, Dent. Mater. 25 (2009) 459–466.
[108] S.B. Mitra, J.D. Oxman, A. Falsafi, T.T. Ton, Fluoride release and recharge behaviour of a nano-filled resin-modified glass ionomer compared with that other fluoride releasing materials, Am. J. Dent. 24 (2011) 372–378.
[109] S.B. Mitra, D. Wu, B.N. Holmes, An application of nanotechnology in advanced dental materials, J. Am. Dent. Assoc. 134 (2003) 1382–1390.

Modern glass-ionomer materials of enhanced properties

8

8.1 Introduction

Conventional glass-ionomers are known to show a modest degree of bioactivity. They release fluoride ions [1], and also sodium, phosphate and silicate, which are beneficial biologically [2]. In saliva, they are capable of taking up both calcium and phosphate ions [3] and at the tooth surface, they are able to exchange ions to develop a strong interfacial bonding region [4,5]. At the bottom of pits and fissures, their structure is altered, probably in association with the uptake of calcium and phosphate, and an enamel-like structure is formed [6].

Despite these observations, both the speed of any ion-exchange processes and the amount of exchangeable ions could be improved. In searching for methods of doing this, there is a difficulty which presents itself immediately, namely that adding substances such as hydroxyapatite, that would improve the bioactivity, slow down the setting reaction and weaken the set cement. The reason for the reduced speed of setting is that candidate additives do not themselves react sufficiently quickly with the polyacid component, if they react at all. Therefore they effectively dilute the proportion of reactive powder in the cement.

Studies have been made of the inclusion of two possible substances to enhance the bioactivity of conventional glass-ionomer cements, hydroxyapatite [7] and bioglass powder [8]. Both were found to reduce the speed of the setting reaction of the cement, with the reduction being greater with larger proportions of additive. In all cases, the set cements were consistently weaker than those with no additive (Table 8.1). This result has also been found with completely inert powders, such as borax [9].

The relationship between the speed of the setting reaction and the strength of the set cement has been widely demonstrated for conventional glass-ionomers based on alumino-silicate glass powders. Any step which extends the working and setting times, including the addition of organic [10] or ionic additives [11], or reducing the powder:liquid ratio [12] results in weaker set cements.

In recent years, a new type of glass-ionomer material has become available that overcomes this problem of the weakening effect of additional fillers designed to enhance the bioactivity of the cement. Known as the glass carbomer®, it overcomes the problem of slow setting by specifying the need to cure with the aid of heat from dental cure lamps.

Another considerable disadvantage of established members of the glass-ionomer family is their brittleness. Including extra filler in the glass carbomer type in and of itself does not help with this drawback; indeed, it makes the situation worse. However, in its final formulation, the glass carbomer also contains a novel component, a silicone oil, which improves the toughness of the set cement and makes the potential durability better.

Materials for the Direct Restoration of Teeth. http://dx.doi.org/10.1016/B978-0-08-100491-3.00008-8

Table 8.1 **Effect on mechanical properties and setting behaviour of hydroxyapatite incorporated into a conventional glass-ionomer cement [7]**

Hydroxyapatite (%)	Working time (min)	Setting time (min)	Compressive strength (MPa)
0	2	9	20 (1)
2.5	3	19	20 (1)
5.0	6	34	18 (1)
10.0	10	55	14 (2)
20.0	10	76	11 (1)

Standard deviations in parentheses.

Another recently launched material of the glass-ionomer type also contains novel components, in particular a patented diurethane monomer capable of polymerizing to give a set material of superior flexural strength and reduced brittleness. It is described as resin-modified glass-ionomer with the added description of 'bioactive ionic resin-based composite'.

Both of these materials are distinctly different from other types of glass-ionomer, and so are discussed separately in the current chapter. In their different ways, they address particular shortcomings of established glass-ionomer materials. Currently, there is one example of the glass carbomer and two of the enhanced performance resin-modified glass-ionomer available, and only one manufacturer currently manufactures each type. Given their early success, it is likely that similar materials will be launched in the future, and that the classes of enhanced performance and enhanced bioactivity glass-ionomers will emerge as distinctive ones in the years to come.

These materials are considered in the succeeding sections of the current chapter, with the conventional glass-ionomer type covered separately from the resin-modified one.

8.2 Enhanced bioactivity conventional glass-ionomer cement

The brand of this type currently available is marketed under the name 'Glass Carbomer®'. Unfortunately, this term has been adopted in the scientific literature to describe these materials [13–16] and, used in this way, implies that the material is of a completely new type. However, it is actually a type of glass-ionomer because it sets by an acid–base reaction between an aqueous polymeric acid and an ion-leachable basic glass. This has been considered for many years to be the defining characteristic of a true glass-ionomer cement [17]. Moreover, recent research confirms the essential soundness of this definition and shows how many chemical and biological properties follow from this feature [18]. For this reason, we prefer to describe this material as an enhanced bioactivity glass-ionomer cement, and to consider the term glass carbomer to be simply the name of the first commercial material of this type.

The material was developed to improve the bioactivity compared with the original conventional glass-ionomer cement and, as already stated, derives partly from the observation that conventional glass-ionomer deep with pits and fissures undergoes a transformation into an enamel-like material [6]. The glass carbomer has been formulated to undergo such a transformation more readily than a conventional glass-ionomer by including hydroxyapatite as additional bioactive filler. In developing the glass carbomer, not only the bioactivity was improved, but additional components have been included and the overall formulation optimized to improve the physical properties [13].

The components of the enhanced bioactivity conventional glass-ionomer (glass carbomer) are as follows:

(i) An aqueous solution of polymeric acid, such as poly(acrylic acid) or acrylic/maleic acid copolymer.

(ii) A glass powder that has been acid washed in a strong acid so that, according to the description in the patent application [19], the surface layers of the particles are substantially depleted in calcium, and the majority of calcium ions lie well inside the particles towards the core. The patent on these materials specifies that the surface layers will contain between half and a quarter of the concentration of calcium ions of the core, a result of acid washing under relatively severe conditions using strong mineral acids, such as hydrochloric acid [19].

(iii) A silicone oil comprising a polydimethylsiloxane that may be either linear or cyclic, though linear appears to be preferred. This substance contains hydroxyl groups, which are able to form hydrogen bonds with some of the other components of the cement, so that it does not leach from the material once it has set.

(iv) A bioactive component that acts as a secondary filler [14]. This has been assumed to be fluorapatite [20], but solid state NMR spectroscopy has demonstrated that it is actually hydroxyapatite [13]. It is included to enhance the possibility of the formation of a structure similar to enamel adjacent to the restoration, as observed for conventional glass-ionomer pit and fissure sealants [6].

The glass used in glass carbomer contains a reasonable amount of strontium [21], as well as a small amount of calcium. It is relatively high in silicon compared with the glasses used in the well-established brands of conventional glass-ionomer Fuji IX and Ketac Molar (see Table 8.2), but contains comparable amounts of aluminium, phosphorus and fluoride.

The glass is subjected to quite extensive acid washing with strong mineral acid, which eventually makes the glass somewhat lacking in reactivity towards poly(acrylic acid) or acrylic/maleic acid copolymer. In addition, the silicone oil is incorporated into the glass powder and becomes adsorbed on the surface. Consequently, the glass powder is very unreactive compared with conventional ionomer glasses. As a result, it is easy to mix with the aqueous acid solution at high powder:liquid ratios, and little or no reaction occurs immediately when these two components are brought together. As a result, the viscosity of the mixture hardly changes in the first few minutes after mixing. This is different from conventional glass-ionomers, where reaction begins immediately on mixing.

Because of this reduced reactivity, the manufacturers recommend that the freshly mixed and placed material should be cured with the application of a dental cure

Table 8.2 Weight percentage composition of glasses in various commercial conventional glass-ionomer cements

	Si	Al	Ca	Na	F	P	Sr	La
Fuji IX	13.7	17.9	0	1.0	10.2	2.2	19.9	0
Ketac Molar	12.4	15.0	10.1	1.7	13.3	2.0	0	17.6
Glass carbomer	20.0	14.1	2.1	1.9	9.0	2.5	13.6	0

Source: N.K. Thanjal, R.W. Billington, S. Shahid, J. Luo, R.G. Hill, G.J. Pearson, Kinetics of fluoride ion release from dental restorative glass ionomer cements: the influence of ultrasound, radiant heat and glass composition, J. Mater. Sci., Mater. Med. 21 (2010) 589–595.

lamp for at least 20 s [15]. This is not because the material is capable of undergoing photo-polymerization, but because dental cure lamps emit heat as well as light. By increasing the temperature of the newly placed cement in this way, the glass carbomer sets to an acceptable extent in a reasonable time. This allows it to be finished by the clinician, and leaves the material sufficiently well set that it is able to function satisfactorily in the mouth.

Effectively the heat treatment overcomes the problems caused by reducing the reactivity of the basic glass and reducing its proportion as a total of the filler within the cement. Heating accelerates the setting reaction so that the material's sluggish setting reaction is overcome. The material therefore attains acceptable strength quickly enough for it to be a practical repair material in dentistry.

The high proportion of glass that can be incorporated as a result its lack of reactivity and also the extra hydroxyapatite filler that is included mean that the glass carbomer would be very brittle. For this reason, the silicone oil is incorporated. It toughens the material, and reduces its brittleness. In this way, glass carbomers are toughened relative to conventional glass-ionomers, and they lack this widely acknowledged drawback of conventional glass-ionomer cements [22]. The hydroxyl functional groups allow the silicone oil to remain bonded within the set cement, so that it is anticipated that these materials will retain a high degree of toughness throughout their service life. However, so far there is no direct evidence to confirm or deny this assumption.

8.2.1 Setting reaction

So far, the setting reaction of glass carbomer cements has only been reported when studied by magic angle spinning nuclear magnetic resonance (MAS-NMR) spectroscopy [13]. This focuses on the inorganic elements aluminium, phosphorus, fluorine and silicon, and gives no information about the polymer component. However, these elements are able to track the distinctive features of glass carbomer chemistry, since they give information about the involvement of the specific acid-washed glass and the hydroxyapatite secondary fillers. It may be assumed that certain aspects of the setting chemistry precisely match those of the setting of conventional glass-ionomer cements, ie, the rise in pH on acid neutralization and the formation of ionic crosslinks based on carboxylate groups. The latter is generated by reaction of the carboxylic acid functional groups of the polymer.

MAS-NMR of the glass in glass carbomer showed it to contain aluminium in predominantly four co-ordinations [13]. It was also shown to occur as Al–O–P [13]. This arrangement is similar to that found in conventional ionomer glasses [23,24], indicating that the extensive acid washing does not influence the structure of the remaining glass substantially. Like conventional glass-ionomers, as setting proceeds so the proportion of four co-ordinate aluminium declines and the proportion of six co-ordinate aluminium increases. Silica tetrahedra were shown to be highly crosslinked by ^{29}Si MAS-NMR, with most of the silicon occurring in the so-called Q4 structures, ie, SiO_4 tetrahedra linked to four other iso-structural tetrahedra. On average, two of these four linked tetrahedra were found to be aluminium-centred [13]. This suggests a slightly greater degree of connectivity in this glass compared to that found in conventional ionomer glasses [23,24]. The significance of this observation is not clear.

From the ^{31}P and ^{19}F MAS-NMR spectra, it was apparent that the adjunct filler was substantially hydroxyapatite rather than fluorapatite. The diminution in the ^{31}P peak due to orthophosphate was taken to indicate that this apatite filler was undergoing a reaction with the polymeric acid, and contributing to setting. This reaction has not been observed previously when synthetic hydroxyapatite was included in a conventional glass-ionomer cement [7], though reaction of poly(acrylic acid) with other calcium phosphate minerals has been observed previously [25].

The conclusion from these studies is that the setting of glass carbomer involves two parallel neutralization reactions, one of the polyacid with the glass and the other of the polyacid with the hydroxyapatite. The resulting material has much in common with a conventional glass-ionomer cement, in that it consists of an ionically crosslinked polyacid matrix with filler embedded in it. In this case, however, the filler is not ion-depleted glass only, but also partially reacted hydroxyapatite. The matrix, too, differs significantly from that which occurs in a conventional glass-ionomer cement in that it also includes the polydimethylsiloxane oil to impart toughness to the set material.

8.2.2 Properties of enhanced bioactivity conventional glass-ionomers

To date, there have been few reported studies of the physical properties of glass carbomers. As a member of the glass-ionomer cement family designed to undergo self-cure (ie, to set by the acid–base reaction only), they are required to meet the specification of the relevant ISO Standard, ISO 9917-1 [26]. The particular mechanical requirement in the Standard is that the material should have a compressive strength of at least 100 MPa. There are, as yet, no published data to confirm that the glass carbomer achieves this value, though equally there are no grounds for doubting that it does.

One study has compared two physical properties of the enhanced bioactivity conventional glass-ionomer with those of a well-established brand of conventional glass-ionomer, Fuji IX (GC Corporation, Leuven, Belgium) [27]. Properties studied were Knoop Hardness, tested ~20 min after setting, and microshear bond strength on both sound and caries-affected dentine. The latter test was carried out after storing the specimens in water at 37°C for 24 h.

Results from the Knoop Hardness experiments are shown in Table 8.3. They show that the conventional glass-ionomer was harder than the glass carbomer by an amount that was statistically significant. Unfortunately, no other mechanical data were reported, so that it is not clear from this finding whether the conventional glass-ionomer is mechanically superior to the glass carbomer, or whether it was simply marginally harder at the time tested.

Microshear bond strengths are shown in Table 8.4. On both substrates, the conventional glass-ionomer gave higher bond strengths than the glass carbomer, but differences were not statistically significant. Both materials showed higher bond strengths to sound dentine than to caries-affected dentine, and the differences were significant for each of them [27].

Table 8.3 Knoop hardness values for glass carbomer and conventional glass-ionomer cement [27]

Material	Knoop hardness value
Fuji IX (GIC)	24.32 (1.21)
Glass carbomer	20.80 (1.61)

Standard deviations in parentheses.

Table 8.4 Microshear bond strengths (MPa) of glass carbomer and conventional glass-ionomer cement [27]

Material	Sound dentine (MPa)	Caries-affected dentine (MPa)
Fuji IX	1.74 (0.40)	1.11 (0.16)
Glass carbomer	1.34 (0.63)	0.89 (0.28)

Standard deviations in parentheses.

Overall, though there were only a limited amount of data reported in this study [27], it was useful because they showed that the properties of glass carbomer are at least comparable with those of a well-known conventional glass-ionomer.

8.2.3 Clinical uses of enhanced bioactivity conventional glass-ionomers

Enhanced bioactivity conventional glass-ionomers (glass carbomers) are intended for use in the same range of applications as conventional glass-ionomers, ie, liners and bases, full restorations of various types, and pit-and-fissure sealants. Because of their similarity to conventional glass-ionomers, it is considered that these materials will prove useful in the restoration of primary dentition [15].

One recent study considered the microleakage and marginal integrity of glass carbomers placed in extracted primary molars and also the effect of placing them with and without a protective coating [15]. In this study, glass carbomer was compared with a conventional glass-ionomer (Ionofil U, Voco, Cuxhaven, Germany) and a polyacid-modified composite resin (Dyract Extra, Dentsply, Konstanz, Germany).

Results showed that, in the uncoated state, the glass carbomer was distinctly inferior to the conventional glass-ionomer [15]. Not only did it show worse marginal leakage, as indicated by dye penetration, the glass carbomer also showed substantial cracking, both on the surface and within the specimens. However, coating improved the performance markedly. Sealing was improved and specimens no longer developed cracks, either at the surface or inside the material [15]. This suggests that glass carbomer possesses a greater degree of sensitivity to moisture loss than the conventional glass-ionomer used in this study, and that sealing the finished restoration with a proprietary photo-cured varnish may be desirable in clinical use. The beneficial effect of using a photo-cured varnish with glass carbomers was also shown in an in vitro study of sealing ability of these materials evaluated by micro-CT [28].

There have been publications on the effectiveness of glass carbomer as a pit-and-fissure sealant. In one [16], the study compared glass carbomer with a resin-based sealant in 48 teeth in 24 patients. After 6 months, both materials showed 100% retention and after 12 months, they both showed 75% retention. This showed that in terms of one important requirement of fissure sealants, namely retention, the glass carbomer performed quite well. However, further work is necessary to establish whether the enhanced bioactivity confers any further or longer term benefits by way of caries inhibition.

These results have been confirmed in a much larger and longer study [29]. The latter study employed 108 children, with follow up examinations for up to 24 months following placement. Assessment involved not only determination of retention but also examination for adjacent caries. At 24 months, retention was good for both materials, and enamel caries was observed in three teeth sealed with glass carbomer. This is a promising finding, despite not being statistically significant. Overall, this result suggests that glass carbomers have the potential to be effective fissure sealants. However, again, this study was not able to identify any benefits specifically attributable to the enhanced bioactivity of the glass carbomer material.

8.3 Enhanced performance resin-modified glass-ionomer cement

Two materials are currently available in this category, namely Activa™ Bioactive Restorative and Activa™ Bioactive Base Liner™, both manufactured by the American company Pulpdent® Corporation. The US Food and Drugs Administration (FDA) gave pre-market approval for these two materials in 2013 [30]. This approval was given on the grounds that these materials can be considered essentially similar to currently available resin-modified glass-ionomers.

As such, they must be able to undergo the same reactions as the well-established resin-modified glass-ionomers [17]. This means that they should be capable of a degree of setting in the dark entirely by an acid–base reaction, as they appear to [30]. Although this reaction is able to occur, in clinical service the setting of these materials can be enhanced by a photo-polymerization reaction that is promoted by irradiation with a dental cure lamp for 20 s [30]. As with the glass carbomer, these materials contain additional components, one a polymer capable of imparting toughness and the other a modified acidic monomer capable of promoting bonding to the tooth.

Properties of the two available enhanced performance resin-modified are summarized in Table 8.5 [30]. From this table, it can be seen that these materials have good compressive strength and the ability to release substantial amounts of fluoride for at least a 28-day period. Moreover, this fluoride release appeared to be sustained well beyond that time.

Table 8.5 Physical properties of enhanced resin-modified glass-ionomers (Activa restorative and Activa Base/Liner) [30]

Property	Activa Restorative	Activa Base/Liner
Light-cure setting time (s)	20	20
Depth of light cure (mm)	4	4
Self-cure setting time at 37°C	2	2
Total filler (%)	56	45
Reactive glass (%)	21.8	19.3
Fluoride release, 1 day (ppm)	230	360
Cumulative fluoride release, 28 days (ppm)	940	1300
Compressive strength (MPa)	280	226
Water sorption, 1 week (%)	1.65	2.30
Polymerization shrinkage (%)	1.7	n/a

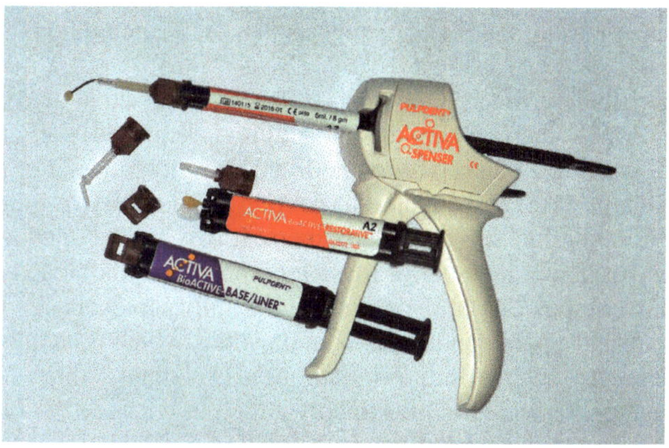

Fig. 8.1 Delivery system for Activa materials.
Courtesy of Pulpdent Corporation, used with permission.

Both materials are supplied as two-paste systems, and the pastes are mixed immediately prior to use [30]. Two possible approaches to mixing are available. One uses the proprietary mixing gun supplied by the manufacturer of the material. This gun is loaded with tubes containing the two pastes, and feeds them into a single nozzle, where an arrangement of baffles promotes mixing as the two pastes are extruded from their respective tubes (Fig. 8.1). Freshly mixed paste is then expressed from the end of the nozzle, where it can be placed as required in the teeth under repair.

Alternatively the two pastes can be extruded onto a conventional mixing pad and blended by hand with a spatula. Even when prepared in this way, it is desirable for the freshly mixed paste to be placed by syringe, so from the mixing pad, it must be loaded into an appropriate tip for delivery. Mixing in this way carries the risk of incorporating air into the paste, which in the form of bubbles can weaken the set material [30].

Neither of these materials contains any of the monomers used in conventional composites, particular bisGMA [30]. In addition, it contains no bisphenol A or its derivatives, so that it is biocompatible for its intended use, and does not contribute to the burden of molecules in the environment that mimic the action of oestrogen.

Much of this information has been provided by the manufacturer, Pulpdent® Corporation. Currently, independent reports on these materials from universities and research institutes are only beginning to appear in the literature. Where possible, this chapter quotes these reports, including accounts of the clinical performance of the materials.

8.3.1 Composition of enhanced performance resin-modified glass-ionomers

Because the two types of material in this category are propriety, there is relatively little information available about their composition, and what there is needs to be inferred from a variety of sources. The fact of their FDA approval as a type of resin-modified glass-ionomer is important, because it suggests that they contain both a reactive basic glass and an acid.

The materials are described by the manufacturer as 'bioactive', but there has been no published information about how this bioactivity is achieved, nor whether it is notably better than that of established resin-modified glass-ionomers. For example, there is no indication about whether the materials contain an additive to promote bioactivity, such as hydroxyapatite, like the glass carbomers. It may be that they are bioactive in just the same way that any member of glass-ionomer family is bioactive, namely because of the ionic composition of the glass and the ability to exchange fluoride.

These materials have been reported to contain silica, which is an inert filler [31], in addition to their reactive glass. Both formulations also contain sodium fluoride (0.75% and 0.9%, respectively), which is presumably added to enhance the fluoride release, a feature which suggests that insufficient fluoride is available from the basic glass. Preliminary indications are that the restorative material has a good fluoride recharge capability [32], and one that is greater than either Ketac Nano resin-modified glass-ionomer or Fuji Triage conventional glass-ionomer over a 3-week period [33].

According to the manufacturers, the acid in these materials is a so-called phosphate acid, ie, based on phosphonic acid groups, $-PO_3H_2$. Such groups are capable of contributing to the bonding of this material to the tooth surface [34], which may protect the restoration from microleakage.

The main novelty of these materials is that they contain a blend of diurethanes, as well as methacrylate monomers such as HEMA. The urethanes have previously been patented for use in novel composite resins [35,36], and as a result, these materials have much in common with composite resins. Indeed, until further work is published, it will not be clear whether these materials have much glass-ionomer character at all, despite the claimed similarity which led to FDA approval.

These materials have been studied for flexural strength and the results compared to those from two conventional glass-ionomer and two resin-modified glass-ionomer cements [31]. Results are shown in Table 8.6.

Table 8.6 Flexural strength of selected glass-ionomer materials [31]

Material	Type	Flexural strength (MPa)
Activa Restorative	Enhanced RMGIC	105.4 (14.3)
Activa Base/Liner	Enhanced RMGIC	99.8 (24.0)
Fuji IX GP Extra	Conventional glass-ionomer	28.1 (5.0)
Fuji Triage	Conventional glass-ionomer	19.7 (4.9)
Ketac Nano	RMGIC	28.4 (10.1)
Vitrebond Plus	RMGIC	24.0 (9.6)

Standard deviations in parentheses.

These results suggest that the materials contain relatively high proportions of resin phase relative to the glass-ionomer one, and both materials have significantly better flexural strengths than any type of glass-ionomer. Indeed, their values exceed the minimum specified for conventional composite resins [37]. This finding suggests that these materials will show good wear in vivo, and may therefore prove durable in clinical service.

8.3.2 *Clinical studies*

The two materials have distinctive applications as a full restorative and liner or base (Activa Restorative and Activa Base Liner, respectively). Experience is beginning to emerge of their uses in these two applications and results are promising. For example, one study gave details of two cases [30]. In one, a 10-year-old boy had a mesio-occlusal lesion in the right primary molar of the maxilla. This was repaired following cavity preparation with a cylindrical diamond bur using a single portion of material injected slowly to fill the cavity from the bottom while avoiding the inclusion of air. The restoration was allowed to self-cure by the acid–base reaction for 20 s, and then cured with visible light for a further 20 s. Then it was finished, giving the result shown in Fig. 8.2.

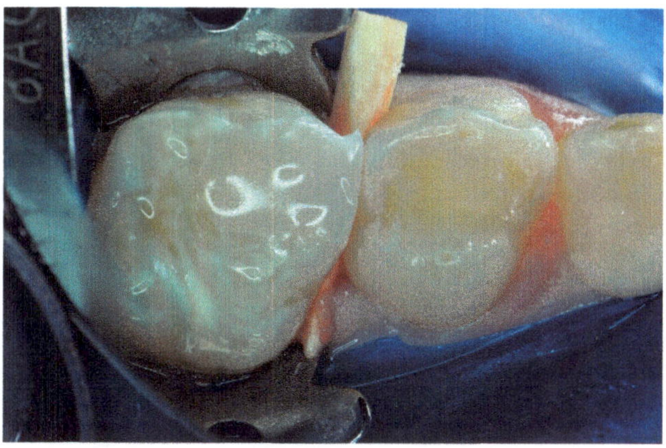

Fig. 8.2 Light-cured Activa Bioactive Restorative, newly placed and after removal of the matrix strip.

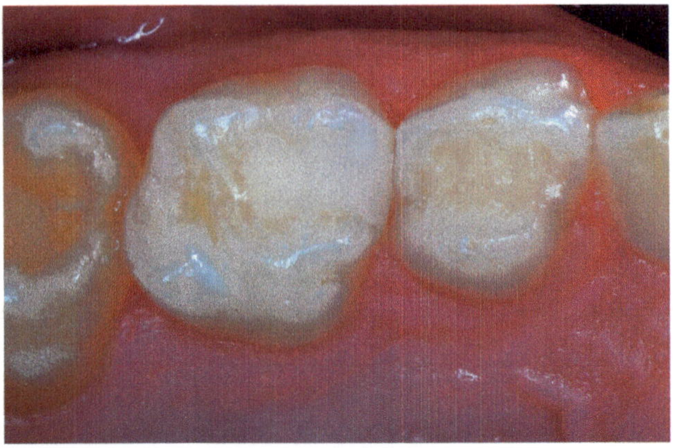

Fig. 8.3 Same restoration as in Fig. 8.2 after 6 months.

After 6 months, there was no detectable wear (Fig. 8.3). All of the margins appeared sound and there were no signs of failure.

In the second case, the material was used to repair an occlusal carious lesion in the right permanent first molar of the mandible of an 11-year-old girl. In this case, cavity preparation included the use of a self-etching bonding agent, which was applied and agitated for 20 s prior to the injection of Activa Restorative. This result was again very sound and aesthetic [30]. However, the fact that a self-etching bonding agent was needed indicates that the material does not show sufficient adhesion to the prepared tooth surface, and feature that is consistent with its high resin content.

These were the two cases described in detail, but a further 390 cases (210 in primary teeth; 180 in permanent teeth) over a 6-month period were also mentioned [30]. In all of these, the material has been found to perform well, handling like an injectable composite resin, and showing no indication of contraction from the margins of the restorations. This was attributed to its low polymerization contraction [30]. The material has also been used without bonding agent, and appears to have bonded to an acceptable extent.

These findings represent the initial reports on the clinical use of these materials. Further work is needed to confirm (or otherwise) the positive findings from these first 6 months of clinical observations. Additional work is also necessary to determine the ideal method of bonding them to the tooth and also the extent to which they can form natural adhesive bonds to the surface of teeth.

Clinical summary

- There are two types of enhanced property glass-ionomers, one of each type (conventional and resin-modified).
- The conventional type is called the *glass carbomer.*
- The resin-modified type is described in this chapter as *enhanced performance resin-modified glass-ionomers.* These are available as a restorative and liner/base grades.
- The glass carbomer has similar properties to conventional glass-ionomers in terms of mechanical strength, adhesion and fluoride release. It is somewhat tougher, though. There do

not appear to be any advantages from the presence of hydroxyapatite within the material, despite claims of improved bioactivity.

- The enhanced performance resin-modified glass-ionomers are high in resin, and as a result appear to have somewhat compromised adhesion. Their bioactivity appears very good.
- Considerable further work is required to know whether or not these materials represent a significant advance in glass-ionomer technology and restorative dentistry.

Clinical use of modified glass-ionomer materials

(a) Glass carbomer

(i) These should be used in the same way as conventional glass-ionomers.

(ii) As for glass-ionomers, cavity preparation can be restricted to removal of caries and unsupported enamel only.

(iii) After cavity preparation, condition the cavity (remove the smear later) using a conditioning solution (typically 10% poly(acrylic acid) or 5% citric acid in water) using a cotton pellet saturated with conditioner placed in the cavity for 15–20 s, after which the surface is rinsed with water for 5 s, lightly dried but not dehydrated. This is achieved by swabbing with dry cotton pellets only.

(iv) In the case of deep caries, protect the pulpal floor with calcium hydroxide setting cement or zinc oxide-eugenol cement.

(v) Mix the glass carbomer cement according to the manufacturer's instructions. For hand-mixed cements, ensure that the correct powder:liquid ratio is used. For capsulated cements, ensure that mixing is carried out for the correct time.

(vi) Completely fill the cavity in one portion, press the cement with an instrument or the finger until the it has hardened, then remove excess using either hand instruments or a bur without water.

(vii) Cover the restoration with varnish, bonding agent or petroleum jelly, and where appropriate cure in accordance with manufacturer's instructions.

(viii) Check occlusion with articulation paper, and correct if necessary.

(ix) The patient should be asked not to eat and drink for 2 h after completion, and preferably to avoid biting on the tooth for 24 h.

(x) If necessary, a final finishing of the restoration can be carried out after a minimum of 24 h following placement. This should use silicone rubber polishing discs and polishing pastes, and should be completed by further varnishing of the restoration.

(b) Enhanced performance resin-modified glass-ionomer (Activa Bioactive Restorative and Activa Bioactive Base Liner)

(i) There is ambiguity about these materials but it is probably safest with the current state of knowledge to employ them as for composite resins, including the use of a bonding agent.

(ii) Prepare the cavity — remove plaque and pellicle from the surface using a non-fluoridated cleaning paste and a rotary brush. Then remove all caries and cut the enamel.

(iii) In the case of deep caries, cover the pulpal wall with calcium hydroxide cement, followed by either zinc polycarboxylate or glass-ionomer cement. Do not use zinc oxide-eugenol, as eugenol is released from this material and it inhibits the polymerization of the material.

(iv) Prepare cut surface and apply appropriate bonding agent, preferably a 4-step one (see Chapter 5).

(v) For a restoration, apply first layer approximately 1 mm thick and light cure for 40 s. Apply subsequent layers, curing each for 40 s.

(vi) Remove excess material (use diamond bur, finishing bur or Arkansas stone). Polish with fluoride-containing paste and silicone discs.
(vii) The patient can eat and drink immediately this procedure is completed.
(viii) For a liner/base, apply only one layer of Activa Bioactive Base Liner, followed by an appropriate full restorative (possibly Activa Bioactive Restorative).

References

[1] L. Forsten, Short- and long-term fluoride release from glass ionomers, Scand. J. Dent. Res. 99 (1991) 241–245.
[2] B. Czarnecka, H. Limanowska-Shaw, J.W. Nicholson, Buffering and ion release by a glass-ionomer cement under near-neutral and acidic conditions, Biomaterials 23 (2002) 2783–2788.
[3] K. Okada, S. Tosaki, K. Hirota, W.R. Hume, Surface hardness change of restorative filling materials stored in saliva, Dent. Mater. 17 (2001) 34–39.
[4] N.G. Ngo, G.J. Mount, M.C.R.B. Peters, A study of glass-ionomer cement and its interface with enamel and dentin using a low-temperature, high-resolution scanning electron microscopic technique, Quintessence Int. 28 (1997) 63–69.
[5] N. Hien-Chi, G. Mount, J. McIntyre, J. Tuisuva, R.J. Von Doussa, Chemical exchange between glass-ionomer restorations and residual carious dentine in permanent molars: an in vivo study, J. Dent. 34 (2006) 608–613.
[6] R.N.B. Van Duinen, C.L. Davidson, A. de Gee, A.J. Feilzer, In situ transformation of glass-ionomer into an enamel-like material, Am. J. Dent. 17 (2004) 223–227.
[7] J.W. Nicholson, S.J. Hawkins, J.E. Smith, The incorporation of hydroxyapatite into glass polyalkenoate ('glass-ionomer') cements: a preliminary study, J. Mater. Sci. Mater. Med. 4 (1993) 418–421.
[8] H. Yli-Urpo, L.V.J. Lassila, T. Harhi, P.K. Vallittu, Compressive strength and surface characterization of glass ionomer cements modified by bioactive glass, Dent. Mater. 21 (2005) 201–209.
[9] R.K. Bansal, U.S. Tewari, P. Singh, D.V.S. Murthy, Modified polylkenoate (glass-ionomer) cement: a study, J. Oral Rehabil. 22 (1995) 533–537.
[10] H.M. Anstice, J.W. Nicholson, Studies in the setting of polyelectrolyte materials, Part 2: the effect of organic compounds on a glass polyalkenoate cement, J. Mater. Sci. Mater. Med. 5 (1994) 299–302.
[11] J.W. Nicholson, Studies in the setting of polyelectrolyte materials, Part 3: effect sodium salts on the setting and properties of glass polyalkenoate and zinc polycarboxylate dental cements, J. Mater. Sci. Mater. Med. 6 (1995) 404–406.
[12] S. Crisp, B.G. Lewis, A.D. Wilson, Characterization of glass-ionomer cements. 2. Effect of powder:liquid ratio on the physical properties, J. Dent. 4 (1976) 287–290.
[13] N. Zainuddin, N. Karpukhina, R.V. Law, Characterisation of remineralising Glass Carbomer® ionomer cement by MAS-NMR spectroscopy, Dent. Mater. 28 (2012) 1051–1058.
[14] U. Menne-Happ, N. Ilie, Effect of gloss and heat on the mechanical behaviour of a glass carbomer cement, J. Dent. 41 (2013) 223–230.
[15] S.B. Cehreli, R.E. Tirali, Z. Yalcinkava, Z.C. Cehreli, Microleakage of newly developed glass carbomer cement in primary teeth, Eur. J. Dent. 7 (2013) 15–21.
[16] K. Gorseta, D. Glavina, A. Borzabadi-Farahani, R.N. Van Duinen, I. Skrinjaric, R.G. Hill, E. Lynch, One-year clinical evaluation of a glass carbomer fissure sealant, a preliminary study, Eur. J. Prosthodont. Restor. Dent. 22 (2014) 67–71.

[17] J.W. McLean, J.W. Nicholson, A.D. Wilson, Proposed nomenclature for glass-ionomer dental cements and related materials, Quintessence Int. 25 (1994) 587–598.
[18] G.J. Mount, M.J. Tyas, J.L. Ferracane, J.W. Nicholson, J.H. Berg, R.J. Simonsen, H.C. Ngo, A revised classification for direct tooth-colored restorative materials, Quintessence Int. 40 (2009) 691–697.
[19] W. Van Duinen, R.N. Van Duinen, Self hardening glass carbomer composition, US Patent application 20060217455 A1, 2004.
[20] X. Chen, M. Du, M. Fan, J. Mulder, M.-C. HuysmNA, J.E. Frencken, Effectiveness of two new types of sealants: retention after 2 years, Clin. Oral Invest. 16 (2012) 1443–1450.
[21] N.K. Thanjal, R.W. Billington, S. Shahid, J. Luo, R.G. Hill, G.J. Pearson, Kinetics of fluoride ion release from dental restorative glass ionomer cements: the influence of ultrasound, radiant heat and glass composition, J. Mater. Sci. Mater. Med. 21 (2010) 589–595.
[22] U. Lohbauer, Dental glass ionomer cements as permanent filling materials? Properties, limitations and future trends, Materials 3 (2010) 76–96.
[23] A. Stamboulis, R.V. Law, R.G. Hill, Characterisation of commercial ionomer glasses using magic angle nuclear magnetic resonance (MAS-NMR), Biomaterials 25 (2004) 3907–3913.
[24] S. Matsuya, A. Stamboulis, R.G. Hill, R.V. Law, Structural characterization of ionomer glasses by multinuclear solid state MAS-NMR spectroscopy, J. Non-Cryst. Solids 353 (2007) 237–243.
[25] K.S. Tenhuisen, P.W. Brown, The formation of hydroxyapatite-ionomer cements at 38 degrees C, J. Dent. Res. 73 (1994) 598–606.
[26] International Organization for Standardization, ISO 9917–1: Dental Water Based Cements, ISO, Geneva, Switzerland, 2007.
[27] I.C. Olegario, A.P.V.F.P. Malagrana, S.S.H. Kim, D. Hess, T.K. Tedesco, A.F.B. Calvo, L.B. Camargo, D.P. Raggio, Mechanical properties of high-viscosity glass ionomer cement and nanoparticle glass carbomer, J. Nanomater. 2015 (2015). Article ID 472401.
[28] X. Chen, V. Cuipers, M. Fan, J.E. Frencken, Marginal leakage of two newer glass ionomer-based sealant materials assessed using micro-CT, J. Dent. 38 (2010) 731–738.
[29] P. Subramaniam, S. Jayasurya, K.L. Girish Babu, Evaluation of glass carbomer sealant and a moisture tolerant resin sealant – a comparative study, Int. J. Dent. Sci. Res. 2 (2015) 42–48.
[30] T.P. Croll, J.H. Berg, K.J. Donly, Dental repair material: a resin-modified glass-ionomer bioactive ionic resin-based composite, Compendium 36 (2015) 60–65.
[31] C.H. Pameijer, F. Garcia-Godoy, B.R. Morrow, S.J. Jefferies, Flexural strength and flexural fatigue properties of resin-modified glass ionomers, J. Clin. Dent. 26 (2015) 23–27.
[32] A.J. Preston, E.A. Agalamanyi, S.M. Higham, L.H. Mair, The recharge of aesthetic dental materials with fluoride in vitro – two years' results, Dent. Mater. 19 (2013) 32–37.
[33] L. Slowikowski, S. John, M. Finkelman, R.D. Perry, M. Harson, G. Krugel, Fluoride ion release and recharge over time by three restoratives, J. Dent. Res. 93 (Special issue A) (2013) Abstract 268.
[34] A. Altin, B. Akgun, Z.S. Bilgici, S.B. Turker, D. Avci, Synthesis, photopolymerization and adhesive properties of novel stable phosphonic acid-containing (meth)acrylamides, J. Polym. Sci., Part A: Polym. Chem. 52 (2014) 511–522.
[35] S. Skaria, K. Berk, Radically curable urethane dimethacrylates and compositions thereof for tougher dental prosthetics, US Patent 8,292,625, 2012.
[36] S. Skaria, K. Berk, Radically curable urethane dimethacrylates and compositions thereof for tougher dental prosthetics, US Patent 8,735,464, 2014.
[37] International Organization for Standardization, ISO4049, Dentistry – Polymer-Based Restorative Materials, ISO, Geneva, Switzerland, 2009.

Materials for pulp capping

9

9.1 Introduction

The pulp of the tooth is a delicate specific tissue and there are severe consequences for its health if it becomes exposed [1]. Several things can lead to its exposure, specifically trauma of the tooth, dental caries and accidents in tooth preparation. Exposure can be followed by infection and inflammation, resulting in considerable pain to the patient and potential morbidity of the pulp itself. When exposure occurs, therefore, the tooth requires treatment. One approach involves complete removal (extirpation) of the pulp and root canal therapy.

Alternatively the pulp may be saved by the process of pulp capping. This involves placing some sort of material over the pulp to protect it and maintain its viability so that more extreme treatment (extraction or endodontic therapy) can be avoided [1]. Two possible approaches are available, namely direct pulp capping, in which a bioactive material is placed directly over the exposed pulp, and indirect pulp capping, in which a cavity liner or sealant material is placed over a residual thin layer of dentine, which may be sound or carious. In the latter approach, the pulp has not been exposed, but it is at risk of becoming so either by the progress of the residual caries or by the process of tooth preparation.

As previous chapters have shown, a number of materials cause adverse reactions to the cells of the pulp, specifically materials that release the monomer HEMA [2]. This monomer has been shown to be capable of diffusing through thin layers of dentine and entering the pulp [3]. Once within the pulp, it proves to be cytotoxic and causes the death of otherwise viable cells within the various parts of the pulp [4,5]. In addition, some light-cure units used in dentistry have been shown to emit sufficient heat to raise the temperature within the pulp to levels at which the cells are destroyed [6,7].

As well as adverse effects of certain types of repair material, pulp can be affected by the entry of bacteria. In fact, this is the main reason for inflammation of the pulp and necrosis. In the presence of bacterial infection, seriously damaging reactions can occur resulting in inflammation and loss of vitality of the pulp [8–10]. In applying any type of pulp capping material, the critical feature needed to ensure survival of the pulp is creation of an adequate seal [11]. A proper durable seal is necessary to prevent invasion of bacteria, and to protect the pulp from the damaging consequences of bacterial infection [1].

9.2 Direct pulp capping

Direct pulp capping involves placing a pulp capping material directly over the exposed pulp with the aim of promoting pulp healing and the generation of reparative dentine [1]. When this procedure is applied successfully, it eliminates the need for alternative, more invasive treatments.

Materials for the Direct Restoration of Teeth. http://dx.doi.org/10.1016/B978-0-08-100491-3.00009-X

There is evidence that the pulp is more likely to survive if exposure occurs by accident during tooth preparation rather than due to the progression of caries [11,12]. This is because caries penetration is inevitably associated with bacterial invasion, and therefore results in infection and inflammation of the pulp [10]. By contrast, exposure due to a mechanical misadventure during tooth preparation does not necessarily result in bacterial invasion. Consequently, the exposed pulp does not become infected or inflamed. As a result, teeth repaired by direct pulp capping following this type of exposure are generally better able to survive with their pulp intact than those whose pulps become exposed due to advancing caries [11].

Clinically, another critical feature for success in direct pulp capping is the extent of pulp bleeding after the pulp has been exposed and before the direct capping agent has been applied [13–15]. Increased bleeding is generally associated with inflammation, so that substantial bleeding may indicate extensive infection, which itself is a sign that there is reduced capacity for induced repair of the exposure [1]. Bleeding also increases the moisture level of the dentine surfaces adjacent to the site of exposure, and leads to increased contamination. As a result, obtaining a sound seal becomes more difficult, and the possibility of bacterial infection is more likely. Bleeding can be controlled by placing a cotton pellet soaked in either saline or dilute sodium hypochlorite solution on the exposed pulp [1,16], and judgement is needed to assess its seriousness and whether it is likely to compromise the quality of the seal obtained when the direct capping material is placed.

Direct pulp capping is generally performed using calcium hydroxide as the main material. This was first introduced to dentistry in 1921 [11], and it is probably the most highly regarded of the available materials. It gives excellent clinical results and is currently typically used in association with some sort of glass-ionomer cement. The literature suggests that either conventional or resin-modified glass-ionomer may be used, though monomer release may occur from the latter type of material, which is potentially damaging, so probably less satisfactory in this application. The cement is used to act as a liner to provide a reliable seal against the ingress of bacteria, and is needed because calcium hydroxide alone is unable to provide an adequate seal [1].

Calcium hydroxide is available as non-setting and setting type. The setting versions of calcium hydroxide materials can be either self-cured or light-cured versions, though light-cured materials are not recommended for direct pulp capping. The non-setting type consists of a pure supersaturated solution of $Ca(OH)_2$ in distilled water or saline. It is by far the oldest type of calcium hydroxide and has a long history of clinical success. Its high alkalinity makes it bactericidal [17] and also bioactive, so that it promotes the formation of reparative dentine in situ.

Mineral trioxide aggregate, MTA, has also been used as a direct pulp capping material, though its primary use in dentistry as an endodontic sealer [18]. It is described in detail in Chapter 10, which deals with materials specifically designed for use in endodontic therapy. However, there has been recent interest in its use as a material for direct pulp capping, and research on this application has been published [19]. It is a hydraulic cement, based on calcium silicate and like calcium hydroxide, it is highly alkaline and this makes it both bactericidal and bioactive. It also has to be used in association with some sort of glass-ionomer liner, in this case to protect the MTA while it undergoes its prolonged setting process [1].

Since 2009, a new material based on hydraulic cement chemistry, Biodentine®, has been available for clinical use [20]. It is also based on calcium silicate but is formulated to set more rapidly than MTA, a change that does not alter its high alkalinity. Consequently, it shares with MTA the features of being both bactericidal and bioactive. Because it sets more quickly than MTA, a protective glass-ionomer liner is not needed with this material. Indeed, it is claimed that Biodentine itself can be used in its own right as a liner, for example, in the open-sandwich technique [21]. However, this approach is controversial, because the alkalinity is potentially damaging to the gingiva, and the material would be expected to erode quickly. In fact, Biodentine is primarily offered as a material for pulp capping, so will be dealt with in detail in the current chapter, though its additional potential uses in clinical dentistry will also be described.

Other materials have been studied for direct pulp capping, but generally without particular success. Zinc oxide-eugenol, resin-modified glass-ionomer and dental adhesives have all been studied, but all proved to have unacceptable cytotoxicity. Zinc oxide-eugenol released eugenol at concentrations capable of damaging pulp cells [22,23], resin-modified glass-ionomer led to chronic inflammation of the pulp that persisted for at least 300 days following placement, and dental adhesives were also been shown to be cytotoxic [24,25]. For the latter materials, their cytotoxicity was attributed to the synergistic effects of the various monomers released by these substances. The overall conclusion is that no material approaches the performance of either calcium hydroxide or calcium silicate materials in this application and that, of the two, non-setting calcium hydroxide remains the best understood and successful material for direct pulp capping.

9.3 Indirect pulp capping

The removal of caries is essential when repairing a tooth damaged by decay. However, when caries is deep this may present a problem, as continued caries removal to prepare the cavity fully may lead to exposure of the pulp. Rather than exposing the pulp in this way, with the risks involved in such a procedure, an alternative approach is to leave the caries-affected demineralized dentine in the region directly adjacent to the pulp and to cover the whole of the affected zone with a cavity liner. This procedure is termed *indirect pulp capping* [1], and it has been shown to be as successful as restoring teeth conventionally with complete caries removal [26–28].

There have been a number of published accounts of the stages that occur when indirect pulp capping is used. These have typically involved re-entering the tooth and reassessing it some 4–12 months or even longer after the initial indirect pulp capping procedure [1]. Findings are generally that where some carious dentine was left in place, the consistency of this carious dentine was initially soft and wet, but it changes to become hard and dry over time following sealing. After this time, cariogenic bacteria are either completely absent or only present in substantially reduced numbers. Though there is typically significant discoloration at the former carious zone, this generally has not progressed at all and, mechanically, the sealed dentine is found to be strong and sound [27,29–31].

Studies have shown that the critical factor in the success of indirect pulp capping is that the restoration should provide an excellent seal [27,29–31]. In this way, further ingress of bacteria is prevented, and any bacteria already present will be unable to remain viable, due to the loss of access to the air. A high quality seal of this type seems to be more important than the choice of material employed [1]. Findings from a variety of studies suggest that, provided the restoration is well sealed, indirect pulp capping gives very favourable outcomes, and that complete caries removal is not needed in order for this procedure to succeed [32]. In addition, there appears to be no increased risk of pulpitis or of premature failure of the restorative in using this technique [32,33]. A long-term, permanent seal can only be obtained by glass-ionomer cements, and conventional glass-ionomers have the additional advantage of having excellent biocompatibility and low irritancy to the pulp.

9.4 Calcium hydroxide

9.4.1 Composition

Calcium hydroxide, $Ca(OH)_2$, has a long history of use in dentistry for pulp capping and it is available in a number of forms. These include as a supersaturated solution, a hard setting cement and also a light-curable material. Its key feature is its high alkalinity (pH 11–12.5), and this can be achieved using calcium hydroxide powder mixed with pure water to the consistency of a light paste [34]. However, used in this way, calcium hydroxide does not set, has no mechanical strength and consequently there is the danger of it being displaced by the forces involved in placing a restorative material over it [35]. Also in this form it cannot be used directly under any resin-based restoration (composite resins, compomers and resin-modified glass-ionomers) because it is hydrophilic and would interfere with bonding systems. To overcome this problem, calcium hydroxide formulations that are capable of undergoing some sort of setting reaction, and thus building up a degree of mechanical strength, are generally used. However, they have slightly different properties and cannot replace supersaturated calcium hydroxide solutions in all clinical situations.

Setting calcium hydroxide cements are typically based on liquid alkyl salicylates, and they are supplied to the clinician as a two-paste pack [36]. Alkyl salicylates that have been used include methyl salicylate, isobutyl salicylate and 1-methyl trimethylene disalicylate [37]. These cements set because the alkyl salicylate contains a phenolic –OH group which has acid character, and this means it can react with the alkaline calcium hydroxide [38].

Calcium hydroxide formulations of this type do not contain water, as the composition shown in Table 9.1 makes clear. This formulation is that of Dycal®, a calcium hydroxide material that has been available for many years and is widely respected.

Despite the absence of water, such formulations are capable of absorbing a small amount of water to initiate their acid–base setting reaction. As reaction proceeds, so water is produced as one of the products, and this sustains the setting process. Studies using infrared spectroscopy have shown that a critical part of the setting reaction involves

Table 9.1 **Composition of Dycal®**

Base paste	Catalyst paste
1,3-Butylene glycol disalicylate	Calcium hydroxide
Zinc oxide	*N*-ethyl-*o*/*p*-toluene sulfonamide
Calcium phosphate	Zinc oxide
Calcium tungstate	Titanium dioxide
Iron oxide (pigment)	Zinc stearate
	Iron oxide (pigment) — dentine shades only

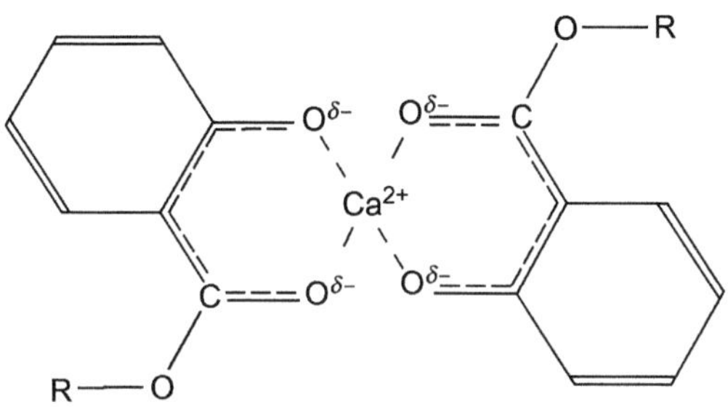

Fig. 9.1 Chelate structure of calcium ion and an alkylsalicylate.

loss of the ester group. This is apparent from the reduction in the band in the region 1675–1695 cm^{-1}. At the same time, there is a corresponding formation of a carboxylate band in the region 1540–1560 cm^{-1}, showing that the product is a salt formed by chelation with the available calcium ions [38]. The typical product of such a reaction is shown in Fig. 9.1.

Chelate materials of this type are products of reaction of a metal base, such as calcium hydroxide or metal oxide, with weakly acidic organic substances with at least two functional groups. The ones used clinically are typically hydrolytically unstable, and this is responsible for their therapeutic effects. Ions released have beneficial properties, reducing inflammation, being bacteriostatic and stimulating the odontoblasts to form secondary dentine. Ideally, calcium hydroxide chelates of this kind dissolve completely with time, and thus have the maximum possible therapeutic effect.

As well as chelate cements of this type, there are also curable calcium hydroxide cements available [39]. These materials have superior mechanical properties to the chelate-type calcium hydroxide cements [40] and also better chemical resistance [41], since they are not affected by treatment with phosphoric acid etchants. A typical example is Biocal®, which has the composition shown in Table 9.2.

The resin component is ethylene urethane dimethacrylate, UDMA [40], a substance of the type used in commercial composite resins. It contains two carbon–carbon double bonds and these are capable of undergoing addition polymerization. This particular reaction is triggered by the photo-initiators present when the material is exposed to light from a dental cure lamp. The calcium hydroxide component effectively serves as filler and is completely enclosed in the polymeric UDMA matrix

Table 9.2 **Composition of Biocal®**

Components
Calcium hydroxide
Ethylene urethane dimethacrylate
Barium sulphate
Inorganic filler
Titanium dioxide
Iron oxide (pigment)
Photo-initiator

after setting. Consequently, it cannot dissociate in water, and any release of Ca^{2+} and OH^- ions must be minimal. This implies that its therapeutic properties are likely to be seriously compromised compared with other types of calcium hydroxide, a point on which further research is clearly needed.

9.4.2 Properties of calcium hydroxide

Calcium hydroxide materials of all types are mechanically weak but disintegrate to provide a local environment that is highly alkaline. Surprisingly, their ability to resist disintegration has been used as an indication of their quality, though the exact details of the test that is best able to evaluate this resistance has been questioned [40]. Studies have varied the conditions, some using pure water and other simulated dentinal fluid, some agitating the specimens and others leaving them still, and some using short durations (1 week) and others long durations (up to 3 months) [40,41]. To an extent, which of these various test regimes is the most appropriate depends on the purpose of the test. Establishing whether a material is likely to be acceptable for clinical service, which is the purpose of the much criticized but relatively simple American Dental Association solubility tests, may be more straightforward than predicting exactly how a material might disintegrate in vivo.

Not surprisingly, disintegration as determined by weight loss is greater in pure water than in simulated dentinal fluid, as the results for the material Dycal® in Table 9.3 show.

Although this test gives much higher values for disintegration in water, water has continued to be the medium most widely used in studies of this type. The caveat here, though, is that results must be considered as preliminary only [41]. A clear concept of

Table 9.3 **Weight loss (%) of Dycal® in aqueous media**

Storage time	1 month	2 months	3 months
In water	35.70 (1.10)	43.18 (3.24)	48.58 (0.42)
In simulated dentinal fluid	21.63 (0.46)	28.55 (0.85)	33.02 (2.04)

Standard deviations in parentheses.

the criterion for deciding which materials are promising in such a test is important, and in particular the notion that they should resist disintegration when this is known to be their mechanism of action is highly questionable.

More recently, the question of the performance of light-cured resin-based calcium hydroxide materials has been considered [41]. In this study, the brand Biocal® was compared with two self-cure calcium hydroxide chelate cements, Dycal and Hidro C. Two criteria were evaluated, namely water sorption and solubility, with pure water being the medium in both cases. Results are shown in Tables 9.4 and 9.5.

From these tables, it can be seen that the resin-based calcium hydroxide shows substantially less water sorption and lower solubility than the two chelate-based cements. It has been suggested that high strength and low solubility are the desirable characteristics of a base or liner material in tooth repair because of the need to resist occlusal forces in service, and also to resist degradation and corresponding loss of function [41]. However, the evidence of the mechanism by which these materials act therapeutically does not support this suggestion, at least as far as resistance to degradation is concerned.

Others have confirmed that light-curable calcium hydroxide materials are resistant to dissolution in water [42]. However, as we have seen, this is not the only criterion to be considered. Given that these materials are known to promote the formation of reparative dentine as a consequence of their high pH, a property which requires at least partial dissolution in order to be manifested, it is likely that the kind of solubility properties shown by the material Dycal makes them more suitable for this particular application. Certainly, a resin-based material that showed absolutely no solubility or degradation in dentinal fluid would not be acceptable clinically, because it could not

Table 9.4 **Mean water sorption values (%) for calcium hydroxide materials**

Material	Supplier	Mean uptake (%)
Biocal®	Biodinamica, Brazil	2.15 (0.36)
Dycal®	Dentsply	5.49 (0.14)
Hidro C®	Dentsply	8.27 (0.99)

Standard deviations in parentheses.

Table 9.5 **Mean water solubility values (%) for calcium hydroxide materials**

Material	Mean solubility (%)
Biocal®	0.72 (0.36)
Dycal®	4.21 (1.30)
Hidro C®	7.65 (0.17)

Standard deviations in parentheses.

increase the local pH at the interface with the pulp. There would therefore be no healing of the exposure and no formation of reparative dentine.

The important findings to emerge from these laboratory studies are that chelate-type calcium hydroxide materials are mechanically weak and also undergo considerable degradation in aqueous conditions. By contrast, light-curable calcium hydroxides are stronger and less susceptible to degradation. To understand their performance, in vivo requires results from clinical and biological studies, and these are dealt with in the following sections.

9.4.3 Use of calcium hydroxide

Calcium hydroxide materials of various kinds are used to cap pulps, both exposed and when still covered by a thin layer of dentine. In carrying out this procedure, it is important that the exposed tissue should be cleaned thoroughly and any bleeding arrested by irrigation with sterile saline [41]. The calcium hydroxide should be placed gently straight onto the pulp, with care being taken to ensure that there is no blood or debris in the way [34].

In clinical use, setting chelate-type calcium hydroxide materials are considered to have the following advantages:

1. They set rapidly in the tooth, partly as a result of the accelerating influence of moisture.
2. They do not interfere with the setting of other materials that may be used to cover them, especially the free-radical polymerization setting reaction of composite resins or resin-modified glass-ionomers.
3. Their high alkalinity has the twin effects of disinfecting the affected region and of promoting the formation of reparative dentine.

As well as being used for direct and indirect pulp capping, calcium hydroxide materials are recommended for use in deep cavities. This is similar to their use in indirect pulp capping, but implies that all of the carious dentine has been removed, leaving behind a thin layer of sound caries-free dentine. Even in this circumstance, the high alkalinity of calcium hydroxide materials is able to stimulate further dentine formation [41,43,44]. Their application where remaining sound dentine is thin will ensure that it does not remain thin. Instead, it will thicken in situ under the influence of the calcium hydroxide to form an improved layer of dentine that is better able to protect the pulp from diffusion of monomers from repair materials or from the effects of bacterial penetration. This process takes time, with typically approximately 2 months time being need to form 0.1 mm of reparative dentine.

Calcium hydroxide has also been used to stimulate the formation of an apical barrier and to promote healing in immature permanent teeth damaged by trauma [45]. Such teeth are especially prone to such damage, as a result of the generally greater physical activity in young adults, with correspondingly greater risk of accidents, including those which damage the teeth. When this type of damage occurs, the teeth may suffer from necrosis of the pulp. Treating such teeth endodontically is complicated because the walls of young permanent teeth are often divergent and their immature apices are difficult to debride and obturate [45]. Introducing a calcium hydroxide material induces apical closure because, under these circumstances too, the high pH stimulates the formation of mineralized tissue and also the repair of periapical tissue. In this way, an apical barrier is formed as a direct result of employing the calcium hydroxide. This process typically takes between 5 and 20 months to complete and has been shown in various studies to have success rates of between 74% and 100% [45]. Failures are generally associated with inadequate control of infection, though cervical root fracture may also be a problem. Either way, any failures that do occur do not seem to be the result of deficiencies in the calcium hydroxide material [45].

The ability of calcium hydroxide to induce the formation of dentine bridges is a clear advantage of these materials. However, there is some doubt about how effective they are over the longer term [46]. In particular, the effectiveness of the seal that they are able to provide against the ingress of bacteria for the lifetime of the overall repair is questionable. Studies have shown that pulps that have been exposed and then capped very often display signs of infection. This infection is a result of microleakage through the material and also due to defects within the dentine brides that are formed. With time, bacteria are able to tunnel through these and infect the underlying pulp [43,47]. This can be avoided by the use of a conventional glass-ionomer, which provides an excellent seal and can be used either as a full restorative material or as the base in the sandwich technique (open or closed).

9.4.4 Biological effects and clinical outcomes

Calcium hydroxide has significant advantages as a material for the direct capping of exposed pulps. Specifically, its high pH acts as an irritant that stimulates the tooth to form reparative dentine when it is placed in contact with healthy pulp tissue. The immediate effect of the high pH is the formation of a superficial layer of necrotic tissue within the pulp which extends to a depth of 2 mm or less [41]. Beyond this tissue, however, there is only a mild inflammatory response and, in the absence of bacterial contamination, this usually goes on to form a barrier of hard tissue, sometimes referred to as a dentine bridge. This structure is formed by calcium ions originally present in the bloodstream of the patient, rather than from the pulp capping material [48]. The calcified material produced in this way seems to be the result of interactions between odontoblasts and connective tissue cells and is called *osteodentine*. This layer of osteodentine is a sign of healing of the exposed pulp, but unfortunately it is porous and it may not cover the site of the exposure completely [34].

The details of the dentine repair mechanism are not known, but it is known to be associated with the release of bioactive molecules by adjacent cells [1]. During the process of development of the dentine, the so-called dentinogenesis, proteins become incorporated into the matrix of the newly formed dentine. Two specific proteins, bone morphogenic protein and transforming growth factor-beta one (TGF-β1) have been shown to stimulate repair of the pulp [46,49–51] and these substances are dissolved from the dentine by the high alkalinity of the calcium hydroxide [51,52]. This suggests that at least part of the mechanism of formation of reparative dentine arises from the presence of important pulp repair proteins and that these occur adjacent to the pulp exposure as a result of the high pH conditions.

Calcium hydroxide not only stimulates the formation of dentine bridges, it is also highly antibacterial [53,54]. This feature also arises from its high alkalinity. It means that bacterial penetration to the pulp is substantially reduced in the presence of calcium hydroxide, and may be eliminated all together.

There have been a number of studies on the antibacterial effects of calcium hydroxide materials, and these materials appear to have the following effects, all of which arise from the ability to provide high local concentrations of hydroxyl ions and the associated high pH [55]:

1. Damage to bacterial cell walls. This arises from the interaction of hydroxyl ions with phospholipids, which are key components of the cell membranes that make up the walls of the bacterial cells. The overall effect of such interaction is massive structural damage to the cell walls, and rapid death of the bacteria.
2. Denaturation of proteins within the bacterial cell, resulting in loss of enzymatic activity and disruption of cellular metabolism.
3. Damage to the DNA, which inhibits replication, thus interfering with cellular activity.

The use of calcium hydroxide therefore tends to create an inherently sterile environment within the region in which the material is placed. Consequent, damaging effects of infection, notably pulp inflammation and even necrosis, are avoided.

9.5 Cements based on calcium silicates

The first calcium silicate cement made available for use in pulp capping was MTA, a material that originated in the building industry and was developed for endodontic therapy [18]. More recently, a modified product of this type, Biodentine®, has become available [20]. The uses of Biodentine overlap with those of MTA, but it has the advantage of faster setting. It has been more widely applied for pulp capping than for endodontic root sealing, but the close similarity in composition and properties with MTA mean that it can be used in both applications.

9.5.1 Mineral trioxide aggregate

MTA is essentially the same as Portland cement, a material widely used in the construction industry. Unlike Portland cement, it contains added bismuth oxide, to impart radiopacity [56,57]. The other principal components are tricalcium silicate, dicalcium silicate and tricalcium aluminate [57,58]. It is available as a grey and a white form. The grey form was the original one, the grey colour being imparted by the presence of tetracalcium alumino ferrate, a dark coloured mineral that is present as a natural impurity in Portland cement. It has the unfortunate potential to darken teeth in which it is used [59]. Because of this, manufacturers have introduced a purification step to their production methods, and this removes the tetracalcium alumino ferrate, and provides a route to a white MTA [60].

White Portland cement has the main components listed in Table 9.6.

Table 9.6 Main components of white Portland cement [61]

Component	Formula
Alite	Ca_3SiO_5
Belite	β-Ca_2SiO_4
Aluminate	$Ca_3Al_2O_6$
Ferrite	$Ca_2(Al/Fe)_2O_5$

In addition to these components, a small fraction of gypsum, $CaSO_4{\cdot}2H_2O$ (up to 5%) is mixed into the powder so that, when water is added, the setting of the aluminate phase is regulated [57]. Mixing with water induces setting of the overall cement, whereupon hydration reactions occur involving the alite and belite components. The product of both reactions is the same, namely a poorly crystalline gel phase comprising calcium silicate hydrate. In addition, some calcium hydroxide is formed and this is crucial for the properties of MTA as a pulp capping material.

The detailed structures of alite and belite are known. Both consist of isolated SiO_4 tetrahedra, the so-called Q^0 species. Following hydration to form Si–OH groups, there is a condensation reaction that results in pairs of SiO_4 tetrahedra becoming joined as dimers, the so-called Q^1 species [57]. Condensation reactions continue and these cause short-chain silicate species to form, with Q^1 end groups and Q^2 mid-chain units (ie, SiO_4 tetrahedra joined at two corners to other SiO_4 tetrahedra [62]). In addition, some of the mid-chain units contain aluminium rather than silicon, and so are $Q^2(1Al)$ species.

As well as the hydration reactions of alite and belite, the components aluminate and ferrite also undergo reactions that contribute to the setting process. In both cases, these reactions also involve the gypsum, with the product formed by aluminate being ettringite, $6CaO{\cdot}Al_2O_3{\cdot}3SiO_3{\cdot}32H_2O$. The product formed by ferrite is the iron substituted counterpart $6CaO{\cdot}Fe_2O_3{\cdot}3SiO_3{\cdot}32H_2O$. This product is stable whereas ettringite is not. Instead it slowly converts to a so-called monosulphate, $4CaO{\cdot}Al_2O_3{\cdot}SiO_3{\cdot}12H_2O$ plus free water, a combination of products that is more stable thermodynamically than the ettringite [61].

One aspect that has proved controversial with this material has been the role of bismuth oxide in the setting process. It has been suggested that bismuth oxide alters the hydration processes of white Portland cement and becomes chemically incorporated into the calcium silicate hydrate phase [63]. This was initially refuted on the grounds that bismuth oxide is very insoluble and has no known reactions under the alkaline conditions that occur within setting white Portland cement [64]. Experimental studies have confirmed this view [57,62]. These have used a variety of experimental techniques, including X-ray diffraction (XRD), magic angle spinning nuclear magnetic resonance, Fourier Transform Infrared spectroscopy and isothermal conduction calorimetry. Findings are quite clear that bismuth oxide is an inert additive and does not participate in the hydration reactions that occur in the setting of white Portland cement [57]. Rather than have any chemical role, it functions purely physically to make the set cement radiopaque. This property is a desirable attribute for a material used in clinical tooth repair.

9.5.2 Biological and clinical effects of MTA

As we have seen, MTA forms calcium hydroxide on reaction with water, so that its resulting effects are similar to those of the older, well-established calcium hydroxide materials. It provides a highly alkaline local environment, which promotes the formation of reparative dentine and it is also strongly antibacterial [18,58,65]. However, it has an advantage over calcium hydroxide materials in that it provides a degree of sealing with the prepared tooth surface and is therefore inherently protective for the pulp when used as a pulp capping agent [1].

Studies of direct pulp capping in patients have shown that there is little to choose between MTA and calcium hydroxide chelate materials [66–69], though some studies report slightly better results for MTA than for calcium hydroxide [70]. Studies of MTA alone and not in comparison with calcium hydroxide show it to have good success in this role over periods of time ranging from 6 months to 4 years [71–74]. MTA is known to seal better than calcium hydroxide materials, but despite this, it should still be used with a liner of conventional glass-ionomer [1]. This provides a full antibacterial seal, which MTA alone is unable to do. MTA has also been found to cause less inflammation than calcium hydroxide and to give a higher quality dentine bridge with fewer defects or other sources of leakage [75].

MTA has been found to have a high solubility in aqueous media, and in one reported study lost 24% of its mass after 78 days storage in water [76]. This is similar to the behaviour of calcium hydroxide chelates, and is the reason that the material is able to generate a high local pH in the surrounding tissues. However, MTA also has disadvantages. Clinically, it is not so easy to use as calcium hydroxide materials because it has a very long setting time, estimated at 2–3 h [18,77]. Because of this, pulp capping with MTA requires a more elaborate technique than with calcium hydroxide. Either a two-step procedure is needed, in which the MTA is placed and followed by a temporary restoration. This allows the MTA to set fully for some time, after which the temporary restoration can be removed and replaced by a permanent one. This may be difficult clinically, and there is the risk that the MTA will be removed along with the temporary restoration. Alternatively, MTA can be used with a carefully chosen quick setting liner, which also allows the MTA time to harden fully while undisturbed within the tooth. Both of these are more demanding clinical procedures than those employed with calcium hydroxide chelate materials and, because of that, may give the material opportunities to behave less than ideally and for the pulp capping procedure to fail.

9.5.3 Biodentine

Biodentine is a specific proprietary brand of calcium silicate cement that has been available to the profession since 2009 [20]. It is manufactured by Septodont, St Maur des Faussés, France. The material is formulated to set more rapidly than MTA or similar calcium silicate cements, and is produced as a dentine replacement material. It is recommended for pulp capping, and also for various aspects of endodontic repair, including root perforations, apexification and retrograde filling [20].

Biodentine is supplied as a powder and a liquid. The main powder components are listed in Table 9.7, which also indicates the function of each component.

Table 9.7 **Composition of Biodentine®**

Substance	Function
Powder	
Tricalcium silicate	Main core material
Calcium oxide	Reactive filler able to react with $CaCl_2$
Calcium carbonate	Reactive filler able to react with $CaCl_2$
Zirconium oxide	Radiopacifier
Iron oxide (trace)	Pigment
Liquid	
Water	Solvent
Calcium chloride	Accelerator
Hydro-soluble polymer	Water reducing agent

Other components may be present, according to the manufacturer, but they are not essential for the material to fulfil its clinical function, and it is apparent from the research literature that they are not generally included in the formulation of Biodentine [20].

The liquid consists of water containing calcium chloride and an unspecified water soluble polymer. Calcium chloride acts as an accelerator in the hydration processes of the tricalcium silicate substance [78]. It forms an acidic solution in water, and its reaction with calcium carbonate, which is basic, also helps to speed up the setting reaction. The overall effect of these components is that Biodentine sets in 9–12 min, which is much faster than MTA materials based on unmodified calcium silicates [79]. The set material has been shown to release calcium ions into aqueous solution [63,80] and this stimulates the deposition of hydroxyapatite in contact with simulated body fluid [81,82].

Setting of Biodentine is partly caused by condensation polymerization of the silicate phase to form a chain structure based on SiO_4 tetrahedra joined at two corners (Q2 structures). This is similar to the setting of Portland cement [61], though it occurs faster due to the accelerating effect of calcium chloride. Setting is accompanied first by a contraction in volume, as the initial solidification occurs. This is followed by expansion as secondary hydration reactions take place to form the various calcium silicate hydrates [83].

The rapid setting of Biodentine results in an initially hardened material. However, chemical reactions continue to take place for some time after this preliminary hardening, as shown experimentally by impedance measurements [84]. Such studies show that there are detectable changes within the Biodentine cement for at least 14 days following hardening, with such changes involving not only hydration reactions, but also reaction of ions exchanged with the surroundings [84].

Set Biodentine material consists substantially of hydrated calcium silicate [79], some of which forms more rapidly in Biodentine than in MTA because of the presence of calcium chloride and calcium carbonate. This latter component, which accounts for 15% of the powder by mass, acts as nucleation sites for the deposition of calcium silicate hydrate. Consequently, the precipitation of calcium silicate hydrate occurs more rapidly within this material, which leads to a shorter setting time [79].

Table 9.8 **Properties of Biodentine® [85,86]**

Property	Value
Setting time	
Dry	9–12 min
Immersed in water	45 min
Compressive strength at 28 days	67.18
Vicker's hardness number	48.4
Initial mass washed out into HBSS, 28 days	23.35%
pH of leachate in deionized water	
3 h	9.14
1 week	8.02

Physical and chemical properties of Biodentine are shown in Table 9.8. The material can be seen to set rapidly, and to have a reasonable compressive strength and Vicker's Hardness Number at 24 h [85,86]. It shows a substantial wash out (solubility) in Hank's balanced salt solution (HBSS), which is presumably at least matched in deionized water. However, the pH of deionized water following storage of set Biodentine is only around 9 at 24 h, rather than the 11–12.5 of traditional calcium hydroxide chelate cements or supersaturated solution. This may suggest that Biodentine is less bioactive than such materials, and hence less effective at promoting the growth of reparative dentine.

9.5.4 Biological properties of Biodentine

To date, only a few reports have appeared in the literature on the biological properties of Biodentine in terms of its effects on the viability of pulp cells [20]. Early results suggest that it has promising results when placed in direct contact with such cells, in that the material appears to show a lack of cytotoxicity and genotoxicity, and to be generally well tolerated by the soft tissue [87,88]. Pulp cells have been shown to remain fully viable and functional when Biodentine has been used for pulp capping, showing that this material is highly biocompatible in this application. This is supported by the finding that human gingival osteoblast cells show similarly positive results when exposed to extracts from Biodentine [88,89]. In another study, Biodentine was shown to induce cell proliferation and biomineralization by immortalized murine pulp cells [90].

In one study where Biodentine was placed over dentine, the elements calcium and silicon (in the form of silicate) were found to be transported into the dentine and also tag-like structures were formed [87]. This was similar to the behaviour of ProRoot MTA, despite the much more rapid hardening reaction of Biodentine. The release of calcium by Biodentine appeared to be well accepted by human fibroblast cells in cell culture studies [91]. The material stimulated the release of increased amounts of TGF-β1 from pulp cells [92], which is probably associated with increased rates of cell differentiation and of mineralization in vivo.

Biodentine has been shown to affect healing positively when placed in direct contact with the pulp [92]. It increased the rate of cell proliferation and migration, which under clinical conditions enhanced the rate of mineralization and healing of the dentine above the exposed pulp. The biological properties of Biodentine are such that it is capable of inducing early and effective formation of reparative dentine [91]. The resulting dentine bridge has a degree of porosity, as does that induced by the presence of MTA, but both are of better quality than that formed by calcium hydroxide [92].

In an animal study with the pig as the animal model, Biodentine was shown to induce the formation of thick calcified layers after 90 days following direct pulp capping [93]. As in previous studies, the underlying soft tissue of the pulp showed no sign of inflammation and the cells remained entirely normal.

9.5.5 Clinical studies of Biodentine

There have been only few reports of clinical studies of the use of Biodentine, because it is a relatively new material. However, a few studies have appeared, and so far findings are generally positive. For example, a study has been described in which Biodentine was used to cap the pulps of intact molars due for extraction for orthodontic reasons [94]. After 6 weeks, it was shown to have induced a substantial depth of dentine bridge. Similar results were also obtained for MTA. However, Biodentine was found to have better handling properties as well as a shorter setting time. Indeed, using MTA has been described as more time-consuming and technically difficult than using Biodentine [95].

Literature provided by the manufacturers suggests that Biodentine can be used for various applications, not only for pulp capping but also for other endodontic applications, such as repair of pulp chamber floor perforations and of lateral root perforations [95]. It can also be used for indirect pulp capping and to line deep carious lesions. However, to date systematic studies are lacking, and there is only limited evidence of clinical success of Biodentine in these applications. Early published results are promising, but more work is necessary before a definitive opinion on this material is possible [95].

Clinical summary

- Pulp capping may be either direct (covering a completely exposed pulp) or indirect (covering very thin dentine, either caries-free or caries-affected).
- Materials used are either calcium hydroxide-based or tricalcium silicate-based (MTA or Biodentine).
- Calcium hydroxide can be used as a supersaturated solution, as chelate cements and as a light-cured resin (in UDMA systems).
- A key requirement is for the material to dissolve/disintegrate to make the surrounding tissue alkaline and thereby to stimulate the production of reparative dentine.
- Both MTA and Biodentine show a high degree of solubility and are able to make the surrounding tissues alkaline, thereby acting as bioactive materials to promote production of reparative dentine.

References

[1] T.J. Hilton, Keys to clinical success with pulp capping: a review of the literature, Oper. Dent. 34 (2009) 615–625.

[2] E. Yoshii, Cytotoxic effects of acrylates and methacrylates: relationships of monomer structures and cytotoxicity, J. Biomed. Mater. Res. 37 (1998) 517–524.

[3] A. Hamid, W.R. Hume, Diffusion of resin monomers through human carious dentin *in vitro*, Endod. Dent. Traumatol. 13 (1997) 1–5.

[4] M. Accorinte, A. Loguercio, A. Reis, A. Muench, V. de Araujo, Adverse effects on human pulp after direct pulp capping with the different components from a total-etch, three-step adhesive system, Dent. Mater. 21 (2005) 599–607.

[5] C. de Souza Costa, A. Lopes do Nascimento, H. Teixeira, U. Fontana, Response of human pulps capped with a self-etching adhesive system, Dent. Mater. 17 (2001) 230–240.

[6] J. Hecbing, E.M. Aparecida Giro, C.A. Costa de Souza, Biocompatibility of an adhesive system applied to exposed human dental pulp, J. Endod. 25 (1999) 676–682.

[7] M. Jontell, C. Hanks, J. Bratel, G. Bergenholtz, Effects of unpolymerized resin components on the function of accessory cells derived from the rat incisor pulp, J. Dent. Res. 74 (1995) 1162–1167.

[8] G. Bergenholtz, J. Lindhe, Effect of soluble plaque factors on inflammatory reactions in the dental pulp, Scand. J. Dent. Res. 83 (1974) 153–158.

[9] M. Brannstrom, K.J. Nordenvall, Bacterial penetration, pulpal reaction and the inner surface of Concise Enamel Bond. Composite fillings in etched and unetched cavities, J. Dent. Res. 57 (1978) 3–10.

[10] P.E. Murray, L.J. Windsor, T.W. Smyth, A.A. Hafez, C.F. Cox, Analysis of pulpal reactions to restorative procedures, materials, pulp-capping and future therapies, Crit. Rev. Oral Biol. Med. 13 (2002) 509–520.

[11] I. Baume, J. Holz, Long-term clinical assessment of direct pulp capping, Int. Dent. J. 31 (1981) 251–260.

[12] A. Al-Hiyasat, K. Barrieshi-Nusair, M. Al-Mari, The radiographic outcomes of direct pulp-capping procedures performed by dental students, J. Am. Dent. Assoc. 137 (2006) 1699–1705.

[13] T. Matsuo, T. Nakanshi, H. Shuimizu, S. Ebisu, A clinical study of direct pulp capping applied to carious-exposed pulps, J. Endod. 22 (1996) 551–556.

[14] H. Stanley, Criteria for standardizing and increasing credibility of direct pulp capping studies, Am. J. Dent. 11 (Spec. No.) (1998) S17–S34.

[15] H. Stanley, Pulp capping: Conserving the dental pulp – can it be done? Is it worth it? Oral Surg. Oral Med. Oral Pathol. Oral Radiol. Endod. 68 (1989) 628–639.

[16] C.A. Costa de Souza, C. Edwards, C. Hanks, Cytotoxic effects of cleansing solutions recommended for chemical lavage of pulp exposures, Am. J. Dent. 14 (2001) 25–30.

[17] K. Stuart, C. Miller, C. Brown Jr., C. Newton, The comparative antimicrobial effect of calcium hydroxide, Oral Surg. Oral Med. Oral Pathol. Oral Radiol. Endod. 72 (1991) 101–104.

[18] M. Torabinejad, C. Hong, F. McDonald, T. Pitt Ford, The chemical constitution and biocompatibility of accelerated Portland cement for endodontic use, Int. Endod. J. 21 (1995) 349–353.

[19] G. Bogen, J.S. Kim, L.K. Bakland, Direct pulp capping with mineral trioxide aggregate, an observational study, J. Am. Dent. Assoc. 139 (2008) 305–315.

[20] O. Malkondu, M.K. Kazandag, E. Kazazoglu, A review on Biodentine, a contemporary dentine replacement and repair material, BioMed Res. Int. 2014 (2014), Article ID 160951.

[21] S. Koubi, G. Elmerini, H. Koubi, H. Tassery, J. Camps, Quantitative evaluation by glucose diffusion of microleakage in aged calcium silicate-based open sandwich restorations, Int. J. Dent. 2012 (2012), Article ID 105863.

[22] W. Hume, An analysis of the release and the diffusion through dentin of eugenol from zinc oxide-eugenol mixtures, J. Dent. Res. 63 (1984) 881–884.

[23] W. Hume, Effect of eugenol on respiration and division in human pulp, mouse fibroblasts, and liver cells in vitro, J. Dent. Res. 63 (1984) 1262–1265.

[24] C. de Souza Costa, M. Vaerten, C. Edwards, C. Hanks, Cytotoxic effects of current dental adhesive systems on immortalized odontoblast cell line MDPC-23, Dent. Mater. 15 (1999) 434–441.

[25] S. Ratanasathien, J. Wataha, C. Hanks, J. Dennison, Cytotoxic interactive effects of dentin bonding components on mouse fibroblasts, J. Dent. Res. 74 (1995) 1602–1606.

[26] J. Foley, D. Evans, A. Blackwell, Partial caries removal and cariostatic materials in primary molar teeth: a randomised controlled clinical trial, Br. Dent. J. 197 (2004) 697–701.

[27] C. Ribeiro, L. Baratieri, J. Pedigao, N. Baratieri, A. Ritter, A clinical, radiographic and scanning electron microscopic evaluation of adhesive restorations on carious dentin in primary teeth, Quintessence Int. 30 (1999) 591–599.

[28] E. Mertz-Fairhurst, J. Curtis, J. Ergle, F. Rueggeberg, S. Adair, Ultraconservative and cariostatic sealed restoratives: results at year 10, J. Am. Dent. Assoc. 129 (1998) 55–66.

[29] L. Bjorndal, A. Thylstrup, A practice-based study on stepwise excavation of deep carious lesions in permanent teeth: a 1-year follow-up study, Community Dent. Oral Epidemiol. 26 (1998) 122–128.

[30] M. Maltz, E. de Oliviera, V. Fontanella, R. Bianchi, A clinical, microbiologic and radiographic study of deep caries lesions after incomplete caries removal, Quintessence Int. 33 (2002) 151–159.

[31] M. Maltz, E. de Oliviera, V. Fontanella, G. Carminatti, Deep caries lesions after incomplete dentine caries removal: 40-month follow-up study, Caries Res. 41 (2007) 493–496.

[32] V. Thompson, R. Craig, F. Curro, W. Green, J. Ship, Treatment of deep carious lesions by complete excavation or partial removal, J. Am. Dent. Assoc. 139 (2008) 705–712.

[33] D. Ricketts, E. Kidd, N. Innes, J. Clarkson, Complete or ultraconservative removal of decayed tissue in unfilled teeth. Cochrane Database Syst. Rev. (3) (2006), Art. No.: CD003808. http://dx.doi.org/10.1002/14651858.CD003808.pub2.

[34] P. Carotte, Endodontics: Part 9, calcium hydroxide, root resorption, endo-perio lesions, Br. Dent. J. 197 (2004) 735–743.

[35] E.C. Combe, Notes on Dental Materials, sixth ed., Churchill Livingstone, Edinburgh, 1992.

[36] H.J. Prosser, B. Stuart, A.D. Wilson, An infra-red spectroscopic study of the setting reaction of a calcium hydroxide dental cement, J. Mater. Sci. 14 (1979) 2894–2900.

[37] H.J. Prosser, D.M. Groffman, A.D. Wilson, The effect of composition on the erosion properties of calcium hydroxide cements, J. Dent. Res. 61 (1982) 1431–1435.

[38] A.D. Wilson, J.W. Nicholson, Acid Base Cements, The University Press, Cambridge, UK, 1993.

[39] Y. Kitasako, S. Shibata, J. Tagami, Migration and particle clearance from hard-setting $Ca(OH)_2$ and self-etching adhesive resin following direct pulp capping, Am. J. Dent. 19 (2006) 370–375.

[40] C.F. Driscoll, G.D. Woolsey, T.G. Reddy, Solubility of zinc oxide-eugenol and calcium hydroxide cements in simulated dentinal fluid, J. Oral Rehabil. 16 (1989) 451–455.

[41] L.F. Francisconi, A.P. de Freitas, P.M.C. Scaffa, R.L.F. Mondelli, P.A.S. Francisconi, Water sorption and solubility of different calcium hydroxide cements, J. Appl. Oral Sci. 17 (2009) 427–431.

[42] F.J.T. Burke, D.C. Watts, Weight loss of three resin-based lining materials containing calcium following a phosphoric acid-etching and washing cycle, J. Dent. 17 (1989) 38–40.
[43] G. Hasselgren, L. Tronstad, Enzyme activity in the pulp following preparation of cavities and insertion of medicaments in cavities in monkeys, Acta Odontol. Scand. 35 (1978) 289–295.
[44] J. Hebling, E.M. Giro, C.A. Costa, Human pulp response after an adhesive system application in deep cavities, J. Dent. 27 (1999) 557–564.
[45] E.C. Sheehy, G.J. Roberts, Use of calcium hydroxide for apical barrier formation and healing in non-vital immature permanent teeth: a review, Br. Dent. J. 183 (1997) 241–246.
[46] A.H. Schuurs, R.J. Gruythuysen, P.R. Wesselink, Pulp capping with adhesive resin-based composite vs calcium hydroxide: a review, Endod. Dent. Traumatol. 16 (2000) 240–250.
[47] J. Ward, Vital pulp therapy in cariously exposed permanent teeth and its limitations, Aust. Endod. J. 28 (2002) 29–37.
[48] I. Sciaky, S. Pisanti, Localised of calcium placed over amputated pulps in dogs' teeth, J. Dent. Res. 39 (1960) 1128–1132.
[49] C. Duque, J. Hebling, A. Smith, M. Giro, M. Freitas, C. de Souza Costa, Reactionary dentinogenesis after applying restorative materials and bioactive dentin matrix molecules as liners in deep cavities prepared in non-human primate teeth, J. Oral Rehabil. 33 (2006) 452–461.
[50] X. Weibo Zhang, F. Walboomers, J. Jansen, The formation of tertiary dentin after pulp capping with a calcium phosphate cement, loaded with PLGA microparticles containing TGF-β1, J. Biomed. Mater. Res. 85A (2007) 439–444.
[51] A. Smith, Vitality of the dentin-pulp complex in health and disease. Growth factors as key mediators, J. Dent. Ed. 67 (2003) 678–689.
[52] L. Graham, P. Cooper, N. Cassidy, J. Nor, A. Sloan, A. Smith, The effect of calcium hydroxide on solubilisation of bio-active dentine matrix components, J. Biomater. 27 (2006) 2865–2873.
[53] C. Barthel, L. Levin, H. Reisner, M. Trope, TNF-α release in monocytes after exposure to calcium hydroxide treated *Escherichia coli* LPS, Int. Endod. J. 30 (1997) 155–159.
[54] J.F. Siqueira, H.P. Lopes, Mechanisms of antibacterial activity of calcium hydroxide: a critical review, Int. Endod. J. 32 (1999) 362–369.
[55] S. Khan, N.K. Inamdar, G.K. Meshram Akash, M.P. Singh, H. Chaurasia, Calcium hydroxide – a great calcific wall, J. Orofacial Res. 1 (2011) 26–30.
[56] J. Camilleri, T. Pitt Ford, Mineral trioxide aggregate: a review of the constituents and biological properties of the material, Int. Endod. J. 39 (2006) 814–817.
[57] Q. Li, N.J. Colemam, The hydration chemistry of ProRoot MTA, Dent. Mater. J. 34 (2015) 458–465.
[58] J. Camilleri, The composition of mineral trioxide aggregate, J. Conserv. Dent. 11 (2008) 141–143.
[59] M. Parirokh, M. Torabinejad, Mineral trioxide aggregate: a comprehensive literature review, Part III: clinical applications, drawbacks and mechanism of action, J. Endod. 36 (2010) 400–413.
[60] J. Song, F. Mante, W. Romaow, S. Kim, Chemical analysis of powder and set forms of Portland cement, gray ProRoot MTA, white ProRoot MTA and gray MTA-Angelus, Oral Surg. Oral Med. Oral Pathol. Oral Radiol. Endod. 102 (2006) 809–815.
[61] H.F.W. Taylor, Cement Chemistry, Academic Press, London, 1990.
[62] Q. Li, N.J. Coleman, Early hydration chemistry of white Portland cement in the presence of bismuth oxide, Adv. Appl. Ceram. 112 (2013) 207–212.

[63] J. Camilleri, Characterization of hydration products of mineral trioxide aggregate, Int. Endod. J. 41 (2008) 408–417.
[64] B.W. Darvell, R.C.T. Wu, 'MTA' – an hydraulic silicate cement: review update and setting reaction, Dent. Mater. 27 (2011) 407–422.
[65] J. Camilleri, F.E. Montesin, L. Di Silvio, T.R. Pitt Ford, The chemical constitution and biocompatibility of accelerated Portland cement for endodontic use, Int. Endod. J. 38 (2005) 834–842.
[66] T. Pitt Ford, M. Torabinejad, H. Abedi, I. Bakland, S. Kariyawasam, Using mineral trioxide aggregate as a pulp-capping material, J. Am. Dent. Assoc. 127 (1996) 1491–1494.
[67] C. de Souza Costa, P. Duarte, P. de Souza, E. Giro, J. Hebling, Cytotoxic effects and pulpal response caused by a mineral trioxide aggregate formulation and calcium hydroxide, Am. J. Dent. 21 (2008) 255–261.
[68] A. Briso, V. Rahal, S. Mestrener, E. dezan Jr., Biological response of pulps submitted to different capping materials, Braz. Oral Res. 20 (2006) 219–225.
[69] M. Dominquez, D. Witherspoon, J. Gutmann, L. Opperman, Histological and scanning electron microscopy assessment of various vital pulp-therapy materials, J. Endod. 29 (2003) 324–333.
[70] J. Mente, B. Geletneky, M. Ohle, M.J. Koch, P.G.F. Ding, D. Wolff, J. Dreyhaupt, N. Martin, H.J. Staehle, T. Pfefferle, Mineral trioxide aggregate or calcium hydroxide direct pulp capping: an analysis of the clinical treatment outcome, J. Endod. 36 (2010) 806–813.
[71] R. Caicedo, P. Abbott, D. Alongi, M. Alarcon, Clinical, radiographic and histological analysis of the effects of mineral trioxide aggregate used in direct pulp capping and pulpotomies of primary teeth, Aust. Dent. J. 51 (2006) 296–305.
[72] N. Farsi, N. Alamoudi, K. Balto, A. Mushayt, Clinical assessment of mineral trioxide aggregate (MTA) as direct pulp capping in young permanent teeth, J. Clin. Pediatr. Dent. 31 (2006) 72–76.
[73] G. Bogen, J. Kim, L. Bakland, Direct pulp capping with mineral trioxide aggregate, J. Am. Dent. Assoc. 139 (2008) 305–315.
[74] M.S. Marques, P.R. Wesselink, H. Shemesh, Outcome of direct pulp capping with mineral trioxide aggregate: a prospective study, J. Endod. 41 (2015) 1026–1031.
[75] M. Aeinehchi, B. Eslami, M. Ghanbariha, A.S. Saffar, Mineral trioxide aggregate (MTA) and calcium hydroxide as pulp-capping agents in human teeth: a preliminary report, Int. Endod. J. 36 (2003) 225–231.
[76] M. Fridland, R. Rosado, MTA solubility: a long-term study, J. Endod. 31 (2005) 376–379.
[77] I. Islam, H. Kheng Chang, A.J. Yap, Comparison of the physical and mechanical properties of MTA and Portland cement, J. Endod. 32 (2006) 193–197.
[78] M.C.G. Juenger, P.J.M. Monteiro, E.M. Gartner, G.P. Denbeaux, A soft X-ray microscope investigation into the effects of calcium chloride on tricalcium silicate hydration, Cement Concrete Res. 35 (2005) 19–25.
[79] J. Camilleri, F. Sorrentino, D. Damidot, Investigation of the hydration and bioactivity of radiopacified tricalcium silicate cement, Biodentine and MTA Angelus, Dent. Mater. 29 (2013) 580–593.
[80] J. Camilleri, P. Kralj, M. Veber, E. Sinagra, Characterization and analysis of acid-extractable and leached trace elements in dental cements, Int. J. Endod. 45 (2012) 737–743.
[81] F.R. Tay, D.H. Pashley, F.A. Rueggeberg, R.J. Loushine, R.N. Weller, Calcium phosphate phase transformation produced by the interaction of the Portland cement component of white mineral trioxide aggregate with a phosphate-containing fluid, J. Endod. 33 (2007) 1347–1351.

[82] L. Han, T. Okiji, S. Okawa, Morphological and chemical analysis of different precipitates on mineral trioxide aggregate immersed in different fluids, Dent. Mater. J. 29 (2010) e20–e28.

[83] L. Grech, B. Mallia, J. Camilleri, Investigation of the physical properties of tricalcium silicate cement for use as root-end filling materials, Int. Endod. J. 46 (2013) 632–641.

[84] C. Villat, V.X. Tran, N. Praddle-Plasse, P. Ponthiaux, F. Wenger, B. Grosgogeat, P. Colon, Impedance methodology: a new way to characterize the setting reaction of dental cements, Dent. Mater. 26 (2010) 1127–1132.

[85] L. Grech, B. Mallia, J. Camilleri, Characterization of set intermediate restorative material, Biodentine, Bioaggregate and a prototype calcium silicate cement for use as root-end filling materials, Int. Endod. J. 46 (2013) 632–641.

[86] S. Rajasekharan, L.C. Martens, R.G.E.C. Cauwels, R.M.H. Verbeeck, Biodentine™ materials characteristics and clinical applications: a review of the literature, Eur. Arch. Paediatr. Dent. 15 (2014) 147–158.

[87] L. Han, T. Okiji, Uptake of calcium and silicon released from calcium silicate-based endodontic materials into root canal dentine, Int. Endod. J. 44 (2011) 1081–1087.

[88] P. Laurent, J. Camps, M. De Meo, J. Dejou, I. About, Induction of specific cell responses to a Ca_3SiO_5-based posterior restorative material, Dent. Mater. 24 (2008) 1486–1494.

[89] H.M. Zhou, Y. Shen, Z.J. Wang, L. Li, Y.F. Zheng, L. Hakkinen, M. Haapasalo, In vitro cytotoxicity evaluation of a novel root repair material, J. Endod. 39 (2013) 478–483.

[90] M. Perard, J. le Clerc, T. Watrin, F. Meary, E. Perez, S. Tricot-Doleux, P. Pellen-Mussi, Spheroid model study comparing the biocompatibility of Biodentine and MTS, J. Mater. Sci. Mater. Med. 24 (2013) 1527–1534.

[91] P. Laurent, J. Camps, M. De Meo, J. Dejou, I. About, Biodentine™ induces TGF-β1 release from human pulp cells and early dental pulp mineralization, Int. Endod. J. 45 (2012) 439–448.

[92] Z. Luo, M. Li, M.R. Kohli, Q. Yu, S. Kim, W.X. He, Effect of Biodentine on the proliferation, migration and adhesion of human dental pulp stem cells, J. Dent. 42 (2014) 490–497.

[93] A. Shayegan, C. Jurysta, R. Atash, M. Petein, A.V. Abbeele, Biodentine used as a pulp-capping agent in primary pig teeth, Pediatr. Dent. 34 (2012) e202–e208.

[94] A. Nowicka, M. Lipska, M. Parafiniuk, K. Sporniak-Tutak, D. Lichota, A. Kosierkiewicz, W. Kaczmarek, J. Buczkowska-Radlinska, Response of human dental pulp capped with biodentine and mineral trioxide aggregate, J. Endod. 39 (2013) 743–747.

[95] S. Rajaseharan, L.C. Martens, R.G.E.C. Cauwels, R.M.H. Verbeeck, Biodentine™ material characteristics and clinical applications: a review of the literature, Eur. Arch. Paediatr. Dent. 15 (3) (2014) 147–158, http://dx.doi.org/10.1007/s403368-014-0114-3.

[96] M. Zanini, J.M. Sautier, A. Berdal, S. Simon, Biodentine induces immortalized murine pulp cell differentiation into odontoblast-like cells and stimulate biomineralization, J. Endod. 38 (2012) 1220–1226.

Materials for root canal filling

10

10.1 Introduction

Endodontic treatment is carried out by practitioners in order to preserve a tooth whose pulp has been damaged in some way [1]. This includes those instants where the injury extends to the peri-radicular tissues. It is carried out because preserving the natural teeth is important in maintaining full function of the dentition, with the associated health benefits that a fully functional set of teeth confers.

The term *endodontic treatment* covers all aspects of repair and treatment of a tooth in which the pulp has been either damaged or exposed as well as the treatment of peri-apical tissues. In the latter case, the pulp is at risk of further damage or destruction. Thus endodontic treatment includes pulp capping, both direct and indirect, as covered in Chapter 8, where the aim is to save the pulp in a viable state and to re-establish the tooth as a fully functioning entity. It also includes the treatment of a tooth whose pulp has become substantially damaged, either by trauma or infection, so that the pulp needs to be extirpated. When this is necessary, it must be followed by sealing of the tooth at the root. This enables the tooth to continue to function structurally, despite no longer being viable.

Endodontic treatment can be so-called non-surgical and surgical, though, in fact, all endodontic treatment is strictly surgical. The so-called non-surgical endodontic treatment has four objectives, namely:

(a) To provide a clean root canal in which the extent of any bacterial ingress is kept low and below a level at which pathological effects occur.
(b) To seal the root at the apex to prevent ingress of fluids that would otherwise act as a source of nutrients for any bacteria remaining inside the root canal. This seal also prevents any irritant substances draining from the root canal into the peri-apical tissues.
(c) To provide a coronal seal, which prevents the pulp chamber from being re-contaminated by oral flora entering from the mouth.
(d) To heal any peri-apical lesion when it is possible with surgical removal of the lesion, ie, without apectomy.

Several different types of material have been employed with varying degrees of clinical success in attempts to create a clinically effective impervious seal at the apex of the tooth root. The most successful and widely used approach is to use a combination of pre-formed obturating points and some sort of canal-sealing material. The latter are placed as high viscosity liquids that set more or less rapidly to form rigid materials that establish a close fit to the interior of the root that ideally seals the root.

A number of features have been identified that should be present in an ideal root canal filling material, both sealers and materials for points. They are that these materials should be:

(a) biocompatible within the root canal and at the root apex;
(b) dimensionally stable;

Materials for the Direct Restoration of Teeth. http://dx.doi.org/10.1016/B978-0-08-100491-3.00010-6

(c) able to conform to the contours of the individual root canals, thereby ensuring that the canals are sealed both apically and laterally;
(d) insoluble in tissue fluids and unaffected by them;
(e) bacteriostatic;
(f) radiopaque;
(g) capable of being removed easily if necessary;
(h) unpigmented, so that the tooth and the gingival tissues do not become stained;
(i) easily manipulated under clinical conditions.

Materials employed as points are usually fabricated from gutta percha, though other materials have been considered (see Sections 10.2 and 10.3). Materials for sealers may be cements, including acid–base cements, or methacrylate monomer-based materials of the type used in composite resins. However, more commonly in modern endodontics, cements based on tricalcium silicate systems that set by hydration processes are used. This chapter discusses the wide variety of possible materials that can be used for this purpose, with some indication of the clinical effectiveness.

There have been extensive studies of the clinical value of endodontic treatment and there is considerable evidence that such treatment is worthwhile and results in generally beneficial outcomes for the patient [1]. A recently published review suggested that the success rate of primary endodontic treatment is 86% [1]. This figure represents the proportion of teeth that remain functional and asymptomatic for at least 2 years after treatment. Such treatment should therefore be employed as the first choice where pulpal damage has occurred, for whatever reason [2]. If this fails, non-surgical re-treatment should be considered as the next step, since this also has a high success rate (78.2%) [1]. As a final step, should re-treatment also fail, surgical treatment can often be performed, even though it has a much lower success rate (63.4%). All of these options are considered preferable to losing the tooth by extraction.

In most parts of the world, endodontics is practised as a postgraduate specialism within dentistry, and there is evidence that specialists obtain better clinical outcomes than those obtained by general dentists [3]. It has also been found that teeth treated in two or more sessions show higher healing rates than those treated in a single session [4], though this effect does not seem to be statistically significant.

Success rates are influenced by several factors. The age of the patient, for example, has been shown to be important, with older patients showing greater failure rates than younger ones [5]. This appears to be also related to the incidence of periodontal disease, which is more prevalent in older people, and capable of causing bone loss around the teeth leading to eventual extraction of the endodontically treated tooth.

10.2 Gutta percha points

The most widely used means of obturating tooth roots following extirpation of the pulp is with gutta percha points which can be compressed into irregularly shaped root canals using either lateral or vertical compaction techniques (Fig. 10.1). These gutta percha points are usually warmed with a heated plugger, with an initial master point placed first, followed by accessory points as necessary to complete obturation [6].

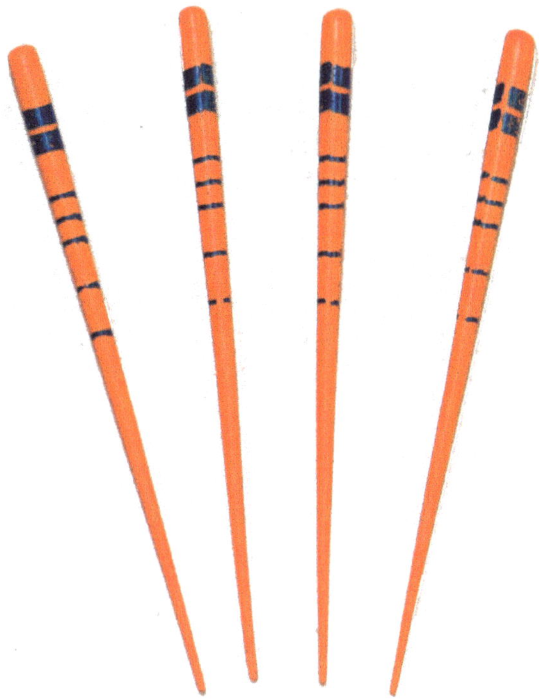

Fig. 10.1 Guta percha points.

Gutta percha fulfils most of the requirements for an ideal point material and, as part of an appropriately formulated composition, is the material of choice for this clinical application. It is considered to be a semi-solid, and as a result is capable of being compressed into irregularly shaped root canals using either lateral or vertical compaction techniques. Gutta percha is dimensionally stable and biocompatible when placed in contact with the root tissues. It becomes plastic on heating to around 60°C and also in the presence of certain solvents, such as xylene, chloroform or eucalyptus oil. It is not naturally radiopaque, but is made so by being formulated with an appropriate inorganic filler, such as barium sulphate [7]. Also, it has sufficient integrity to allow it to be removed from the root canal under circumstances where this becomes necessary [6].

Because of its thermoplastic character, gutta percha cannot be sterilized by heating. Instead, where disinfection is necessary, a dilute solution of sodium hypochlorite (typically 5%) should be used.

Gutta percha is obtained from the sap of trees of the Sapotaceae family, mainly *Pallaquium gutta* [8]. These trees occur mainly in the Malaysian and Indonesian archipelago of South East Asia [9]. Material obtained by coagulating their sap was used centuries ago by inhabitants of the Malaysian archipelago for making objects such as knife handles and walking sticks. Having been introduced to the western world by the plant hunter John Tradescant in the 17th century, the material was eventually proposed for use in root canal filling by Dr G.R. Bowman, a clinician from Missouri, in 1867 [8].

Commercial production of gutta percha points for endodontics began in 1887, when the S.S. White Company introduced these products [8]. However, it was not until 1959 that the concept of using standardized root canal instruments in association with standard sized gutta percha points was proposed [10]. This occurred at the second International Conference of Endodontics, held in Philadelphia, and from this beginning, a range of standardized endodontic files and points have now become available to the profession. Gutta percha points of various types are now offered, including solid core points, thermo-compactable and medicated versions [8].

The sap from which gutta percha is derived is collected from the trees in which it occurs by tapping the juice from the trunks. This involves making v-shaped or concentric cuts, and allowing the sap to drain into cups. Following this, the gutta percha is purified by a complicated series of steps involving coagulation and purification to produce 'Final ultra pure' gutta percha which can be formulated into the final product for endodontic use [8].

10.2.1 Structure and composition of gutta percha for endodontics

Gutta percha consists primarily of the polymer of trans-1,4-isoprene (Fig. 10.2). It is a structural isomer of natural rubber, which is *cis*-1,4-polyisoprene, and the structure of gutta percha means that it has greater linearity and crystallizes more readily than natural rubber. These features mean that gutta percha is harder, less tough and more brittle than its structural isomer [11].

At room temperature, gutta percha is a rigid material, but it softens slightly at 25–30°C and generally becomes pliable and capable of taking up the shape of root canals on heating above this temperature range [12]. Gutta percha changes its properties on ageing, becoming more brittle and less elastic due to oxidation. To maintain its properties and to slow down any effects of ageing, gutta percha should be stored in a cool place and out of the light prior to use [7].

For endodontic use, gutta percha is formulated to include other components in addition to its polymeric ingredient. These include waxes and resins, as well as finely divided inorganic fillers (zinc oxide and typically barium sulphate). Zinc oxide is added as reinforcing filler, aimed at giving the material improved strength and rigidity. Barium sulphate, where present, is there to confer increased radiopacity, though other radiopacifiers may be used in other brands [7], and zinc oxide itself confers a degree of radiopacity. Small amounts of anti-oxidants may also be present. A typical composition is shown in Table 10.1.

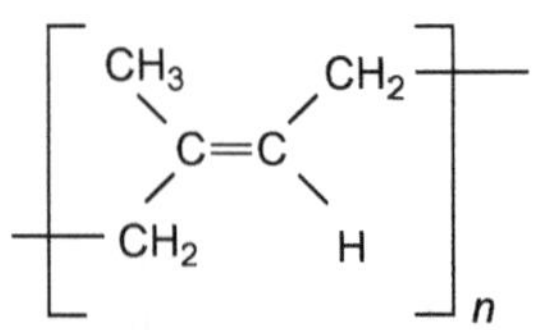

Fig. 10.2 Chemical structure of gutta percha (*trans*-1,4-polyisoprene).

Table 10.1 Composition of typical commercial gutta percha points [7]

Component	Proportion by mass (%)
Gutta percha polymer	14.5
Wax/resin	1.2
Barium sulphate	28.0
Zinc oxide	56.3

Studies have shown that the composition of gutta percha points varies between manufacturers [7]. In particular, the proportions of gutta percha polymer and zinc oxide filler may differ widely. These differences may lead to variations in mechanical properties and also in the ease of flow on heating between different proprietary brands.

10.3 Alternative materials for endodontic points

Gutta percha is the most widely used material for endodontic points, for the reasons already described. However, other materials have been used, of which until recently, silver was the most important [13], and silver points had the advantage of being inherently bactericidal.

However, as a metal, silver has significant disadvantages compared with gutta percha. Mechanically, it is much more rigid than gutta percha, and therefore less able to deform to fully obturate awkwardly shaped root canals. This meant that it could not be easily adapted to the canal walls. This in turn placed greater demands on the sealants used in association with these points if a reliable seal was to be created at the root apex. Obtaining satisfactory seals proved challenging and limited the success of endodontic treatment with silver points.

Silver points also had the significant disadvantage that they undergo corrosion in the presence of serum and blood [14]. The corrosion products caused serious and irreversible staining of the tooth and the surrounding tissues, a feature that was clearly unacceptable for patients.

In view of these clinical problems, since 2013 the American Association of Endodontists has recommended that silver points should no longer be used in endodontic therapy. However, despite this, the Association does not advocate the prophylactic removal of silver points unless there is evidence of some sort of clinical problem, such as corrosion and/or discolouration. This view of the clinical value of silver points appears to be widespread, and few, if any, manufacturers throughout the world continue to offer these items. This suggests that they are now of historical interest only.

Endodontic points based on synthetic polymers are also available. One relatively new material is supplied as Resilon, manufactured by the Penton Clinical company, USA [15], and comprises a blend of polycaprolactone polymer with small amounts of dimethacrylate monomer (3–10%). It is filled with a mixture of bioactive glass, bismuth oxychloride and barium sulphate [16]. The latter are included to make the material radiopaque.

Resilon is designed to be used in association with a resin sealer material. Its physical properties resemble those of gutta percha, as does its biocompatibility [15]. Studies suggest that the quality of the obturation that can be obtained is also similar to that of gutta percha, and preliminary clinical reports suggest that outcomes are much the same. Unlike gutta percha, however, there is some evidence that Resilon is susceptible to degradation in the presence of oral fluids [15,16] though the extent to which this can occur in vivo has not been reported.

Resilon is expensive compared with gutta percha, and the results reported to date suggest that it may not offer any particular clinical advantages over the latter material. Moreover, further studies are needed to confirm its efficacy in service, and to determine how its long-term properties compare with those of gutta percha.

10.4 Root canal sealers

Pre-formed endodontic points are not, in themselves, sufficient to create a sound clinical seal in a tooth from which the pulp has been extirpated. In addition, it is necessary to use some sort of sealer. This is applied as a high viscosity paste, and while still able to flow, it can adapt to the canal wall and to the obturating point to produce a seal that can prevent the passage of bacteria. This sealer sets by some sort of chemical process to create a rigid solid that remains in position and provides a continuing seal to prevent the admission of bacteria.

Sealant materials cannot be used alone to obturate root canals because of the setting process, which typically results in the material undergoing some sort of shrinkage. The significance of such shrinkage is minimized by the presence of the semi-solid point. However, the fact that shrinkage occurs prevents the sealer material alone from providing a completely impervious seal. Also, mixing such sealants tends to incorporate air, which means that the set material contains voids through which leakage may occur. The lack of a purely mechanical barrier means that the sealer should ideally have some inherent anti-bacterial properties. The combination of a reasonable but incomplete barrier with anti-bacterial character allows the sealer to perform its clinical function of maintaining the empty pulp chamber in an acceptably sterile condition.

It should be noted in passing that the possibility of using only one of the materials (eg, gutta percha points or sealer paste) has been considered for endodontic therapy [17]. The concept has been called ‘monoblock’. However, though it would be advantages in the clinic if it were feasible, it has not proved possible to develop the approach for practical use. Either gutta percha or sealer alone cannot produce a seal of sufficient soundness or durability to give acceptable clinical results.

Sealing materials are currently available to the profession in a wide variety of chemical types, as shown in Table 10.2. Some current brands of each type are also listed. These materials are described in the following sections of this chapter.

Table 10.2 **Types of endodontic sealer materials**

Type	Commercial examples (manufacturer)
Zinc oxide-eugenol	Tubiseal (Kerr)
Calcium hydroxide cements	Apexit (Ivoclar), Sealapex (Kerr)
Glass-ionomer cements	Ketac Endo (3M-ESPE, Endion (Voco)
Silicones	RSA RoekoSeal (Roeko)
Epoxy resins	AH Plus (Dentsply), Diaket (3M-ESPE)
Dimethacrylate resins	EndoREZ (Ultradent), Epiphany (Pentron Clinical)
Tricalcium silicate hydraulic cements	ProRoot MTA (Dentsply)

The essential features of some of them have already been described in other chapters, and these details are not repeated. Rather, what follows emphasizes the application of these materials as endodontic sealers.

10.4.1 Zinc oxide-eugenol

Zinc oxide-eugenol is a somewhat old-fashioned material, but it is widely used as an endodontic sealer [18]. It has relatively poor mechanical properties, but is easy to use in the dental clinic [19] and outcomes are good, which explains its continuing popularity. When set, it is biocompatible towards dental hard tissues, though it is cytotoxic towards soft tissues [20]. Zinc oxide-eugenol is susceptible to hydrolysis, which causes the material to decompose and release eugenol. It is this latter substance which is responsible for the cement's adverse effects on soft tissues, but which also makes the material bactericidal.

Zinc oxide-eugenol is a type of acid–base cement, and forms by reaction of eugenol with zinc oxide powder. The matrix of the cement is a chelate substance consisting of zinc eugenolate. For this reaction to occur, at least a trace of water is essential [21].

Eugenol is a type of phenol, and as such is weakly acidic. Its systematic chemical name is 4-allyl-2-methoxy phenol, and it has the structure shown in Fig. 10.3 [22]. Like all acids, it can only manifest its acidic character in the presence of water. In principle, the mixture of zinc oxide with eugenol can obtain its water from the moisture present in the mouth but in practice, if it does so, it sets only slowly [19]. To obtain a cement with more rapid and reliable setting behaviour, small amounts of accelerator

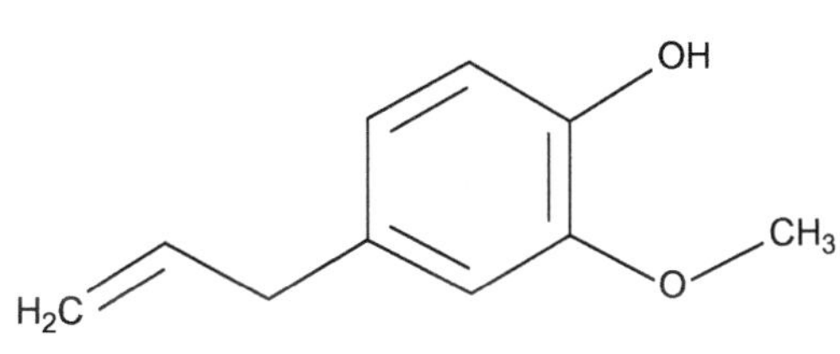

Fig. 10.3 Structure of eugenol.

Table 10.3 Composition of Grossman's sealer

Powder component	Liquid
Zinc oxide (42%) Staybellite resin (27%) Bismuth sub-carbonate (15%) Barium sulphate (15%) Sodium borate (1%)	Eugenol (100%)

are added. A number of substances have been shown to be capable of accelerating the setting reaction of zinc oxide-eugenol cements and these can either be added to the eugenol liquid or to the zinc oxide powder. The original composition that was found to be clinically acceptable, and which has been available for over 70 years, is known as Grossman's sealer after its inventor, and this contains a trace of sodium borate in the zinc oxide base powder as accelerator (Table 10.3).

Current proprietary brands of zinc oxide-eugenol may contain a variety of alternative accelerators. Acetic acid (0.1–2%) can be included in the eugenol, and some sort of zinc salt, such as zinc propionate [23], zinc succinate [23] or zinc acetate [24] blended with the zinc oxide. These combinations result in cements that set more rapidly than zinc oxide with eugenol alone, and at least part of the effectiveness of these accelerators arises from their highly hydrophilic nature, which causes the newly mixed cement pastes to absorb water from the surroundings more readily. Water has been shown to be an essential component of the reaction mixture [25,26], and high ambient humidity therefore improves the speed of the setting reaction [25].

The zinc oxide used in zinc oxide-eugenol cements is not the deactivated substance used in zinc phosphate cements [19]. Instead, it needs to be as reactive as possible, a state that is achieved by omitting the heat-treatment stage during manufacture [19], and ensuring that the particle size is as fine as possible [26].

Zinc oxide-eugenol cement is mechanically weak, with compressive strengths in the range 13–38 MPA at 24 h [19]. Setting times are reasonably rapid, ranging from 4 to 14 min, depending on the details of the formulation [27]. Resulting cements show a substantial degree of plastic character and, for this reason, are able to provide a good seal at the root apex, despite having a high setting shrinkage [28]. These cements also have good bactericidal properties [29], which is a further benefit when they are used as endodontic sealers. However, they are irritants towards the peri-apical tissues if extruded beyond the tooth apex, and where this happens, the reaction may so severe that is has to be removed by apectomy.

Overall, despite not having completely ideal properties as sealing materials, zinc oxide-eugenol is an effective material. Its many years of satisfactory clinical service demonstrate this, and outcomes with it are generally good. There is little current research on zinc oxide-eugenol endodontic sealers, but this is a reflection on the fact that it is a mature material with a proven track record. It remains one of the most widely used materials for endodontic sealing [18], and is likely to remain so for the foreseeable future.

10.4.2 Calcium hydroxide cements

As described in Chapter 9, the main use of calcium hydroxide is as a pulp capping material. It is also used as a medicament for intra-canal treatment and in some apexification procedures [30]. In addition, following pioneering studies in the late 1970s [31], it has also become used as the main active component of a group of proprietary root canal sealers.

Calcium hydroxide materials have a number of advantages when used in this application. Their high pH makes them anti-bacterial [32] and also promotes repair around the sealer through calcification and stimulation of hard tissue development [33]. Calcium hydroxide sealers need to maintain a high degree of integrity in order to remain in place for the necessary time, and ideally should not disintegrate in situ. However, there is evidence that they are not always able to fulfil this requirement, and studies have shown a significant degree of disintegration of these materials [30]. There is also an important question concerning the relationship between in situ stability and the leaching of calcium and hydroxyl ions. The latter is necessary to both raise the local pH and to promote hard tissue regeneration, in other words, to confer therapeutic benefits.

Leakage around calcium hydroxide sealers has been studied experimentally, and findings have generally been satisfactory [34–36]. However, there have been some adverse reports [37], and these variations have been attributed to crucial differences in experimental methods [38]. Leakage appears to be related to both the solubility of the material and the questionable adhesion to both the dentine walls and the gutta percha points. The calcium hydroxide sealer Apexit, for example, was found to have a high solubility when set compared with other types of endodontic sealer [39] and, in some studies, sealer particles have been found to occur with the tissues at a considerable distance from the sample [40,41].

A particular advantage of calcium hydroxide sealers is their anti-bacterial nature, a feature which is related to their high pH. Several in vitro studies have demonstrated that these show considerable anti-bacterial activity [42–44]. Despite their biocidal character, these materials are less toxic than zinc oxide-eugenol sealers towards human periodontal ligament cells [40,41].

The physical properties of calcium hydroxide materials are acceptable for their use as endodontic sealers. They flow well in their unset state, so they can reach and seal the apical foramen of the affected tooth, and also adapt to the shape of any irregularities of the dentinal wall.

Calcium hydroxide materials have variable setting times. For example, Apexit sets in about 2 h at 100% relative humidity [39], whereas Sealapex takes 2–3 weeks to set under the same conditions [45,46]. Set materials have good dimensional stability [29], though they have some capacity for expanding at high humidity [46], which probably promotes good sealing.

Overall, calcium hydroxide materials appear satisfactory as endodontic sealers in clinical service [47,48], though they are not outstanding in this application [30]. Established brands continue to be made available for practitioners, and clearly find favour with certain members of the profession. They must be used carefully, and in particular all the moisture must be removed from the root canal using paper points of the correct number and width. Any traces of moisture left behind will speed up the setting of calcium hydroxide sealer, allowing it to harden within a few seconds, thus making the insertion of gutta percha points impossible.

10.4.3 Glass-ionomer cements

The essential nature of conventional glass-ionomers has been covered in detail in Chapter 5. As was described in that chapter, these materials undergo a hardening reaction in reasonable time arising from the attack of a basic glass powder by an aqueous solution of polymeric acid [49]. They have two particular features that make them attractive as potential endodontic sealers, namely their low setting shrinkage and their ability to form a true adhesive bond to both enamel and dentine [50]. Both of these features suggest that a glass-ionomer cement should form an excellent seal at the tooth apex and therefore be the basis of a satisfactory endodontic sealer.

However, in practice there were problems to be overcome before a glass-ionomer cement could function as a sealer in this way [51]. In particular, improvements were necessary in the working time, which from a practical point of view in endodontics was too short [50,52]. Partly because of the short setting time, transporting the cement to the root apex in a sufficiently fluid state proved to be challenging.

These problems were overcome by the early 1990s when the product Ketac Endo was launched. It was formulated with the consistency of a luting cement, which meant it had a relatively low powder to liquid ratio. This enabled it to flow into place and to adapt well to the contours of the root canal, including as quite thin films where necessary. It included a radiopacifying agent, which overcame another problem of glass-ionomers in this application, namely their X-ray transparency [51].

Since the launch of Ketac Endo, other glass-ionomer products for use as endodontic sealers have appeared on the market. They typically have reasonable physical properties [50,52], certainly better than those of zinc oxide-eugenol cements and they are less susceptible to hydrolytic degradation.

The good adhesion of glass-ionomers to enamel and dentine has been confirmed for these cements when formulated for use as endodontic sealers [50,51]. However, despite this, these materials are less good at providing a sound seal than was anticipated. The reason for this is not clear. Nonetheless, they have been shown to reduce coronal ingress of micro-organisms in teeth where glass-ionomer had been used to seal the canal orifices and also placed on the floor of the pulp chamber [53–56]. They are thus capable of maintaining the treated tooth in an appropriate sterile condition, as required for successful endodontic treatment.

Glass-ionomers are known to have strong anti-bacterial properties when newly placed [57], a feature which is attributed to the combined effects of their low early pH and their ability to release fluoride in an 'early burst' shortly after forming [58]. These effects have been confirmed for glass-ionomer endodontic sealers [59], but anti-bacterial effects were transient, and had disappeared after 24 h. This contrasts with zinc oxide-eugenol cement, which has been shown to maintain its anti-bacterial activity for several days after setting [59], and was probably able to do so for considerably longer than this.

Clinical results are generally good when glass-ionomers are used as endodontic sealers [49], and support the use of glass-ionomers in this application [60]. As well as straightforward endodontic sealing, glass-ionomers have been reported in other endodontic applications. For example, in vitro studies of their use to repair root perforations or root resorption cavities have been published [50,61], though the positive results still lack the support of in vivo findings. From these published studies, however, it is possible to conclude that glass-ionomer cements have good biocompatibility towards apical tissues, and that these acceptable biological findings support the use of glass-ionomers in this application.

10.4.4 Silicones

The root canal sealers based on silicone are a variation on the addition-polymerized silicone used clinically as an impression material [62]. They have been modified to improve their flow, but their essential chemistry is the same. They consist of two-paste systems comprising a base and a catalyst paste. The silicone components are a polydimethylsiloxane polymer blended with paraffin oil and filled with finely divided zirconium dioxide. This latter substance both reinforces the set silicone material and confers radiopacity.

Silicone-based endodontic sealers have to be mixed immediately prior to use [62,63], and this is done using a mechanical delivery system that ensures complete mixing of both pastes without the incorporation of air. Also present in one of the pastes is a trace of platinum to act as catalyst for the setting reaction. Setting involves pendant unsaturated groups on one of the polymer chains reacting with a hydrogen atom attached directly to a silicon atom (Fig. 10.4). The reaction results in cross-links between the polysiloxane chains, and these cause the material to set to a resilient rubbery solid [13].

Silicone endodontic sealers are formulated with very small particle size particles of zirconium oxide. This means that the unset silicone paste is able to achieve very thin film thickness, typically of the order of 5 μm. This ensures good flow into surface irregularities and also good adaption to the walls of the root canal.

Silicone endodontic sealers in their set state are insoluble materials with good dimensional stability [62,63]. They undergo a slight expansion on setting, which

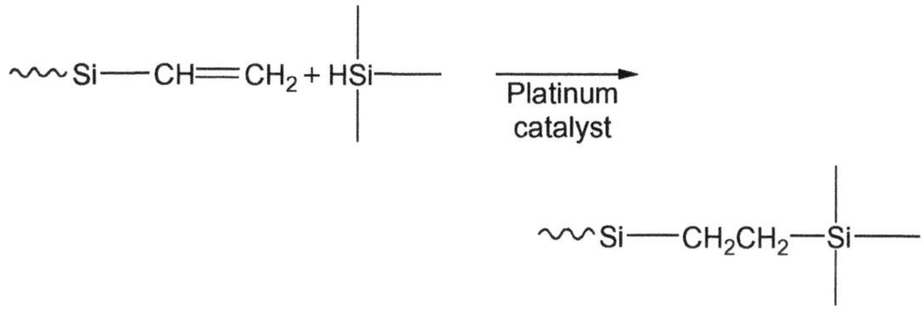

Fig. 10.4 Setting of polysiloxane addition polymer.

improves their adaptation to the root canal walls, and hence enhances the quality of the seal that they provide. However, in spite of this, studies have suggested that the seal achieved under conditions designed to model those in the clinic is not as good as that of Grossman's sealer based on zinc oxide-eugenol [63].

Studies have confirmed that addition silicones are biocompatible at the root apex [64], though they lack anti-bacterial properties. They therefore rely on providing a high-quality seal in order to prevent bacterial colonization of the sterile pulp chamber.

10.4.5 Epoxy resins

Epoxy resin-based materials are available for use as endodontic sealers [64]. They set by a ring-opening polymerization reaction between hexamethylene tetratramine (Fig. 10.5), which is part of the powder component, and *bis*-phenol resin monomer, which comprises the liquid component [13]. In addition to the reactive molecule, the powder contains bismuth oxide (50%) to impart radiopacity and titanium dioxide (5%) as a pigment. The powder also contains silver particles (10%) to make the set material anti-bacterial.

Outcomes with epoxy sealers appear good [65]. The set epoxy resin has good physical properties, providing an acceptable seal with gutta percha points [66] and being resistant to degradation in aqueous conditions [67]. However, studies have shown that these materials leak more than other sealers, especially those of the dimethacrylate resin type, which seal exceptionally well [68]. For epoxy sealers, most of the leakage has been shown to occur between the sealer and the wall of the root canal [69]. This probably arises from polymerization shrinkage within these materials and also because they are too hydrophobic to bond to the walls of the tooth.

The epoxy sealer AH26 Plus has been shown to have reasonable anti-bacterial properties [43]. In a comparative study of several different types of endodontic sealer, it was found to be as effective as Grossman's sealer in reducing the number of cultivable cells of *Enterococcus faecalis*. By contrast, the calcium hydroxide sealers Apexit and Sealapex were not effective at all in reducing the number of these cells.

An important property of an endodontic sealer is that it should be biocompatible with the tissues at the apex of the tooth [70]. Epoxy sealers do not fulfil this requirement particularly well. For example, although it gives reasonable results, AH26 has been shown to release formaldehyde, with the maximum release occurring 2 days after mixing [71]. Formaldehyde arises from the disinfectant, methenamine, which is used in this material. Unfortunately, it can undergo hydrolysis in situ to generate both formaldehyde and ammonia, both of which can lead to adverse biological reactions in the patient. These adverse reactions include paraesthesia (ie, abnormal sensation, such as tingling) in the alveolar nerve [72]. AH26 Plus, by contrast, is claimed not to suffer from this disadvantage, presumably because of subtle differences in composition that have not been explained in the literature [72].

Both AH26 and AH26 Plus are epoxy-based endodontic sealers that have been used for some years. They set hard, making them difficult to remove, but despite this, they remain in use and overall their properties appear acceptable if not ideal for this application.

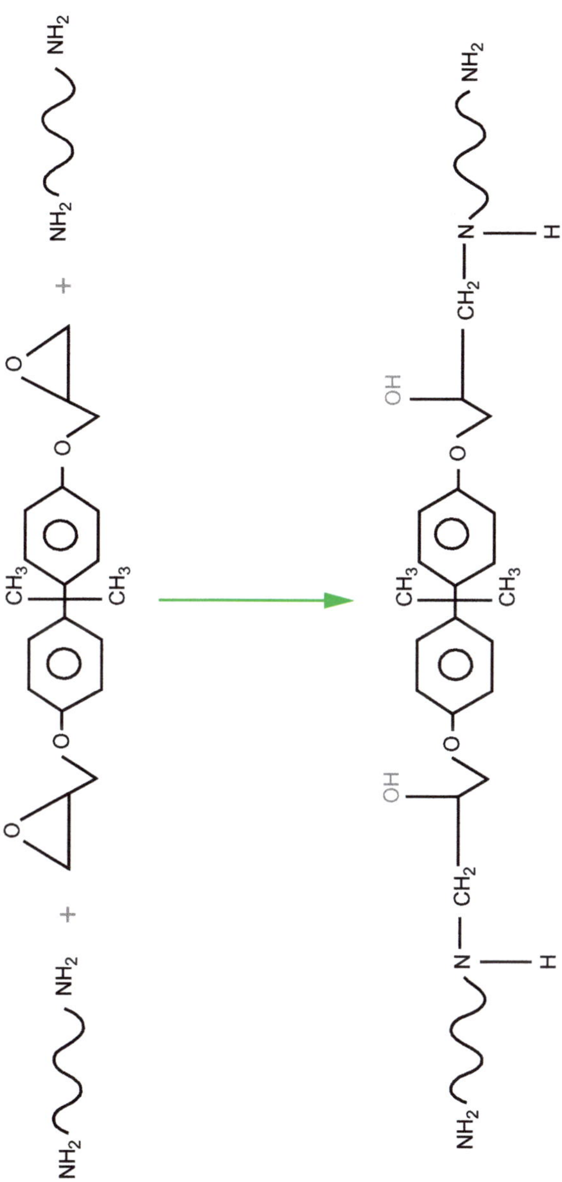

Fig. 10.5 Setting of epoxy resin.

10.4.6 Dimethacrylate resin-based sealers

Dimethacrylate resin-based endodontic sealers are based on the same kind of methacrylate chemistry as composite resins. They differ from composite resins, though, in that the filler is not quartz or silicate glass, and not present to provide good aesthetics. Rather the filler is a blend of zinc oxide and barium sulphate, and these have the combined functions of improving strength, reducing setting shrinkage and conferring radiopacity [73,74].

Resin-based sealers harden by an addition polymerization between unsaturated methacrylate groups at the ends of the monomer molecules [75]. These materials are supplied as two-paste systems, each of which contains a component of the free radical initiator. Mixing of the two pastes brings about combination of these initiator components, with the result that free radicals are generated, the addition polymerization takes place and the material sets.

Over the years, a number of brands of this type of endodontic sealer have become available [75]. In recent years, there has been considerable interest in two brands, which have been widely studied. These are EndoREZ (Ultradent Products, Utah) and Epiphany (Penton Clinical, Connecticut), though other materials of this type are also discussed in recent publications [76]. The brand Epiphany has been designed specifically to be used in conjunction with the polycaprolactone endodontic points marketed under the brand name Resilon. The good adhesion obtained between the resin and these points has led to the suggestion that this system may be capable of behaving effectively as a monoblock [75], though experimental results do not really support this concept.

Endodontic resin systems are based on a variety of monomers containing methacrylate groups, and typically comprise substantial amounts of urethane dimethacrylate. Some of these materials may also contain HEMA, which imparts a degree of hydrophilic character [75]. In general, whatever the formulation, resin-based endodontic sealers are capable of being used in slightly moist root canals, and their filler loading is sufficiently low that they are able to flow into surface irregularities, including dentinal tubules, and form resin tags.

Studies of the sealing ability of these materials have given highly variable results. For example, one study compared the Epiphany/Resilon system with that based on AH Plus (epoxy) with gutta percha, and found the fluid leakage of both systems to be comparable [73]. By contrast, other studies have found the leakage in the methacrylate resin system to be significantly less ($p<0.05$) [74,77]. Contradictory results have also been found for bacterial leakage studies, with some studies reporting no differences between Epiphany/Resilon and AH Plus/gutta percha [78,79], and others reporting superior results for the methacrylate resin system [80,81]. There is thus no consensus on whether or not these systems give reduced leakage and, given their composition and the known lack of bonding ability of composite resins, this is not surprising. It may be that they should ideally be used with bonding agents, though this would make their use clinically very cumbersome. Even within the literature published so far, it is clear that they are very technique-sensitive.

There have been several studies of the biological effects of resin-based endodontic sealers [82–85]. As with other types of endodontic sealer, adverse reactions are reported, including cytotoxicity and damage to the DNA when these materials were placed in contact with primary cell cultures of human periodontal ligament cells [82,83]. However, results were no worse than for materials such as AH26 or zinc oxide-eugenol, and also adverse reactions subsided over time, once irritating substances stopped being eluted from the specimens.

These biological findings suggest that these resin-based endodontic sealers are acceptable for clinical use, a result that has been confirmed by clinical evaluations [86–88]. In one 5-year study involving 129 patients, results showed that root canals were adequately filled in 76.66% of cases (92) and were short in 10.83% (13) of cases. In 15 cases (12.50%), there was evidence of slight resorption of the sealer at the apex within the lumen of the root canal. These clinical results show that resin-based sealers compare well with sealers based on other types of material, and that they are satisfactory for use in endodontics [48,89].

10.4.7 Tricalcium silicate hydraulic cements

The main tricalcium silicate cements used in endodontic sealing and related applications are MTA, which has already been mentioned in Chapter 8. MTA was introduced to the profession in 1993 for use in clinical endodontics and there are currently two main products on the market, namely ProRoot MTA, grey and white (Tulsa Dental Products, Tulsa, USA), and MTA-Angelus (Angelus Soluções Odontológicas, Londrina, Brazil). There are also the related products Biodentine (Septodont, St Maur des Faussés, France) and Bioaggregate (Verio Dental, Vancouver, Canada), where the main component is refined tricalcium silicate, so that the setting chemistry is essentially the same as for the MTA materials. In all cases, the main reason for employing them in endodontics is that they have good sealing ability [90–92] and have excellent biocompatibility with the tissues of the root apex [91,93].

As shown in Chapter 9, MTA consists of Portland cement with added bismuth oxide as radiopacifying agent [94]. This latter substance does not participate in the setting reaction, but remains as an essentially inert filler within the set MTA matrix [95].

Although it used in the commercial brands of MTA, bismuth oxide may not be the ideal radiopacifying agent [96]. It increases the porosity of the base Portland cement and this may increase the rate of dissolution and disintegration of the material [97,98]. Other radiopacifying agents have been investigated [99]. These include zirconium oxide, calcium tungstate [99], gold powder and silver/tin alloy [100,101], but these are not yet included in commercially available formulations of MTA.

The setting reactions of the various tricalcium silicate cements are very similar, as described in Chapter 8. They also resemble the setting of Portland cement. The initial setting involves the hydration of the alite (Ca_2SiO_5) and belite (β-Ca_2SiO_4) phases to form a poorly crystalline gel phase consisting of calcium hydroxide in calcium silicate hydrate (approximate formula: $Ca_3Si_2O_7$) [102]. After the initial hardening, further condensation reactions occur which improve the strength and give rise to short silicate chains within the structure [103].

The presence of calcium hydroxide within the set MTA cement makes the material alkaline [104,105]. For example, the material ProRoot MTA has been found to have a pH of 10.2 when stored for 1 day in water. This is slightly lower than the value for pure Portland cement (11.8), but sufficient to make the material bioactive when placed in the root canal.

There have been numerous studies of the interaction of MTA with various types of cell, and the general conclusion is that this material is biocompatible for its intended application [106]. The most significant of these studies have evaluated MTA against gingival fibroblasts [107–110] and against periodontal ligament fibroblasts [107,108,110]. However, other cell types, such as mouse L929 [111,112] and rat bone marrow cells [113] have also been used, again with very positive outcomes.

MTA has been found to give good biological results when used for root-end filling in vivo. It promotes only low peri-radicular inflammation [114] and frequently causes cementum to form on its surface [115]. It has also been found to induce the formation of apical hard tissue [116] and, in non-infected teeth, to support almost complete regeneration of the peri-radicular periodontum [117]. Thus, MTA is not only biocompatible, it is also bioactive and generally promotes a positive response in the tissues with which it comes into contact [106,118].

MTA has a wide variety of clinical uses within endodontics. The main one is a root-end filling material [116–120], but it is also used for pulp capping, pulpotomy and to repair lateral root perforations [121–125]. It can be used for apical barrier formation in teeth with open apexes [126]. Its relatively long setting time may be a disadvantage, but this has been addressed in related products such as Biodentine by the inclusion of calcium chloride as an accelerator.

In recent years, numerous accounts have been published on case reports in which MTA has been used on one or other of these endodontic applications [127]. However, few properly designed research studies have appeared. Nevertheless, published clinical findings are consistently good and there is evidence that the material is acceptable for use within endodontics. As a consequence of these favourable findings, MTA is now widely used in endodontics.

The material does suffer from some disadvantages. As already mentioned, MTA itself has a long setting time, and is also quite difficult to handle [128,129]. It is also difficult to remove once set [128,129]. However, these disadvantages are more than compensated for by the advantages, and this material is likely to be used in a variety of endodontic applications for many years to come.

Clinical summary

- Two broad types of material are used: pre-formed points and sealers.
- Gutta percha is the most widely used material for points. It is a semi-solid with excellent biocompatibility properties.
- Other materials have been used, of which currently the polycaprolactone-based material, ‘Resilon’, has become available and is finding some use by practitioners.
- A variety of sealers are available, with differing advantages and disadvantages. They are placed as high viscosity pastes and set to provide seals of varying degrees of rigidity. These are:
  zinc oxide-eugenol;
  calcium hydroxide chelates;
  glass-ionomer cement (conventional);

silicones;
epoxy resins;
dimethacrylate resins;
tricalcium silicate cements (MTA).

References

[1] R.F. Elemam, I. Pretty, Comparison of the success rate of endodontic treatment and implant treatment, ISRN Dent. 2011 (2011), article 640509.
[2] S. Rahbaran, M.S. Gilthorpe, S.D. Harrison, K. Gulabivala, Comparison of clinical outcome of peri-apical surgery in endodontics and oral surgery units of a teaching dental hospital: a retrospective study, Oral Surg. Oral Med. Oral Pathol. Oral Radiol. Endod. 91 (2001) 700–709.
[3] B.S. Alley, G. Gray Kitchens, L.W. Alley, P.D. Eleazer, A comparison of survival of teeth following endodontic treatment performed by general dentists or by specialists, Oral Surg. Oral Med. Oral Pathol. Oral Radiol. Endod. 98 (2004) 115–118.
[4] S. Friedman, S. Abitbol, H.P. Lawrence, Treatment outcomes in endodontics: the Toronto study. Phase 1: initial treatment, J. Endod. 29 (2003) 787–793.
[5] T. Dammaschke, D. Steven, M. Kaup, K.H.R. Ott, Long-term survival of root-canal-treated teeth: a retrospective study over 10 years, J. Endod. 29 (2003) 638–643.
[6] P. Carotte, Endodontics: Part 8. Filling the root canal system, Br. Dent. J. 197 (2004) 667–672.
[7] E.D. Gurgel-Filho, J.P. Andrade Feitosa, F.B. Teixeira, R.C. Monteiro de Paula, J.B. Araujo Silva Jr., F.J. Souza-Filho, Chemical and X-ray analyses of five brands of dental gutta-percha cones, Int. Endod. J. 36 (2003) 302–307.
[8] R. Prakash, V. Gopikrishna, D. Kandaswamy, Gutta-percha – an untold story, Endodontology 17 (2005) 32–36.
[9] B.J. Borthakur, Search for indigenous gutta-percha, Endodontology 14 (2002) 24–27.
[10] J.I. Ingle, L.F. Bakland, Obturation of the radicular space, Ch 11 in: Textbook of Endodontics, B.C. Dekker, Hamilton, ON, 2002, pp. 598–636.
[11] J.W. Nicholson, The Chemistry of Polymers, fourth ed., Royal Society of Chemistry, Cambridge, 2012.
[12] C.E. Friedman, J.L. Sandrick, M.A. Heuer, G.W. Rapp, Composition and physical properties of gutta-percha endodontic filling materials, J. Endod. 3 (1977) 304–308.
[13] J.F. McCabe, A.W.G. Walls, Applied Dental Materials, ninth ed., Blackwell Munsgaard, Oxford, 2008.
[14] J.M. Brady, C.E. del Rio, Corrosion of endodontic silver cones in humans: a scanning electron microscope and X-ray microprobe study, J. Endod. 1 (1975) 205–210.
[15] M. Lofti, N. Ghasemi, S. Rahimi, S. Vosoughhoseini, M.A. Saghiri, A. Shahidi, Resilon: a comprehensive literature review, J. Dent. Res. Dent. Clin. Dent. Prospects 7 (2013) 119–130.
[16] P. Borbely, K. Gulabivala, J. Knowles, Degradation properties and ion release characteristics of Resilon and phosphate glass/polycaprolactone composites, Int. Endod. J. 12 (2008) 1093–1100.
[17] F.R. Tay, D.H. Pashley, Monoblocks in root canals – a hypothetical or tangible goal? J. Endod. 33 (2007) 391–398.
[18] J. Camps, L. Pommel, F. Bukiet, I. About, Influence of the powder/liquid ratio on the properties of zinc oxide-eugenol-based root canal sealers, Dent. Mater. 20 (2004) 915–923.

[19] A.D. Wilson, J.W. Nicholson, Acid Base Cements, The University Press, Cambridge, 1993.

[20] Y.C. Ho, F.M. Huang, Y.C. Chang, Mechanism of cytotoxicity of eugenol in human osteoblastic cells *in vitro*, Int. Endod. J. 39 (2006) 389–393.

[21] G.M. Brauer, A review of zinc oxide-eugenol type filling materials and cements, Rev. Belge Med. Dent. 20 (1965) 323–364.

[22] A.D. Wilson, R.J. Mesley, Zinc oxide eugenol cements. III. Infrared spectroscopic studies, J. Dent. Res. 51 (1972) 1581–1588.

[23] K.J. Anusavic, Chapter 16 in: Phillips' Science of Dental Materials, 11th ed., W.B. Saunders, Philadelphia, 2003.

[24] A.D. Wilson, R.F. Batchelor, Zinc oxide eugenol cements. II. Study of erosion and disintegration, J. Dent. Res. 49 (1970) 593–598.

[25] S. Crisp, M. Ambersley, A.D. Wilson, Zinc oxide eugenol cements. V. Instrumental studies of the catalysis and acceleration of the setting reaction, J. Dent. Res. 59 (1980) 44–54.

[26] H.J. Prosser, A.D. Wilson, Zinc oxide eugenol cements. VI. Effect of zinc oxide type on the setting reactions, J. Biomed. Mater. Res. 16 (1982) 585–598.

[27] C.G. Plant, I.H. Jones, H.J. Wilson, Setting characteristics of lining and cementing materials, Br. Dent. J. 133 (1972) 21–74.

[28] S. Civjan, G.M. Brauer, Physical properties of cements based on zinc oxide, hydrogenated resin, *o*-ethoxybenzoic acid and eugenol, J. Dent. Res. 42 (1964) 281–299.

[29] G.S. Beagrie, J.H.P. Main, D.C. Smith, Inflammatory reaction evoked by zinc polyacrylate and zinc eugenate cements: a comparison, Br. Dent. J. 132 (1972) 351–357.

[30] L.S. Desai, N. Chandler, Calcium hydroxide-based root canal sealers: a review, J. Endod. 35 (2009) 475–480.

[31] F. Goldberg, J. Gurfunkel, Analysis of the use of Dycal with gutta percha points as an endodontic filling technique, Oral Surg. Oral Med. Oral Pathol. 47 (1979) 78–82.

[32] A. Bystrom, R. Claesson, G. Sundqvist, The antibacterial effect of camphorated *para*-monochlorophenol, camphorated phenol and calcium hydroxide in treatment of infected root canals, Endod. Dent. Traumatol. 1 (1985) 170–175.

[33] M. Manhart, The calcium hydroxide method of endodontic sealing, Oral Surg. Oral Med. Oral Pathol. 54 (1982) 219–224.

[34] I. Hovland, T. Dumsha, Leakage evaluation *in vitro* of the root canal sealer cement Sealapex, Int. Endod. J. 18 (1985) 179–182.

[35] F. Sleder, M. Ludlow, J. Bohacek, Long-term sealing ability of a calcium hydroxide sealer, J. Endod. 17 (1991) 541–543.

[36] K. Lim, B. Tidmarsh, The sealing ability of Sealapex compared with AH26, J. Endod. 12 (1986) 564–566.

[37] I. Miletic, S. Ribaric, Z. Karlovic, S. Jukić, A. Bošnjak, I. Anić, Apical leakage of five root canal sealers after one year of storage, J. Endod. 28 (2002) 431–432.

[38] J. Ingle, C. Newton, J.G. West, Obturation of the radicular space, in: J. Ingle, L. Bakland (Eds.), Endodontics, BC Decker, Hamilton, ON, 2002, pp. 571–668.

[39] F. McMichen, G. Pearson, S. Rahbaran, K. Gulabivala, A comparative study of selected physical properties of five root canal sealers, Int. Endod. J. 36 (2003) 629–635.

[40] I. Tronstad, F. Barnett, M. Flax, Solubility and biocompatibility of calcium hydroxide containing root canal sealers, Endod. Dent. Traumatol. 4 (1988) 152–159.

[41] I. Soares, F. Goldberg, E. Massone, I.M. Soares, Periapical tissue response to two calcium hydroxide containing endodontic sealers, J. Endod. 16 (1990) 166–169.

[42] Z. Fuss, E. Weiss, M. Shalhav, Antimicrobial activity of calcium hydroxide containing endodontic sealers in *Enterococcus faecalis in vitro*, Int. Endod. J. 30 (1997) 397–402.

[43] G. Kayoglu, H. Erten, T. Alacam, D. Ørstavik, Short-term antibacterial activity of endodontic sealers to *Enterococcus faecalis*, Int. Endod. J. 38 (2005) 483–488.
[44] A. Abdulkader, R. Guduid, E. Saunders, The antimicrobial activity of endodontic sealers to anaerobic bacteria, Int. Endod. J. 29 (1996) 280–283.
[45] N. Allan, M. Williams, M. Schaeffer, Setting times for endodontic sealers under clinical usage and *in vitro* conditions, J. Endod. 27 (2001) 421–423.
[46] M. Partovi, A. Al-Havvaz, B. Soleimani, In vitro computer analysis of crown discoloration from commonly used endodontic sealers, Aust. Endod. J. 32 (2006) 116–119.
[47] D. Ørstavik, Materials used for root canal obturation: technical, biological and clinical testing, Endod. Topics 12 (2005) 25–38.
[48] D. Ørstavik, K. Kerekes, H. Eriksen, Clinical performance of three endodontic sealers, Endod. Dent. Traumatol. 3 (1987) 178–186.
[49] G.J. Mount, Color Atlas of Glass Ionomer Cement, second ed., Martin Dunitz, London, 2002.
[50] J. Camilleri, Glass-ionomers in contemporary endodontics, Chapter 5, in: S.K. Sidhu (Ed.), Glass-Ionomers in Dentistry, Springer International Publishing, Switzerland, 2016.
[51] H. Ray, S. Seltzer, A new glass-ionomer root canal sealer, J. Endod. 17 (1991) 598–603.
[52] R.A. Buck, Glass ionomer endodontic sealers – literature review, Gen. Dent. 50 (2002) 365–368.
[53] Z. Mohammadi, S. Shalavi, Clinical applications of glass ionomers in endodontics: a review, Int. Dent. J. 62 (2012) 244–250.
[54] P. Chailertvanitkul, W.P. Saunders, D. MacKenzie, An evaluation of microbial coronal leakage in the restored pulp chamber of root-canal treated multirooted teeth, Int. Endod. J. 30 (1997) 318–322.
[55] C.R. Barthel, J. Moshonov, G. Shuping, D. Ørstavik, Bacterial leakage versus dye leakage in obturated root canals, Int. Endod. J. 32 (1999) 370–375.
[56] C.R. Barthel, S. Zimmer, R. Wussogk, J.-F. Roulet, Long-term bacterial leakage along obturated roots restored with temporary and adhesive fillings, J. Endod. 27 (2001) 559–562.
[57] J.P. Loyola-Rodriguez, F. Garcia-Godoy, R. Lindqvist, Growth inhibition of glass ionomer cements on mutans streptococci, Pediatr. Dent. 16 (1994) 346–349.
[58] E.J. DeSchepper, R.R. White, W. von der Lehr, Antibacterial effects of glass ionomers, Am. J. Dent. 2 (1989) 74–78.
[59] M. Shalhav, Z. Fuss, E.I. Weiss, In vitro antibacterial activity of a glass ionomer endodontic sealer, J. Endod. 23 (1997) 616–619.
[60] M.A.A. De Bryne, R.J.G. De Moor, The use of glass ionomer cements in both conventional and surgical endodontics, Int. Endod. J. 37 (2004) 91–104.
[61] S. Friedman, C. Lost, M. Zarrabian, M. Trope, Evaluation of success and failure after endodontic therapy using a glass ionomer cement sealer, J. Endod. 21 (1995) 384–390.
[62] P. Jain, V. Pruthi, V.K. Sikri, An *ex vivo* evaluation of the sealing ability of polydimethylsiloxane-based root canal sealers, Indian J. Dent. Res. 25 (2014) 336–339.
[63] J.V. Barbizam, M. Souza, D. Cecchin, J. Dabbel, Effectiveness of a silicon-based root canal sealer for filling of simulated lateral canals, Braz. Dent. J. 18 (2007) 20–23.
[64] A. Chandra, H. Rahman, A. Agarwal, A. Verma, Toxicity of root canal sealers in vitro, Oral Biol Dent. 2 (2014) 2, http://dx.doi.org/10.7243/2053-5775-2-2.
[65] H. Singh, S. Markan, M. Kaur, G. Gupta, 'Endodontic sealers': current concepts and comparative analysis, Dent. Open J. 2 (2015) 32–37.
[66] D. Ørstavik, Weight loss of endodontic sealers, cements and pastes in water, Scand. J. Dent. Res. 91 (1983) 316–319.
[67] L.M. Resende, F.J. Rached-Junior, M.A. Versiani, A.E. Souza-Gabriel, C.E. Miranda, Y.T. Silva-Sousa, M.D. Sousa Neto, A comparative study of AH Plus, Epiphany and Ephiphany SE root canal sealers, Int. Endod. J. 42 (2009) 785–793.

[68] F. Paque, G. Sirtes, Apical sealing ability of Resilon/Epiphany versus gutta percha/AH Plus: immediate and 16-months leakage, Int. Endod. J. 40 (2007) 722–729.
[69] V.A. Mahajan, A.I. Kamra, An in vitro evaluation of apical sealing of three epoxy resin based commercial preparations, Endodontology 19 (2007) 7–11.
[70] T.H. Huang, J.J. Yang, H. Li, C.T. Kao, The biocompatibility evaluation of epoxy resin-based root canal sealers in vitro, Biomaterials 23 (2002) 77–83.
[71] L.S. Spangberg, S.V. Barbosa, M. Trope, F. Barnett, B. Hammond, Controlled release of medicaments in endodontic therapy, Endod. Dent. Traumatol. 1 (1985) 130–134.
[72] M.R. Leonardo, L.A. Bezerra da Silva, M.T. Filho, R. Santana da Silva, Release of formaldehyde by 4 endodontic sealers, Oral Surg. Oral Med. Oral Pathol. Oral Radiol. Endod. 88 (1999) 221–225.
[73] E.O. Onay, M. Ungor, H. Orucoglu, An *in vitro* evaluation of the apical sealing ability of a new resin-based root canal obturation system, J. Endod. 32 (2006) 976–978.
[74] U. Tunga, E. Bodrumlu, Assessment of the sealing ability of a new root canal obturation material, J. Endod. 32 (2006) 876–878.
[75] Y.K. Kim, S. Grandini, J.M. Ames, L.-S. Gu, S.K. Kim, D.H. Pashley, J.L. Gutmann, F.R. Tay, Critical review on methacrylate resin-based root canal sealers, J. Endod. 36 (2010) 383–399.
[76] R.V. Kumar, C.S. Shruthi, Evaluation of the sealing ability of resin cement used as a root canal sealer: an in vitro study, J. Conserv. Dent. 15 (2012) 274–277.
[77] R.K. Stratton, M.J. Apicella, P. Mines, A fluid filtration comparison of gutta-percha versus Resilon, a new soft resin endodontic obturation system, J. Endod. 32 (2006) 642–645.
[78] E. Pitout, T.G. Oberholzer, E. Blignaut, J. Molepo, Coronal leakage of teeth root filled with gutta-percha or Resilon root canal filling material, J. Endod. 32 (2006) 879–881.
[79] S.G. Biggs, K.I. Knowles, J.L. Ibarrola, D.H. Pashley, An *in vitro* assessment of the sealing ability of Resilon/Epiphany using fluid filtration, J. Endod. 32 (2006) 759–761.
[80] G. Shipper, D. Ørstavik, F.B. Texeira, M. Trope, An evaluation of microbial leakage in roots filled with a thermoplastic synthetic polymer-based root canal filling material (Resilon), J. Endod. 30 (2004) 342–347.
[81] C. Maltezos, G.N. Glickman, P. Ezzo, J. He, Comparison of the sealing of Resilon, ProRoot MTA and Super-EBA as root-end filling materials: a bacterial leakage study, J. Endod. 32 (2006) 324–327.
[82] F. Huang, K. Tai, M. Chou, Y. Chang, Cytotoxicity of resin zinc oxide-eugenol and calcium hydroxide based root canal sealers on human periodontal ligament cells and permanent V79 cells, Int. Endod. J. 35 (2002) 153–158.
[83] T.H. Huang, H. Lee, C.T. Koa, Evaluation of the genotoxicity of zinc oxide eugenol-based, calcium hydroxide-based and epoxy resin-based root canal sealers by comet assay, J. Endod. 27 (2001) 744–748.
[84] E.A. Koulaouzidou, K.T. Papazisis, P. Beltes, G.D. Geromichalos, A.H. Kortsaris, Cytotoxicity of three resin-based root canal sealers: an *in vitro* evaluation, Endod. Dent. Traumatol. 14 (1998) 182–185.
[85] J.E. Key, F.G. Rahemtulla, P.D. Eleazer, Cytotoxicity of a new root canal filling material on human gingival fibroblasts, J. Endod. 32 (2006) 756–758.
[86] O. Zmener, C.H. Pameijer, Clinical and radiographic evaluation of a resin-based root canal sealer, Am. J. Dent. 17 (2004) 19–22.
[87] O. Zmener, C.H. Pameijer, Clinical and radiographical evaluation of a resin-based root canal sealer: a 5-year follow-up, J. Endod. 33 (2007) 676–679.

[88] M. Pawinska, A. Kierklo, G. Marczuk-Kolada, New technology in endodontics – the Resilon-Epiphany system for obturation of root canals, Adv. Med. Sci. 51 (Suppl. 1) (2006) 154–157.
[89] D.B. Swartz, A.E. Skidmore, J.A. Griffin, Twenty years of endodontic success and failure, J. Endod. 9 (1983) 198–202.
[90] S.J. Lee, M. Monsef, M. Torabinejad, Sealing ability of a mineral trioxide aggregate for repair of lateral root perforations, J. Endod. 11 (1993) 541–544.
[91] M. Torabinejad, M. Parirokh, Mineral trioxide aggregate: a comprehensive review – Part II: leakage and biocompatibility investigations, J. Endod. 36 (2010) 190–202.
[92] H.W. Roberts, J.M. Toth, D.W. Berzins, D.G. Charlton, Mineral trioxide aggregate material use in endodontic treatment: a review of the literature, Dent. Mater. 24 (2008) 149–164.
[93] R. Holland, V. de Souza, M.J. Nery, J.A. Otoboni Filho, P.F. Bernabé, E. Dezan Jr., Reaction of rat connective tissue to implanted dentin tube filled with mineral trioxide aggregate, Portland cement or calcium hydroxide, J. Endod. 25 (1999) 161–166.
[94] C. Estrela, L.L. Bammann, C.R. Estrela, R.S. Silva, J.D. Pecora, Antimicrobial and chemical study of MTA, Portland cement, calcium hydroxide paste, Sealapex and Dycal, Braz. Dent. J. 22 (2000) 3–9.
[95] Q. Li, N.J. Coleman, The hydration chemistry of ProRoot MTA, Dent. Mater. J. 34 (2015) 458–465.
[96] M. Tanomaru-Filho, V. Morales, G.F. da Silva, R. Bosso, J.M.S.N. Reis, M.A.H. Duarte, J.M. Guerreiro-Tanomaru, Compressive strength and setting times of MTA and Portland cement associated with different radiopacifying agents, ISRN Dent. 2012 (2012).
[97] K.S. Coomaraswamy, P.J. Lumley, M.P. Hofmann, Effect of bismuth oxide radioopacifier content on the material properties of an endodontic Portland cement-based (MTA-like) system, J. Endod. 33 (2007) 295–298.
[98] J. Camilleri, The physical properties of accelerated Portland cement for endodontic use, Int. Endod. J. 41 (2008) 151–157.
[99] M.A. Hungaro Duarte, G.D. de Oliveira El Kadre, R.R. Vivian, J.M. Guerreiro Tanomaru, M.T. Filho, I.G. de Moraes, Radiopacity of Portland cement associated with different radiopacifying agents, J. Endod. 35 (2009) 737–740.
[100] M. Tanomaru-Filho, G.F. da Silva, M.A. Duarte, M. Gonçalves, J. Tanomura, Radiopacity evaluation of root-end filling materials by digitization of images, J. Appl. Oral Sci. 16 (2008) 376–379.
[101] J. Camilleri, M. Ganolfi, Evaluation of the radiopacity of calcium silicate cements containing different radiopacifiers, Int. Endod. J. 43 (2010) 21–30.
[102] H.F.W. Taylor, Cement Chemistry, Academic Press, London, 1990.
[103] Q. Li, N.J. Coleman, Early hydration of white Portland cement in the presence of bismuth oxide, Adv. Appl. Ceram. 112 (2013) 207–212. .Chemistry of ProRoot MTA, Dent. Mater. J. 34 (2015) 458–465.
[104] J. Camilleri, Hydration mechanisms of mineral trioxide aggregate, Int. Endod. J. 40 (2007) 462–470.
[105] M. Fridland, R. Rosado, MTA solubility: a long term study, J. Endod. 31 (2005) 376–379.
[106] J. Camilleri, T.R. Pitt Ford, Review of constituents and properties of mineral trioxide aggregate, Int. Endod. J. 39 (2006) 747–754.
[107] M. Osorio, A. Hefti, F.J. Vertucci, A.L. Shawley, Cytotoxicity of endodontic materials, J. Endod. 24 (1998) 91–96.
[108] A. Pistorius, B. Willerhausen, B. Briseno Marroquin, Effect of apical root-end filling materials on gingival fibroblasts, Int. Endod. J. 36 (2003) 610–615.

[109] M.A. Camp, B.G. Jeansonne, T. Lallier, Adhesion of human fibroblasts to root-end filling materials, J. Endod. 29 (2003) 602–607.
[110] S. Bonson, B.G. Jeansonne, T.E. Lallier, Root-end filling materials alter fibroblast differentiation, J. Dent. Res. 83 (2004) 408–413.
[111] M. Torabinejad, C.U. Hong, T.R. Pitt Ford, J.D. Kettering, Cytotoxicity of four root-end filling materials, J. Endod. 21 (1995) 489–492.
[112] Q.G.M. Yaltirik, H. Ozbas, K.E. Safavi, L.S. Spangberg, Adhesion of human osteoblasts on root-end filling materials, J. Endod. 26 (2000) 404–406.
[113] A. Nakayama, B. Ogiso, N. Tanabe, O. Takeichi, K. Matsuzaka, T. Inoue, Behaviour of bone marrow osteoblast-like cells on mineral trioxide aggregate morphology and expression of type I collagen and bone-related protein mRNAs, Int. Endod. J. 38 (2005) 203–210.
[114] M. Torabinejad, C.U. Hong, S.J. Lee, M. Mousef, T.R. Pitt Ford, Investigation of mineral trioxide aggregate for root-end filling in dogs, J. Endod. 21 (1995) 603–608.
[115] M. Torabinejad, T.R. Pitt Ford, D.J. McKendry, H.R. Abedi, D.A. Miller, S.P. Kariyawasam, Histologic assessment of mineral trioxide aggregate as root end filling material in monkeys, J. Endod. 23 (1997) 225–228.
[116] S. Shabahang, M. Torabinejad, P.P. Boyne, H. Abedi, P. McMillan, A comparative study of root-end induction using osteogenic protein-I, calcium hydroxide and mineral trioxide aggregate in dogs, J. Endod. 25 (1999) 1–5.
[117] J.D. Regan, J.L. Gutmann, D.E. Witherspoon, Comparison of Diaket and MTA when used as root-end filling materials to support regeneration of the periradicular tissues, Int. Endod. J. 35 (2002) 840–847.
[118] M.-G. Aminozarbian, M. Barati, I. Salehi, S.B. Mousavi, Biocompatibility of mineral trioxide aggregate and three new endodontic cements: an animal study, Dent. Res. J. (Isfahan) 9 (2012) 54–59.
[119] M. Toribinejad, C.U. Hong, F. McDonald, T.R. Pitt Ford, Physical and chemical properties of a new rootend filling material, J. Endod. 21 (1995) 349–353.
[120] M. Toribinejad, T.R. Pitt Ford, D.J. McKendry, H.R. Abedi, D.A. Miller, S.P. Kariyawasam, Histologic assessment of mineral trioxide aggregate as a root-end filling in monkeys, J. Endod. 23 (1997) 225–228.
[121] B.S. Chong, T.R. Pitt Ford, M.B. Hudson, A prospective clinical study of mineral trioxide aggregate and IRM when used as root-end filling materials in endodontic surgery, Int. Endod. J. 36 (2003) 520–526.
[122] W.P. Saunders, A prospective clinical study of periradicular surgery using mineral trioxide aggregate as a root end filling, J. Endod. 34 (2008) 660–665.
[123] G. Casella, S. Ferlito, The use of mineral trioxide aggregate in endodontics, Minerva Stomatol. 55 (2006) 123–143.
[124] T.R. Pitt Ford, M. Toribinejad, D.J. McKendry, C.U. Hong, S.P. Kariyawasam, Use of mineral trioxide aggregate for repair of furcal perforations, Oral Surg. Oral Med. Oral Path. Oral Radiol. Endod. 79 (1995) 756–763.
[125] S.J. Lee, M. Monsef, M. Toribinejad, Sealing ability of a mineral trioxide aggregate for repair of lateral root canal perforations, J. Endod. 19 (1993) 541–544.
[126] M. Parirokh, M. Torabinejad, Mineral trioxide aggregate: a comprehensive review – Part I: chemical, physical and antibacterial properties, J. Endod. 36 (2010) 16–27.
[127] M. Parirokh, M. Torabinejad, Mineral trioxide aggregate: a comprehensive review – Part III: clinical applications, drawbacks and mechanism of action, J. Endod. 36 (2010) 400–413.

[128] S.I. Kratchman, Perforation repair and one-step apexification procedures, Dent. Clin. North Am. 48 (2004) 291–307.
[129] J. Camilleri, F.F. Montesin, K. Brady, R. Sweeney, R.V. Curtis, T.R. Pitt Ford, The constitution of mineral trioxide aggregate, Dent. Mater. 21 (2005) 297–303.

Index

Note: Page numbers followed by *b* indicate boxes, *f* indicate figures, *t* indicate tables and *s* indicate schemes.

Edwards Brothers Malloy
Ann Arbor MI. USA
November 10, 2016